GRAINGER & ALLISON'S DIAGNOSTIC RADIOLOGY

The Musculoskeletal System

SIXTH EDITION

GRAINGER & ALLISON'S DIAGNOSTIC RADIOLOGY

SIXTH EDITION

The Musculoskeletal System

EDITED BY

Andrew J. Grainger, BM, BS, MRCP, FRCR

Philip O'Connor, MBBS, MRCP, FRCR, FFSEM(UK)

ELSEVIER

London   New York   Oxford   Philadelphia   St Louis   Sydney   Toronto

ELSEVIER

ISBN: 978-0-7020-6936-9

Executive Content Strategist: Michael Houston
Content Development Specialist: Louise Cook
Project Manager: Andrew Riley
Design: Christian Bilbow
Marketing Manager: Rachael Pignotti

Working together to grow libraries in developing countries

www.elsevier.com • www.bookaid.org

Contents

Preface, vi
List of Contributors, vii

1 Imaging Techniques and Fundamental Observations for the Musculoskeletal System, 1
Philip W.P. Bearcroft • Melanie A. Hopper

2 Internal Derangements of Joints: Upper and Lower Limbs, 24
Robert S.D. Campbell • Andrew J. Dunn • Eugene McNally • Ahmed Daghir

3 Bone Tumours (1): Benign Tumours and Tumour-Like Lesions of Bone, 54
Asif Saifuddin

4 Bone Tumours (2): Malignant Bone Tumours, 79
A. Mark Davies • Steven L.J. James • Asif Saifuddin

5 Soft Tissue Tumours, 99
Paul O'Donnell

6 Metabolic and Endocrine Skeletal Disease, 121
Thomas M. Link • Judith E. Adams

7 Arthritis, 156
Andrew J. Grainger • Philip O'Connor

8 Appendicular and Pelvic Trauma, 182
Nigel Raby • Philip M. Hughes • James Ricketts

9 Bone, Joint and Spinal Infection, 213
Balashanmugam Rajashanker • Richard W. Whitehouse

Index, 251

PREFACE

The 9 chapters in this book have been selected from the contents of the Musculoskeletal System section in *Grainger & Allison's Diagnostic Radiology, Sixth Edition.* These chapters provide a succinct up-to-date overview of current imaging techniques and their clinical applications in daily practice and it is hoped that with this concise format the user will quickly grasp the fundamentals they need to know. Throughout these chapters, the relative merits of different imaging investigations are described, variations are discussed and recent imaging advances are detailed. Please note that imaging techniques of the spine are considered in the separate section 'The Spine' in *Grainger & Allison's Diagnostic Radiology, Sixth Edition.*

Grainger & Allison's Diagnostic Radiology has long been recognized as the standard general reference work in the field, and it is hoped that this book, utilizing the content from the latest sixth edition of this classic reference work, will provide radiology trainees and practitioners with ready access to the most current information, written by internationally recognized experts, on what is new and important in the radiological diagnosis of musculoskeletal disorders.

LIST OF CONTRIBUTORS

Judith E. Adams, MBBS, FRCR, FRCP, FBIR
Professor of Clinical Radiology, Department of
Radiology and Manchester Academic Health Science
Centre, The Royal Infirmary, Central Manchester
University Hospitals NHS Foundation Trust,
Manchester, UK

Philip W.P. Bearcroft, MA, MB, BChir, FRCR, FRCP
Consultant Radiologist, Department of Radiology,
Cambridge University Hospitals NHS Foundation,
Cambridge, UK

Robert S.D. Campbell, MB, ChB, FRCR
Consultant Musculoskeletal Radiologist, Department of
Radiology, Royal Liverpool University Hospital,
Liverpool, UK

Ahmed Daghir, MRCP, FRCR
Clinical Fellow, Department of Radiology, Nuffield
Orthopaedic Centre, Oxford, UK

A. Mark Davies, MBChB, DMRD, FRCR
Consultant Radiologist, MRI Centre, Royal
Orthopaedic Hospital NHS Foundation Trust,
Birmingham, UK

Andrew J. Dunn, MBChB, FRCR
Consultant Musculoskeletal Radiologist, Department of
Radiology, Royal Liverpool University Hospital,
Liverpool, UK

Andrew J. Grainger, BM, BS, MRCP, FRCR
Consultant and Honorary Clinical Associate Professor,
Musculoskeletal Radiology, Leeds Teaching Hospitals
and Leeds Musculoskeletal Biomedical Research
Centre, Leeds, UK

Melanie A. Hopper, MB ChB, MRCS, FRCR
Consultant Radiologist, Department of Radiology,
Addenbrooke's Hospital, Cambridge University
Hospitals NHS Foundation Trust, Cambridge, UK

Philip M. Hughes, MBBS, MRCP, FRCR
Consultant Radiologist, Radiology, Plymouth Hospitals
Trust, Plymouth, Cornwall, UK

Steven L.J. James, MB, ChB, FRCR
Consultant Musculoskeletal Radiologist, The Royal
Orthopaedic Hospital NHS Foundation Trust,
Birmingham, UK

Thomas M. Link, MD, PhD
Professor of Radiology; Chief, Musculoskeletal
Imaging; Clinical Director Musculoskeletal and
Quantitative Imaging Research, Department of
Radiology and Biomedical Imaging, University of
California San Francisco, San Francisco, CA, USA

Eugene McNally, MB BCh, BAO, FRCPI, FRCR
Consultant Musculoskeletal Radiologist and Clinical
Lead, Nuffield Orthopaedic Centre and University of
Oxford, Oxford, UK

Philip O'Connor, MBBS, MRCP, FRCR, FFSEM(UK)
Musculoskeletal Radiologist, Clinical Radiology, Leeds
Teaching Hospitals Trust, The University of Leeds,
West Yorkshire, UK

Paul O'Donnell, MBBS, MRCP, FRCR
Consultant Radiologist, Royal National Orthopaedic
Hospital; Honorary Senior Lecturer, University
College London, London, UK

Nigel Raby, MB ChB, MRCP, FRCR
Consultant Radiologist, Department of Radiology,
Western Infirmary, Glasgow, UK

Balashanmugam Rajashanker, MBBS, MRCP, FRCR
Consultant Radiologist, Clinical Radiology, Central
Manchester Foundation Trust, Manchester, UK

James Ricketts, BMBS
Radiology Registrar, Derriford Hospital, Plymouth, UK

Asif Saifuddin, BSc(Hons), MB ChB, MRCP, FRCR
Consultant Musculoskeletal Radiologist, Imaging
Department, The Royal National Orthopaedic
Hospital, Stanmore, Middlesex, UK

Richard W. Whitehouse, MB, ChB, MD, FRCR
Consultant Radiologist, Clinical Radiology, Manchester
Royal Infirmary, Manchester, UK

CHAPTER 1

IMAGING TECHNIQUES AND FUNDAMENTAL OBSERVATIONS FOR THE MUSCULOSKELETAL SYSTEM

Philip W.P. Bearcroft • Melanie A. Hopper

CHAPTER OUTLINE

INTRODUCTION

IMAGING TECHNIQUES AVAILABLE

NORMAL IMAGING APPEARANCES

SPECIFIC RADIOLOGICAL SCENARIOS

INTRODUCTION

There are numerous imaging investigations available to clinicians and radiologists for the assessment of musculoskeletal disease. This chapter will describe the individual investigations, concentrating on the strengths and weaknesses of each technique. Variations will be discussed and recent imaging advances detailed. A working knowledge of the normal appearance of musculoskeletal structures is essential and these will then be described. Finally, three common imaging scenarios will be explained: calcification in soft tissues, gas in soft tissues and periosteal reaction.

IMAGING TECHNIQUES AVAILABLE

Radiography

Radiography has an important role in the preliminary evaluation of musculoskeletal disorders and for many conditions no further imaging is required. The technique relies upon the differing absorption of ionising radiation by tissues within the body. As a result, radiography provides excellent contrast between tissues such as fat and muscle and bone. It does not, however, provide contrast between soft tissues and has limited ability to demonstrate bone loss compared to cross-sectional techniques.

To aid diagnosis, two views of a body part are typically taken. Conventionally these are in the lateral plane and the anteroposterior (AP) plane, which is termed dorsopedal (DP) in the feet and dorsopalmar (DP) in the hands. Particularly in trauma, two views, preferably orthogonal, are important to minimise misinterpretation of overlapping structures (Fig. 1-1).

In complex anatomical areas or when specific information is needed, additional or alternative views are frequently obtained.

Benefits

Radiographs are readily available as an imaging technique. Traditionally viewed as hard copy film, technological advances now mean that in the majority of institutions radiographs are obtained, viewed and stored digitally. The picture archiving and communication system (PACS) provides immediate access to previous radiographs for comparison not just for radiography but for all imaging investigations.

Radiographs also provide initial soft-tissue assessment and can demonstrate soft-tissue swelling as well as joint effusions, which can be particularly useful in areas where bony abnormality may be radiographically occult (Fig. 1-2).

Disadvantages

An awareness of the limitations of radiographic evaluation is crucial. As in other areas of the body, artefact from external structures such as clothing and from overlapping structures can be misinterpreted as an abnormality. Some sites can be difficult to appreciate fully using radiographs. The medial end of the clavicle, for example, can be problematic due to multiple overlying structures and an abnormality may be more difficult to detect. It is important that radiographs, as with other imaging investigations, are interpreted in light of the clinical details and additional imaging should be undertaken if concern persists. The lack of radiographic soft-tissue evaluation is well recognised as the attenuation of X-rays by most soft-tissue structures lies within a narrow range and this limits the interrogation of soft-tissue structures.

One of the main drawbacks of radiography is its reliance upon ionising radiation and the potential resulting side effects. However, particularly in the extremities, the dose involved is minimal and although the hazards of

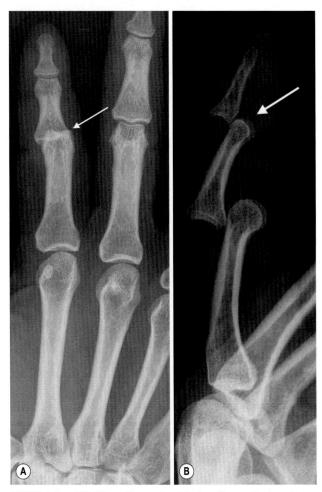

FIGURE 1-1 ■ (A) AP radiograph of index finger demonstrates dislocation of the proximal interphalangeal joint (arrow). (B) Dislocated distal interphalangeal joint is only evident on the orthogonal view (arrow).

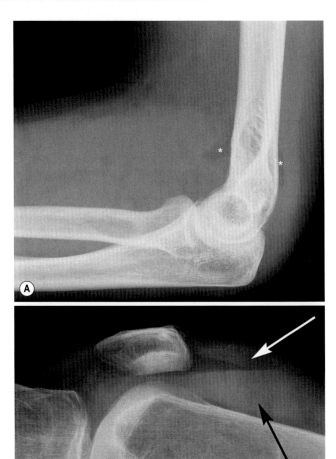

FIGURE 1-2 ■ (A) Lateral radiograph of the elbow shows joint effusion displacing the fat pads (*) indicating intra-articular injury. (B) Horizontal beam lateral radiograph of the knee shows lipohaemarthrosis due to occult fracture with a linear fat (white arrow)/fluid (black arrow) level.

ionising radiation should never be ignored, the diagnostic benefits generally outweigh the possible risk when radiographs are correctly used.

Advances and Variations

Stress Views. Standard radiographs allow static evaluation of musculoskeletal structures. Imaging a joint under passive or active stress may also provide indirect assessment of ligamentous injury.[1,2] For example, comparative flexion and extension views of the cervical spine provide valuable information regarding stability of the atlanto-axial joint (Fig. 1-3).

Fluoroscopy. Fluoroscopic techniques have a wide range of uses across radiological specialties. They utilise an X-ray source similar to standard radiographs but provide real-time dynamic video images that are typically used in the radiology department and in orthopaedic surgery to guide interventional procedures such as needle placement and fracture reduction. Images are viewed on

a digital unit and are amplified to enable them to be seen in normal light, especially useful in the operating theatre.

Arthrography. The basic premise of arthrography is the injection of a radio-opaque contrast medium into a joint usually guided by fluoroscopy, although US guidance can be used as an alternative. Distension of the joint provides indirect information about the soft tissues which can be deduced from the distribution of the injected contrast medium (Fig. 1-4). Fluoroscopic evaluation also allows an element of dynamic assessment. With the advent of more sophisticated cross-sectional imaging which provides detailed and direct assessment of the internal joint structures, arthrography is now more frequently used in combination with MRI and, occasionally, CT following the injection of gadolinium-based or iodine-based contrast medium, respectively. Arthrography is frequently combined with the injection of local anaesthetic to

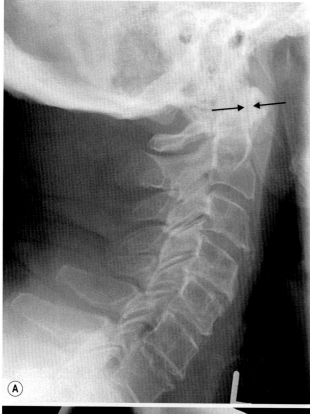

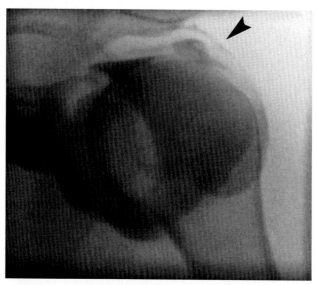

FIGURE 1-4 ■ Fluoroscopic image of the shoulder shows contrast medium within the glenohumeral joint extending into the subacromial bursa (arrowhead) indicating a rotator cuff tear.

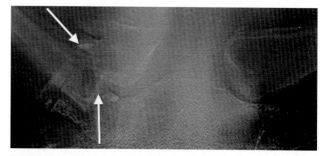

FIGURE 1-5 ■ Tomographic image of medial right medial clavicle fracture (arrows), normal left side.

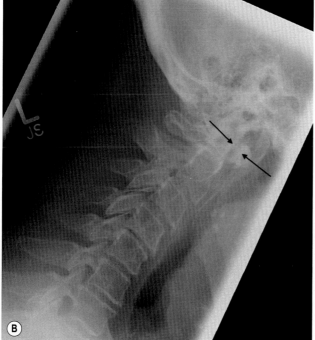

FIGURE 1-3 ■ **Lateral radiographs of the cervical spine in (A) extension and (B) flexion.** Atlantoaxial subluxation due to disruption of the transverse ligament is demonstrated on the view taken in flexion with widening of the atlantoaxial distance (black arrows).

provide additional diagnostic information in patients with possible joint symptoms, helping distinguish assymtpomatic and symptomatic abnormalities; corticosteroid may be introduced as a therapeutic agent.

Tomosynthesis. Digital tomosynthesis represents a modification of the conventional radiographic technique to acquire multiple low-dose images of a body part across a range of projection angles of the X-ray tube. Currently well established in breast imaging, interest in the application of tomosynthesis to other areas, including the musculoskeletal system, is growing.[3] The radiation dose is greater than that of conventional radiography but less than CT and preliminary studies suggest it has a role in the imaging of orthopaedic prostheses as the metallic-related streak artefacts encountered with CT is reduced.[4] Digital tomosynthesis also reduces the difficulty of composite shadow, showing promise in the assessment of anatomically complex areas (Fig. 1-5).

Ultrasound (US)

In current clinical practice US has an important role in the diagnosis and management of musculoskeletal disease,

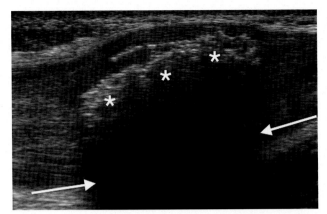

FIGURE 1-6 ■ **Sonographic image of the medial thigh shows heterotopic calcification (*) and posterior acoustic shadowing (arrows) within the adductor musculature not evident on radiographic assessment.**

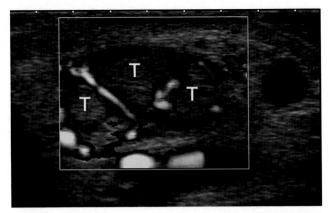

FIGURE 1-7 ■ **Transverse PD sonogram of the first extensor compartment tendons (T) at the wrist.** Abnormal vascularisation, particularly within the tendon sheath surrounding the tendons, indicates tenosynovitis.

providing high-resolution assessment of soft tissues. Evaluation of bone is limited, but US can afford information regarding the bony surface and periosteum. Typically, musculoskeletal US requires a linear array high-frequency probe of at least 7 MHz, and greater than 10 MHz is preferred. This is ideal for superficial abnormalities; deeper lesions necessitate a lower-frequency probe to provide adequate depth, albeit at reduced spatial resolution.

Benefits

US main benefits lie in its ability to give real-time, high-resolution and dynamic diagnostic information. In general the technique is fast and well tolerated by patients and allows direct clinical correlation of symptoms and abnormalites by the operator. Importantly, there is no ionising radiation. The ability of US to differentiate between solid and cystic structures is particularly useful in the musculoskeletal system. Soft-tissue calcification is evident earlier on US than on radiographs (Fig. 1-6).

Doppler assessment of vascularity is important in soft-tissue masses and also in the assessment of inflammatory and degenerative disorders where the presence of new blood vessel formation, known as neovascularisation, can be used to indicate disease activity and healing (Fig. 1-7). For the assessment of the majority of musculoskeletal conditions, the direction of vascular flow is not particularly useful and so the more sensitive power Doppler (PD) is favoured over colour Doppler techniques, as PD maximises spatial resolution and flow sensitivity at the expense of directional information.

The ability of US to demonstrate the movement of tissues in real time underpins one of its main advantages during review of musculoskeletal disorders. Abnormalities such as tendon subluxation and impingement may be clinically suspected but confirmation using real-time US can be invaluable diagnostically and as an aid to treatment. There is widespread use of US guidance for interventional techniques. The anatomy of the extremities in particular allows excellent needle visualisation as it is nearly always possible to position the needle parallel to

the transducer, maximising the clarity with which a needle is seen.

Disadvantages

Ultrasound is operator dependent and there is a steep learning curve. Artefacts can be challenging in musculoskeletal scanning.[5] Anisotropy describes the artefactual loss of tissue reflectivity when the US beam is applied at an oblique course to the tissue fibres under examination. The highly structured and fibrillar arrangement of tissues such as tendons and muscle makes this a particular problem in musculoskeletal US (Fig. 1-8A) and the resultant hypoechogenicity can simulate an abnormality such as tendinosis or tearing of a muscle or tendon. Beam edge artefact is evident at the edge of larger tendons such as the Achilles, with loss of normal signal and posterior acoustic shadowing that can mimic or conceal abnormal findings.

Advances and Variations

Beam steering of the transducer array produces tilting of the beam electronically of up to 40° from the main beam direction. When utilised instead of, or in addition to, manual angulation of the probe, this allows image generation from differing angles and provides a reduction in or even elimination of anisotropic artefact (Fig. 1-8).

Extended field-of-view (EFOV) or panoramic ultrasound gives a continuous image greater than the size of the ultrasound probe and although this does not necessarily improve the diagnostic ability of US, it provides images which more readily demonstrate the relevant abnormal findings than on the static images obtained by the operator (Fig. 1-9).

Elastography. The US assessment of tissue elasticity as an aid to diagnosis is well established in other radiological sub-specialities such as breast imaging and early studies suggest that there will be a role for the technique in musculoskeletal scanning. Elastography provides an assessment of tissue stiffness and requires the operator to

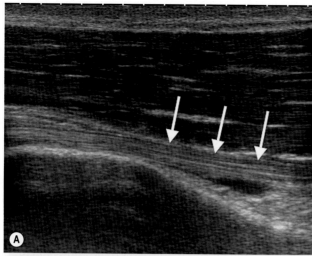

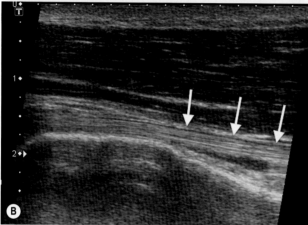

FIGURE 1-8 ■ **Longitudinal ultrasound images of the long head of biceps tendon (arrows).** (A) Distal anisotropic artefact. (B) Artefact eliminated using beam steer.

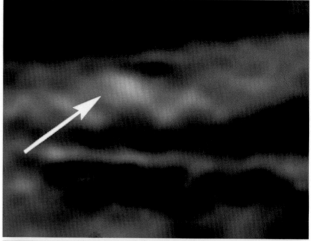

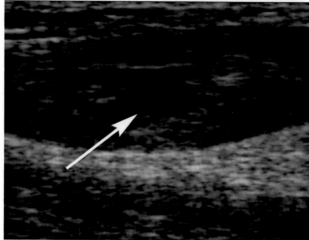

FIGURE 1-10 ■ **Partial thickness tear of the Achilles tendon.** B-mode US shows focal hypoechogenicity (lower arrow). Elastogram shows decreased tendon stiffness (upper arrow).

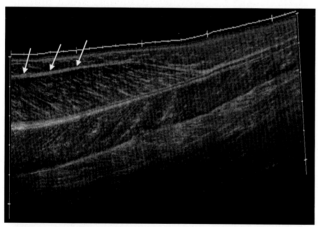

FIGURE 1-9 ■ **EFOV sonogram of the lower calf shows hypoechoic fascicle bundles covered by hyperechoic perimysium.** Echogenic epimysium surrounds each muscle (arrows).

gently compress the tissues under evaluation beneath the transducer. The strain or displacement of the tissues is determined by their hardness or softness. Normal ligaments and tendons are resistant to compression but tissue softening occurs in several conditions including

degeneration and trauma.[6] The potential of elastography does not lie in the replacement of traditional B-mode US imaging but rather as a complementary technique. There is particular potential in the assessment of soft-tissue conditions which on B-mode imaging have an isoechoic appearance to the normal surrounding tissues such as early tendon degeneration or tearing (Fig. 1-10).

Contrast-enhanced US. Development of abnormal new blood vessels in musculoskeletal pathology is accompanied by the formation of abnormal nerves and there is good scientific correlation between these changes and pain.[7] Therefore, the early identification of new vessels is important in the diagnosis of disease and potentially provides a target for treatment (Fig. 1-7).

Contrast media-enhanced US (CEUS) detects low blood flow that may not be detectable by more traditional Doppler techniques. The intravenous injection of microbubble contrast media has been shown to allow more accurate assessment of synovial vascularity, which in turn correlates with disease activity in rheumatological disorders.[8] How this will influence patient management in the clinical setting is not fully understood and currently the use of CEUS in the assessment and follow-up of rheumatological disease remains at the research level.

Computed Tomography (CT)

Benefits

CT is ideally suited for the evaluation of bony structures and soft-tissue calcification and provides excellent spatial resolution and demarcation of bony structure and detail. Typically, images are acquired in the axial plane but it is a noteworthy strength that CT images can be reconstructed into any other plane. Surface 3D-rendered reformatting can also be a useful aid to surgical planning.

Despite its limitations in assessment of muscle and fat, CT has a role in imaging patients in whom MRI is contraindicated and can be combined with the injection of intra-articular iodinated contrast media in a similar way to the more widely utilised MR arthrography.

Disadvantages

As with radiography, CT relies upon ionising radiation. CT, even of an extremity, is associated with a radiation dose many times that of conventional radiography. This is more of a consideration in CT of the axial skeleton where radiation is also directed through the thoracic and abdominal organs. For the evaluation of musculoskeletal conditions, the main weakness of CT lies in the poor differentiation of soft-tissues structures as, even when abnormal, their attenuation values remain similar to adjacent normal structures and so are relatively poorly demonstrated. Despite the structural bony detail afforded, CT is not the optimum imaging investigation for infiltrative bone marrow disorders as alterations in the water/fat content are generally more usefully demonstrated using MRI. Artefact from metallic devices such as orthopaedic prostheses is arguably less problematic for CT than MRI but may still limit diagnostic performance.

Advances and Variations

Many advances in modern CT imaging are directed towards maintaining image quality whilst reducing dose and a variety of techniques such as multiplanar image acquisition and iterative reconstruction have been employed.[9] CT is widely used for detailed evaluation of bony trauma and fracture assessment. The exquisite bone detail it provides allows for review of focal bony metastases, be they lytic, sclerotic or mixed. These are generally more conspicuous on MR images but CT crucially provides important information regarding cortical breach and potential pathological fracture risk.

Dual-energy CT. Utilising two X-ray tubes positioned at 90° to each other with corresponding detectors allows the simultaneous acquisition of images with different energy levels. Analysis of the data sets can differentiate, for example, uric acid crystals from gout against calcium within soft tissues and thus reliably detect gouty tophi.[10,11] Dual-energy CT also has been shown to demonstrate post-traumatic bone bruising due to changes in marrow composition,[12] previously an area where CT has not been helpful.

The role of CT is continuously expanding; for example, in many centres radiographic skeletal surveys for multiple myeloma have been successfully replaced with vertex-to-knee low-dose CT.[13]

Magnetic Resonance Imaging (MRI)

The advent of MRI revolutionised the imaging of musculoskeletal structures, providing unequalled direct assessment of soft tissues and joints.

Benefits

MR images are generated by the effect of a strong magnetic field on the hydrogen nuclei in water molecules, thereby avoiding the potential risks of ionising radiation. Like CT, MRI provides excellent spatial resolution but its ability to distinguish between two similar tissues (contrast resolution) is far superior. MRI is a rapidly progressing technology; particular interest has evolved in functional MRI techniques, enabling the visualisation of physiological processes and their changes in different disease states.

Disadvantages

The contraindications of MRI apply to imaging musculoskeletal structures as to any body system. Because of the strong magnetic field strength, many implantable medical devices such as cardiac pacemakers are considered to be unsafe. Ferrous materials also cause significant difficulty for the radiologist due to susceptibility artefact from image distortion and signal voids. Modern orthopaedic prostheses produced from titanium and other non-ferrous materials are less problematic than older devices but can still provide a challenge. Much time has been invested in the development and improvement of metal artefact reduction sequences (MARS) to limit this problem.[14] MRI is highly sensitive but findings are not always specific. High signal within bone marrow on fluid-sensitive sequences, for example, may be due to a range of clinical entities from trauma to infection or tumour. It is therefore important to interpret imaging findings in the context of clinical history and examination. MR is not a stand-alone technique and correlation with other investigations is important.

Advances and Variations

MR Arthrography. Performing arthrography with gadolinium contrast medium and combining with MRI provides joint distension and additional information about the internal joint structures.[15] Used principally in the shoulder and hip, MR arthrography has a particular use for the assessment of labral injury.

Cartilage Imaging. MRI is an excellent investigation for non-invasive assessment of articular cartilage. As advances develop in the treatment of chondral injury, so the interest in accurate cartilage-specific sequences increases. As yet, no single sequence has proven to be perfect and advances have concentrated on assessment of morphological changes and biochemical alterations in early chondral damage.

Imaging sequences such as fluid-sensitive fast spin-echo (FSE) and 3D T1-weighted spoiled gradient-recalled echo (SPRG) provide excellent review of morphological changes such as surface fissuring and cartilage loss. Biochemical changes relate mainly to variation in cartilage water content and abnormalities of proteoglycan composition and distribution which have been shown to correlate with cartilage degeneration. Anomalies in water content can be assessed by T2 mapping and techniques such as delayed gadolinium-enhanced MR imaging cartilage (dGEMRIC) identify abnormality of chondral structure before morphological abnormalities become evident. Newer techniques assessing cartilage sodium content (Na MRI) show promise in the early identification of cartilage injury.[16]

MR Elastography (MRE). Changes in muscle structure and/or composition can occur in a range of conditions causing alteration of tissue stiffness. MRE gives a quantitative and non-invasive assessment of tissue stiffness by measuring the propagation of mechanical waves through the tissue. MRE has already proven useful in liver and breast disease. Studies have shown the technique can evaluate changes in the mechanical properties of muscle due to conditions such as neuromuscular disease and malignancy but the role of MRE in routine practice has yet to be established.[17]

Diffusion-weighted MRI. Diffusion-weighted MRI (DWI) provides tissue characterisation visualising the movement of water molecules. Diseased tissues demonstrate altered diffusion capacity and several studies have indicated improved sensitivity in the detection of skeletal metastases when comparing DWI to conventional MRI. MR can also assess the direction of water diffusion; this provides diffusion tensor imaging and tractography.[18] Initial results in musculoskeletal diseases have been promising as it is now possible to appreciate directly variations in fibre microarchitecture in, for example, muscles rather than secondary change.

Nuclear Medicine

All nuclear medicine scintigraphic procedures require the introduction of a radiopharmaceutical into the patient; the emitted radiation is then detected by a camera and displayed in much the same way as a standard radiograph. The skeletal scintogram is the most commonly encountered nuclear medicine technique for the evaluation of musculoskeletal abnormalities. This utilises technetium-99m-labelled methylene diphosphonate (^{99m}Tc-MDP), which identifies increased osteoblastic activity and therefore areas of high bone turnover (Fig. 1-11).

Benefits

Bone scintigraphy is widely available and is highly sensitive for a broad spectrum of osseous conditions as changes in bone metabolism predate alterations in morphology.

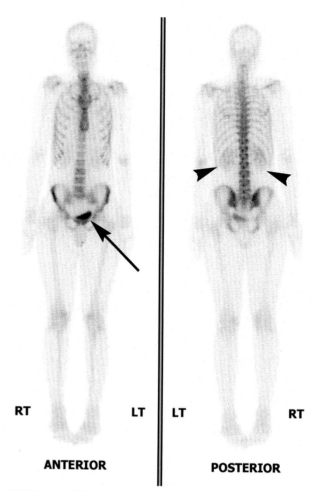

FIGURE 1-11 ■ **^{99m}Tc-MDP bone scintogram shows normal distribution of radiotracer within the skeleton and urinary tract.** The renal outlines are visible (arrowhead) and radiotracer is evident within the urinary bladder (arrow).

It delivers a functional assessment of bone metabolism of the entire skeleton at the same time. Triple-phase scintigraphy obtains images at three different time periods after injection of the radiotracer and improves the differentiation of bony and soft-tissue disease.

Disadvantages

Although highly sensitive, bone scintigraphy has low specificity. Increased bone turnover is evident in a wide spectrum of bone disorders, including degeneration, infection, trauma and malignancy. Lytic lesions without increase in osteoblastic activity such as multiple myeloma are occult. Accurate localisation can be difficult, particularly in anatomically complex locations. The radiation dose of the injected radiotracer is high compared to radiography and is applied to the entire body rather than limited to the area under review. The spatial resolution of standard scintigraphy is several times less than other imaging investigations.

Advances and Variations

Single photon emission computed tomography (SPECT) can be utilised in musculoskeletal disease using similar

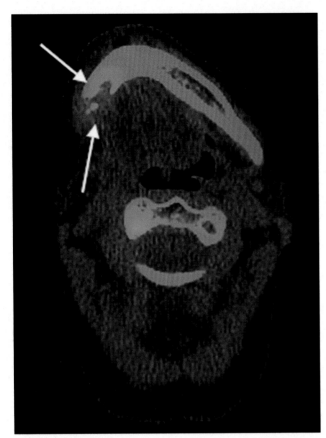

FIGURE 1-12 ■ **SPECT CT of the mandible.** Axial image shows increased radiotracer uptake (arrows) due to osteonecrosis of the jaw; increased uptake posteriorly is due to degeneration within the cervical spine.

radiopharmecuticals to traditional bone scintigraphy. The benefit lies in the multiplanar data acquired, which can be reformatted to provide 3D images. Side-by-side comparison with CT or overlying both data sets with software-based fusion can give anatomical correlation, but this is being superseded by hybrid SPECT CT superimposing the scintigraphic findings on high-resolution CT images to give functional anatomical mapping (Fig. 1-12). Studies suggest this may be useful in assessment of a range of musculoskeletal disorders such as infection, trauma and osteoarthrosis, particularly in areas such as the spine and other anatomically complex locations.[19]

NORMAL IMAGING APPEARANCES

Radiography

Bones and Joints

Radiographs provide an excellent primary assessment of bone and joint conditions. In the case of trauma, radiographs reliably identify fractures and dislocation. They provide useful assessment of painful bones and joints and are invaluable for the review of bony deformity and anatomical variation. Normal bone has a dense cortex of varying thickness. Radiographs demonstrate a distinct corticomedullary junction and within the medulla trabecular structure should be appreciated. Different bones have differing ratios of cortex and medullary cavity; this affects their radiographic appearance and how readily abnormality is radiographically visualised when diseased.

Soft Tissues

Air, fat and skeletal muscle have differing absorption characteristics for ionising radiation and it is possible to discriminate between them on radiographs. In general, however, radiographs have poor sensitivity for the detection of soft-tissue abnormalities.

Ultrasound

Bone and Joints

Ultrasound is unable to provide diagnostic information regarding internal bone structure but periosteal reaction may be seen and US can be used to confirm fractures of superficial bones such as metatarsal stress fractures or fractures in children. The growth plate can be identified as a distinct hypoechoic interruption to the hyperechoic cortex in the skeletally immature skeleton and should not be mistaken for a fracture.

There is increasing interest in the use of US as an aid to clinical assessment of joint disease.[20] US is highly sensitive for the detection of joint fluid. Simple joint fluid is hypoechoic and compressible and posterior acoustic enhancement can be appreciated. Internal echoes within joint fluid may be seen due to debris, proteinaceous fluid, crystal arthropathy and even loose bodies. Normal synovium is not visible at US. Abnormal synovium has a wide range of appearances from anechoic to hyperechoic intra-articular tissue. Internal vascularity can be helpful and, unlike joint fluid, thickened synovium may be deformed by probe pressure but is not displaced.

Hyaline cartilage has a uniform hypoechoic appearance similar to joint fluid. It may be necessary to displace adjacent joint fluid with probe pressure to fully appreciate the underlying cartilage. The bone cortex should be clearly evident as a continuous hyperechoic structure. Near the articular surfaces, in particular, normal grooves in the cortex should not be mistaken for bony erosions; this is particularly prominent over the dorsal aspect of the metacarpal heads.

Soft Tissues

Fat. Subcutaneous fat is clearly defined as a separate layer deep to the dermal tissues. Predominantly hypoechoic, there are multiple linear hyperechoic connective tissue septa within the fat. The majority of these lie parallel to the skin surface.

Muscle, Tendons and Ligaments. The majority of skeletal muscle is superficial and therefore readily assessed using a linear array high-frequency transducer.

A lower-frequency linear probe or even a curvilinear probe may be used for deeper structures such as the gluteal musculature. Skeletal muscle is generally less echogenic than subcutaneous fat with a highly organised configuration. Muscle fibres are arranged as separate hypoechoic fascicles wrapped by a thin connective tissue endomysium which is not readily visualised. Groups of fascicles are bundled together by a thicker, echogenic perimysial sheath, clearly distinguished at US. Each muscle is encompassed by a dense and irregular connective tissue echogenic epimysium; this layer forms a continuation with the tendon and with the endomysium and perimysium (Fig. 1-9). Finally there is a fascial integument covering the epimysium; this is not defined as a separate structure at imaging. The echogenicity of muscle can change, depending upon its state; relaxed muscle is often more echogenic than when contracted.

Muscle fibres frequently lie obliquely to the skin surface and this, combined with their linear arrangement, makes anisotropic artefact a consideration when evaluating for abnormality. It is important to appreciate the underlying muscle structure and to image transverse and longitudinal to the muscle not just to the limb.

Tendons possess a fibrillar arrangement of echogenic fascicles which lie parallel to the longitudinal axis of the tendon (Figs. 1-8 and 1-13). The surrounding tendon sheath can be identified as a highly echogenic thin line lying immediately adjacent. When present, the synovial sheath is usually anechoic and not identified as a separate layer. In certain areas such as the wrist and ankle a small amount of synovial fluid is normal and acts to cushion the tendon during movement. It is important to assess a tendon in both a relaxed state and under tension. Generally, under tension, the tendon becomes taut, reducing anisotropy and providing more reliable assessment of internal hypoechoic foci. However, this also temporarily obliterates small abnormal blood vessels within the tendon which are more fully appreciated with the tendon relaxed.

Dynamic assessment of the muscle tendon unit can provide useful diagnostic information. Injury to the tendon itself or to surrounding structures can allow the tendon to sublux or dislocate within the normal range of movement.

Ligaments. Similar to tendons, ligaments are composed of type 1 collagen fibres which are arrayed in an echogenic and fibrillar distribution. Normal ligaments vary in size and comparison with the contralateral side is often useful. Injury causes loss of the linear structure and disruption of fibres with hypoechoic foci. Evaluation with the ligament under tension is preferred.

Nerves. Even small distal neural structures are exquisitely demonstrated using US (Fig. 1-13). Each nerve is enveloped by its epineurium, a loose connective tissue matrix. The multiple hypoechoic neural fascicles are individually covered by echogenic layers of dense connective tissue, termed the perineurium. Imaging transverse to the nerve allows the operator to identify the fascicles as separate discreet round bundles. Longitudinal evaluation shows the parallel fascicular arrangement.

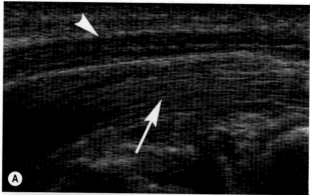
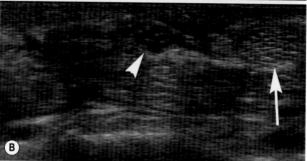

FIGURE 1-13 ■ (A) Longitudinal and (B) transverse ultrasound images of the median nerve (arrowheads) showing hypoechoic fascicles differing from the fibrillar pattern within adjacent tendons (arrows).

Computed Tomography

Bone

Bony cortex is a dense high-attenuation layer thinning at the metaphyses and epiphyses of long bones. Individual trabeculae can be appreciated within the medullary cavity on CT. Bone is a dynamic organ and alterations in bone morphology can indicate disease processes: for example, the presence of osteophytes in osteoarthrosis.

Soft Tissues

Even by adjusting the window and level parameters to maximise contrast between adjacent soft-tissue elements, it is not usually possible to differentiate normal from abnormal soft-tissue structures in musculoskeletal disease. Conversely, although the attenuation values of fat and skeletal muscle differ enough that they can be distinguished as separate tissues, this is seldom useful clinically.

MRI

Bone and Joints

With its ability to differentiate fatty and haematopoietic marrow, MRI is a valuable technique for non-invasive marrow assessment.

It is essential to remember that bone is a dynamic organ. Age-dependent variation in both composition and distribution of bone marrow is well recognised. At birth the entire skeleton contains red haematopoietic marrow

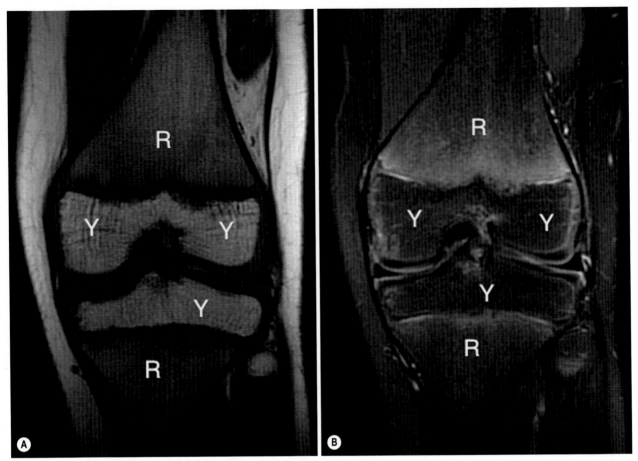

FIGURE 1-14 ■ **Coronal MR images of a skeletally immature patient.** (A) T1-weighted and (B) proton density fat-saturated images showing yellow marrow in the epiphyses (Y) and red marrow in the metadiaphyses (R).

and over the next two decades there is a predictable conversion to yellow fatty bone marrow. Conversion is a symmetrical process, beginning in the peripheral long bones, and follows a centripetal course to the axial skeleton. Within each bone, conversion starts around the vessels within the mid-diaphysis, expanding out towards the metaphyses. As the epiphyses and apophyses ossify, they contain yellow marrow (Fig. 1-14). By the end of the third decade conversion is complete and bone marrow has an adult distribution; the majority of the adult skeleton contains yellow marrow and red marrow persists only in the skull, spine, clavicles, scapulae, pelvis and proximal humeral and femoral metaphyses (hence the predilection of bloodborne metastases to these sites in adults).

An increase in functional demand can trigger reconversion of fatty to haematopoietic marrow. This process can arise secondary to benign conditions such as heavy smoking and is seen in chronic anaemia whatever the underlying cause. Reconversion occurs in a predictable pattern exactly reversing the conversion process occurring from axial to distal. Although this appears straightforward, the interpretation of marrow signal abnormalities is complex with a wide spectrum of normal variation; it can be difficult to differentiate red marrow hyperplasia from malignant infiltration.

The appearance of normal bone marrow on MRI is determined by the pulse sequence parameters and the marrow constituents, particularly the proportion of fat cells but also the relative quantities of water and trabecular matrix. Differentiation between fatty and haematopoietic marrow is best appreciated on T1-weighted sequences. Yellow or fatty marrow has signal characteristics similar to those of subcutaneous fat on T1-weighted imaging. On T2-weighted sequences fatty marrow signal intensity is typically higher than muscle and similar to or slightly lower than subcutaneous fat. The appearance of yellow marrow using gradient-echo sequences is variable and predominantly dependent upon the quantity of trabecular bone. Trabeculae produce susceptibility and the higher the density of trabeculae, the greater the artefact and signal loss seen on gradient-echo sequences.

On T1-weighted imaging, haematopoietic marrow signal is lower than yellow marrow but still higher than that of the intervertebral discs and muscle (Fig. 1-14A). Red marrow has a similar or slightly higher signal than skeletal muscle on both T1- and T2-weighted imaging. This is a useful comparison as, outside the neonatal period, decreased signal relative to muscle is a sensitive indicator of non-physiological marrow infiltration.

Red marrow returns intermediate signal similar to skeletal muscle, whereas yellow marrow signal is lower than muscle on fluid-sensitive, fat-suppression sequences such as STIR or fat-saturated T2 (T2fs) sequences (Fig. 1-14B). These sequences can be used to emphasise the conspicuity of abnormal processes as the majority will cause increased fluid signal. Use of gadolinium-based contrast medium can also be used to accentuate the presence of abnormalities, as normal adult marrow does not significantly enhance but many malignancies will demonstrate increased signal intensity. Care must be taken in interpretation of the paediatric skeleton following contrast medium as normal enhancement of the vertebral marrow in infants and even young children can be striking.

Unlike other imaging investigations, MRI allows direct evaluation of the internal joint soft-tissue structures. As techniques for the treatment of chondral injury improve, accurate assessment of cartilage becomes more important. Proton density fat-supressed and T2-weighted sequences are widely used in routine practice and show hyaline cartilage as a discreet intermediate signal layer separate to high signal fluid and low signal bony cortex (Fig. 1-14B). Increased cartilage signal indicates increased fluid content and is indicative of chondral softening or chondromalacia. More advanced injury such as fissuring, irregularity or cartilage defect can be assessed. Further sequences optimised for assessment of morphological and biochemical changes within articular cartilage have been developed and are discussed earlier in the chapter.

Soft Tissues

Normal fat returns returns high signal on both T1- and fast spin-echo (FSE) T2-weighted sequences and signal should be uniformly saturated (decreased) using fat suppression sequences such as STIR or spectral fat suppression (Fig. 1-15). Internal connective tissue septation can be appreciated but is less conspicuous than on US evaluation. The deep fascia is evident as a discrete low signal band demarcating subcutaneous fat from the underlying muscle compartments.

Generally, muscle abnormalities can be grouped into abnormal masses, muscle atrophy, disorders causing muscle oedema and anatomical variations. It is critical to employ sequences which will demonstrate these conditions and normally a combination of T1-weighted and fluid sensitive T2 fat-suppressed (T2fs) or STIR sequences are used.

Normal skeletal muscle signal is slightly higher than water and much lower than fat on T1-weighted sequences. On T2-weighted sequences skeletal muscle signal is much lower than both fat and fluid and on STIR or T2fs sequences normal muscle signal is higher than fat and lower than fluid (Fig. 1-15). Skeletal muscles are symmetrical when compared to the contralateral side; this is particularly useful when assessing for subtle findings such as focal scarring or anomalous muscles. The fat distribution within a muscle generally conforms to a predictable and often characteristic pattern. The musculotendinous junction does not represent a discreet cutoff between muscle fibres and the tendon; instead, there is a gradual coalescence of tendon fibres. Denervation and disuse fat

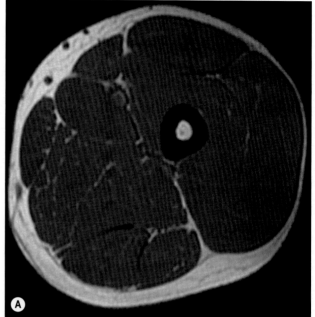

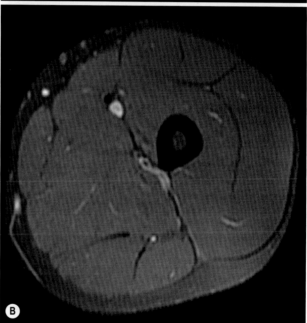

FIGURE 1-15 ■ **Axial MR images through the mid-thigh.** (A) T1- and (B) T2-weighted fat-saturated images showing skin, normal fat distribution, muscle and bone.

atrophy of a muscle begins first around this myotendinous junction.

Tendons and ligaments are both chiefly composed of type 1 collagen and have a similar MR appearance, being of low signal on all conventional sequences.

SPECIFIC RADIOLOGICAL SCENARIOS

Soft-tissue Calcification and Ossification

Soft-tissue mineralisation is frequently encountered in routine radiological practice. It is important to

TABLE 1-1   Soft-Tissue Calcification
Dystrophic calcification
Metabolic calcification
Calcium pyrophosphate deposition disease
Tumoral calcinosis
Malignant calcification

differentiate between calcification and ossification to aid with diagnosis, although this can be difficult in small lesions and calcification can progress to ossification over time.

Ossified foci have a cortex and internal medullary trabeculation mirroring normal bone structure. Soft-tissue calcification can occur in a myriad of abnormalities (Table 1-1); over 95% of lesions, however, are due to dystrophic calcification. Metabolic calcification, calcium hydroxyapatite deposition disease, tumoral calcinosis and malignant causes of calcification/ossification are much less common.

Dystrophic Calcification

By far the most common cause of soft-tissue calcification, dystrophic calcification occurs in damaged or devitalised tissues with formation of amorphous calcified deposits which may evolve into ossification. Importantly, dystrophic calcification is not related to abnormalities of serum calcium or phosphate. The misnomer myositis ossificans has previously been used to describe soft-tissue mineralisation particularly secondary to trauma. As this often does not occur in muscle, does not always have an inflammatory aetiology and may not always be ossified, the term has generally been replaced with heterotopic calcification or ossification.

Arterial Vascular Calcification. Although previously considered to be a passive process, recent studies have indicated that the underlying mechanisms of vascular calcification are active and highly regulated. Arterial calcification is a reliable clinical marker for atherosclerosis and the extent of calcification strongly correlates with the severity of arterial disease.[21] Vascular calcification models divide aetiology into two main categories. Subintimal lipid deposition occurring in atherosclerotic disease triggers a cascade similar to that occurring in soft-tissue calcification. The extent of arterial calcification ranges from irregular plaques to extensive tramline calcification predominantly affecting the aorta, pelvic and lower extremity arteries. Non-atherosclerotic calcification affects the media of the arterial wall and is believed to be triggered by interaction with toxins such as in diabetes, hyperparathyroidism and uraemia. This causes a finer and sometimes granular calcific pattern. In practice, the processes involved in medial calcification are also implicated in accelerated atherosclerosis and so there is considerable overlap in their radiological appearance (Fig. 1-16).

Venous Vascular Calcification. Calcification around a venous valve is relatively common and has the

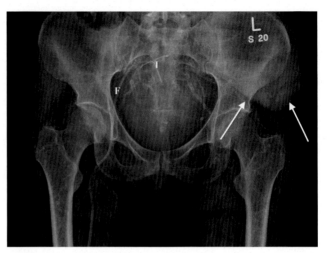

FIGURE 1-16 ■ **Pelvic radiograph of a patient with chronic renal failure.** Extensive vascular calcification and soft-tissue calcification. External artefact from ileostomy bag (arrows), IUCD (I) and right femoral line (F).

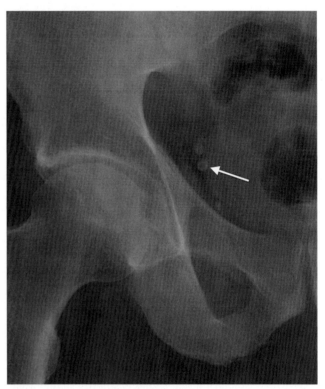

FIGURE 1-17 ■ **Hip radiograph shows phleboliths of the pelvis venous plexus.** One phlebolith is en face and so has a central lucency (arrow).

characteristic appearance of lamellation with central lucency visible when viewed en face. These phleboliths are most often encountered related to the pelvic venous plexus or lower limb veins (Fig. 1-17) but may also be seen in chronic varicosities and less frequently within soft-tissue haemangiomas. The combination of multiple enchondromas (Ollier's disease) and soft-tissue haemangiomas is seen in Maffucci's syndrome (Fig. 1-18).

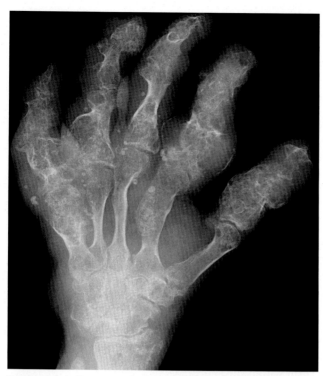

FIGURE 1-18 ■ Hand radiograph of patient with Maffucci's syndrome shows extensive multiple enchondromas with phleboliths in soft-tissue haemangiomas.

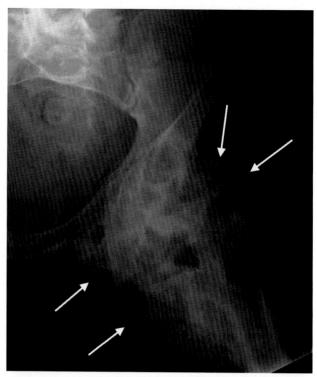

FIGURE 1-19 ■ Extensive heterotopic ossification with ankylosis (arrows) of the left hip in a patient with post-traumatic quadriplegia.

Trauma. Calcification is commonly seen related to previous soft-tissue injury. Even seemingly minor trauma such as subcutaneous or intramuscular injections can stimulate the development of dense calcifications occurring at the characteristic injection sites such as the upper arm and buttocks. Post-traumatic heterotopic mineralisation is recognised as a common complication following closed head injuries, burns and in paraplegia.[22] Ossification can be extensive and ankylosis is not infrequent if calcification bridges across the joint. Classically the shoulder and pelvic girdles and elbows are affected (Fig. 1-19). US can be a useful diagnostic tool for focal calcification as it will show calcification not yet visible on plain film (Fig. 1-6).

Calcium Hydroxyapatite Deposition Disease. Calcium hydroxyapatite deposition disease (HADD) should be differentiated from the other crystal deposition disorders, calcium pyrophosphate dihydrate deposition disease (CPPD) and monosodium urate crystal deposition disease (gout). HADD represents the formation of calcium hydroxyapatite crystals within the periarticular soft tissues and usually manifests as amorphous, dystrophic calcification within the tendons of the rotator cuff (Fig. 1-20). Typically affecting the middle-aged and elderly, HADD generally has a mono-articular presentation and can be very painful, mimicking infection or conditions such as frozen shoulder. The underlying aetiology is thought to be linked to minor repetitive trauma causing necrosis and inflammation. Over time the calcific deposits may regress, remain stable or mature. Ultrasound can be of value in assessing the maturity of these deposits; in general, dense

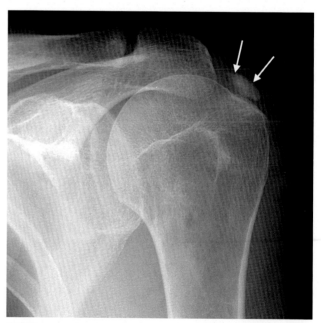

FIGURE 1-20 ■ AP radiograph of shoulder showing dense hydroxyapatite deposit (arrows) in the superior rotator cuff in a patient with calcific tendinosis.

fragmented deposits with distal acoustic shadowing are indicators of more long-standing calcification.

Congenital Causes for Soft-tissue Calcification. Fibrodysplasia ossificans progressiva (FOP) is a rare, autosomal dominant disorder with variable penetrance causing replacement of normal muscle and connective tissue by profuse heterotopic ossification. The initial manifestation is swelling of the muscular fascial planes, usually affecting the neck and shoulder planes first. This is followed by multifocal calcification progressing into ossification. Over time, mobility becomes restricted and respiration is constrained by bands of extraseletal bone formation within the thorax. CT, MRI and scintigraphy can identify early changes.[23] FOP is associated with short first metacarpals and metatarsals along with small cervical vertebral bodies with relative prominence of the pedicles. The condition is usually fatal in early life.

Infection

Bacterial and Fungal Infection. Calcification is a rare feature of bacterial infection but may occur in the cavity of an abscess. Extensive calcified lymphadenitis is highly suggestive of previous tuberculous infection. A similar appearance is seen in fungal infection with histoplasmosis and coccidioidomycosis where these are endemic. Neural calcification is reported almost exclusively in leprosy and so is a significant finding.[24] Calcification most frequently occurs as linear opacification, typically of the ulnar nerve (Fig. 1-21).

Parasitic Infection. Soft-tissue calcification related to parasitic infection often has a distinctive morphology indicative of the pathogen involved. Most of these infections are rare in the developed world but are encountered occasionally in visitors or migrants from endemic areas.

Cysticercosis can develop in the brain and skeletal muscle following exposure to the eggs of *Taenia solium* (pork tapeworm) and should be differentiated from infection by the adult tapeworm, which affects the gut. The disease is endemic in Central and South America, Africa, Asia and parts of Eastern Europe. Within muscle, cysticercosis is seen as multiple foci of intramuscular calcification, which are orientated longitudinally along the muscle fibres and measure up to 1 cm in length; these characteristically have the appearance of grains of rice (Fig. 1-22). *Dracunculus medinensis* (guinea worm) causes a parasitic infection (dracunculiasis) found throughout tropical Africa, the Middle East, India, the Far East and the northern countries of South America. Larvae are ingested in contaminated drinking water and pass through the intestinal wall to mature in the subcutaneous tissues where the calcification of the dead adult female guinea worm has a distinctive long coiled or curled appearance (Fig. 1-23). Infection with the filarial *Loa loa* may also give calcification of the adult worm within the subcutaneous soft tissues. In loiasis the calcification has a fine linear or coiled thread-like appearance and is best seen in the extremities. *Loa loa* is endemic in West and Central Africa. Infection occurs from a fly bite, with the larvae maturing into the adult worm within the subcutaneous tissues.

Autoimmune

Dermatomyositis. Dermatomyositis is an inflammatory muscle disorder of unknown aetiology modulated by

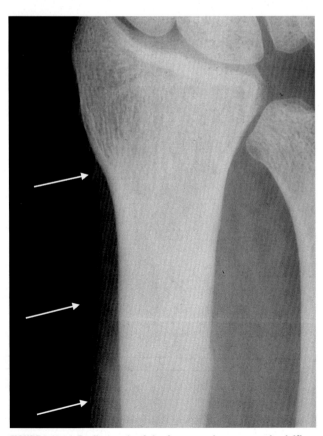

FIGURE 1-21 ■ Radiograph of the forearm shows neural calcification (arrows) in leprosy.

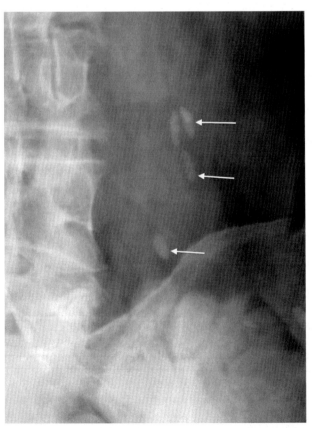

FIGURE 1-22 ■ Rice-like calcification of cysticercosis (arrows) affecting the psoas muscle.

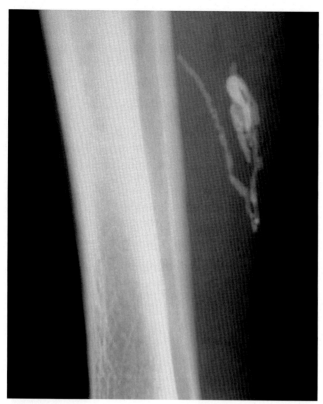

FIGURE 1-23 ■ Coiled calcification within the subcutaneous tissues of the lower leg in guinea worm infection.

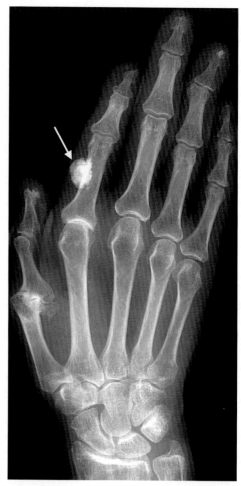

FIGURE 1-24 ■ Radiograph of the hand in a patient with progressive systemic sclerosis. Calcinosis circumscripta (arrow), soft-tissue loss of the tip of the index finger and thumb MCP joint arthritis are present.

the immune system. Several infectious agents such as Coxsackie virus and *Toxoplasma* have been implicated as possible triggers. The disorder can occur at any age and may affect either sex, but is most common in adult women, although there is a severe juvenile form. Skin and muscle involvement is typically seen but patients may also develop joint disease and debilitating oesophageal and cardiopulmonary disease. Dermatomyositis is frequently associated with non-specific subcutaneous calcinosis appreciated on radiographs; the formation of sheet-like calcification along muscle and fascial planes is characteristic but much less common. In the adult form, there is a strong association with malignancy, particularly of the bronchus, breast, stomach and ovary.[25]

Progressive Systemic Sclerosis (Scleroderma). This is a generalised autoimmune disorder of unknown cause which is characterised by extensive fibrosis and widespread small vessel vasculopathy. Scleroderma refers to the cutaneous manifestation but there is frequent visceral involvement, particularly of the oesophagus, kidneys, heart and lungs. Typical features in the hands are resorption of the terminal phalanges (acro-osteolysis), discrete soft-tissue calcification (calcinosis circumscripta) (Fig. 1-24) and occasionally intra-articular calcification. Erosions can occur due to overlap with rheumatoid arthritis and other connective tissue diseases.

Neoplastic. Dystrophic localised intratumoral calcification can be seen in both benign and malignant lesions due to haemorrhage and necrosis. In malignant disease this can occur due to treatment response. This differs from those tumours that mineralise due to the presence

of osteoprogenitor cell populations; these are discussed later in the chapter. The pattern of soft-tissue mineralisation can point towards the underlying cause. Punctate or 'ring and arc' calcification is seen with soft-tissue chondromas; phleboliths are classically seen in haemangiomas. Lipomas, particularly when parosteal, can ossify.

Metabolic Calcification. Metabolic calcification, also known as metastatic calcification, is the accumulation of calcium salts in normal tissue and occurs as the result of elevated serum calcium-phosphate product. When the calcification is evident at radiography, there is a diffuse deposition of fine granular calcification. There are a range of causes, but chronic renal failure is the most common (Fig. 1-16). Other causes to consider include hyperparathyroidism, sarcoidosis and certain drugs. Metabolic calcification due to primary hyperparathyroidism is rarely encountered in modern medical practice as it is generally diagnosed and treated before the development of radiographic abnormality but it can cause arterial and periarticular calcification as well as chondrocalcinosis. Secondary hyperparathyroidism is typically seen in relation to chronic renal disease. Periarticular and soft-tissue calcification can be a prominent feature, particularly in association with long-term renal dialysis where it has a dramatic negative impact on prognosis.[26] Chondrocalcinosis is infrequently seen in secondary hyperparathyroidism.

Hypoparathyroid states such as hypoparathyroidism, pseudohypoparathyroidism and pseudopseudohypoparathyroidism can also cause abnormal soft-tissue calcification. Primary deficiency of parathormone (PTH) occurs usually due to surgical excision of, or trauma to, the parathyroid glands. Calcification, when it occurs, is typically subcutaneous. Premature closure of the epiphyses, osteosclerosis and basal ganglia calcification may also be evident. Pseudohypoparathyroidism has several subtypes but is an X-linked dominant disorder caused by intrinsic resistance to PTH. Radiographic features are similar to hypoparathyroidism but there are characteristic phenotypic changes including rounded facies, and short fourth and fifth metacarpals/metatarsals. Pseudopseudohypoparathyroidism is also an inherited disorder; the imaging appearances are identical to those of pseudohypoparathyroidism but the serum calcium and phosphate levels are normal.

Abnormal soft-tissue calcification related to drug excess is now rarely encountered as a solitary abnormality but metabolic calcification can occur with drugs which impact upon the complex inter-regulation of calcium, phosphate and vitamin D. Hypervitaminosis D is generally seen in chronic renal failure in those reliant on dialysis but is also seen due to the treatment of rickets and osteomalacia. The radiological features relate to the formation of smooth, lobulated masses of calcium hydroxyapatite within and around joints, and within tendon sheaths and bursae. In children hypervitaminosis D causes the development of dense metaphyseal bands and diffuse cortical thickening, which may be associated with generalised osteosclerosis. In the mature skeleton most of these features are absent and osteosclerosis may be the only skeletal manifestation.[27] Excessive intake of alkali, usually calcium carbonate and milk, is reported in patients with renal impairment and peptic ulcer disease can result in the deposition of soft-tissue calcification, which is similar in appearance to that seen in hypervitaminosis D and can mimic other disorders such as renal osteodystrophy, collagen vascular disorders and idiopathic tumoral calcinosis.

Calcium Pyrophosphate Dihydrate Deposition Disease (CPPD)

CPPD is the umbrella term for the abnormal accretion of calcium pyrophosphate dihydrate crystals in and around joints. There is thought to be an association between CPPD and many other conditions such as diabetes, hyperparathyroidism, haemachromatosis, hypomagnesaemia and gout. CPPD can manifest as acute intermittent synovitis (pseudogout), chronic pyrophosphate arthropathy or chondrocalcinosis. Pyrophosphate arthropathy is radiologically similar to osteoarthrosis (OA) and may be indistinguishable on imaging. Suggestive features include an unusual pattern of joint involvement such as the radiocapitellar articulation of the elbow, large subchondral cysts and a relative paucity of osteophytes. Pyrophosphate arthropathy can be rapidly destructive and bone fragmentation may be a feature. Chondrocalcinosis is most commonly seen in the knee and can affect hyaline (articular) cartilage and fibrocartilage (menisci, triangular fibrocartilage, symphysis pubis and annulus fibrosus).

Tumoral Calcinosis

Tumoral calcinosis is a rare hereditary dysfunction of phosphate metabolism occurring particularly in patients of African descent. Biochemistry shows normal serum calcium but there may be mild hyperphosphataemia. Radiologically there is deposition of characteristic large, globular soft-tissue calcification around joints, predominantly affecting the extensor surface where there is generally bursal involvement. CT may demonstrate the lesions to be cystic with internal layering of calcium.

Malignant Calcification

The soft-tissue malignancies that classically mineralise are extraskeletal osteosarcoma, extraskeletal chondrosarcoma and synovial sarcoma as well as metastases from bone forming tumours (Fig. 1-25). In the latter, calcification is seen in up to 30% of cases and can range from fine non-specific calcified foci to dense eccentric calcification.

Rarely, disseminated malignancy such as leukaemia, myeloma or bony metastases can manifest with widespread soft-tissue calcification due to hypercalcaemia from extensive bone destruction.

Gas in the Soft Tissues

Air or gas within the soft tissues is indicated by radiolucency on radiographs or CT; this can take the form of locules or can be more linear, outlining the soft-tissue planes. Small locules of gas can be difficult to appreciate on MRI and returns low signal on all sequences (Fig. 1-26). Soft-tissue gas may form directly within the soft tissues or, more commonly, is seen following perforation of the skin or a body cavity.

Vacuum phenomenon occurs in synovial joints, intervertebral discs and vertebral bodies due to the accumulation of gas, mainly nitrogen, in the adjacent soft tissues. The appearances can be accentuated by traction on the effected joint: hence the term 'vacuum phenomenon' despite no true vacuum being present. The gas appears as radiolucent lines that can be seen using radiography. The majority of cases are attributed to degeneration but more rarely vacuum phenomenon related to fracture non-union, infection or tumour is described.[28]

Soft-tissue gas occurring secondary to infection is most frequently seen in the extremities of patients with diabetes or peripheral vascular disease (Fig. 1-27). Gas is typically produced by anaerobic bacteria; the classic example is gas gangrene caused by several species of *Clostridium*. This can be life-threatening and in its most severe form causes critical sepsis, extensive oedema and soft-tissue necrosis with gas formation which may be palpable as subcutaneous crepitus. Other anaerobic

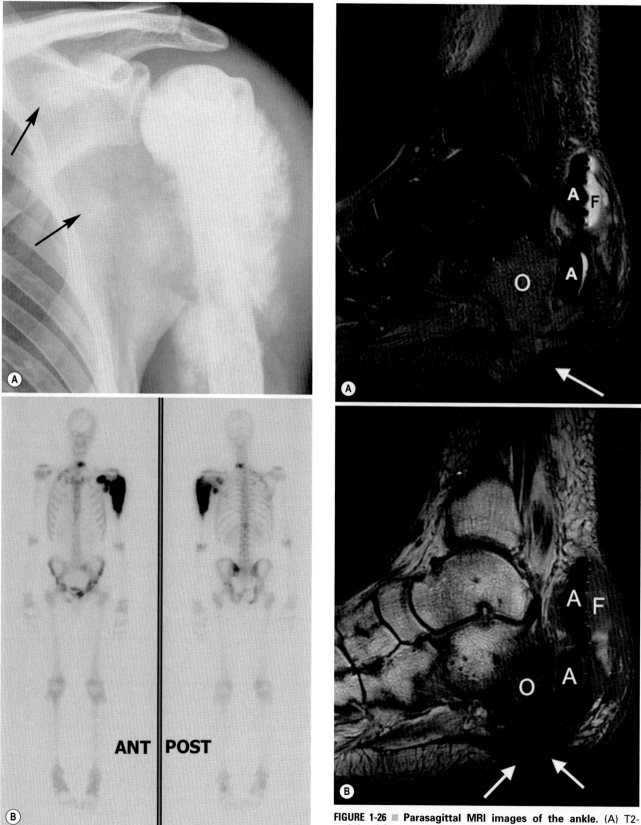

FIGURE 1-25 ■ Osteosarcoma of the proximal humerus. (A) Radiograph shows dense new bone formation and aggressive periosteal reaction. Ossified lymph node metastases (arrows). (B) ^{99m}Tc-MDP bone scintigraphy shows increased radiotracer uptake within the primary humeral lesion, malignant lymph nodes within the axilla and spinal and pelvic bone metastases.

FIGURE 1-26 ■ Parasagittal MRI images of the ankle. (A) T2-weighted fat-saturated and (B) T1-weighted images show fluid (F) and air (A) collections posteriorly tracking from a plantar ulcer (arrows). There is osteomyelitis within the calcaneus with intraosseous gas and surrounding bone oedema (O).

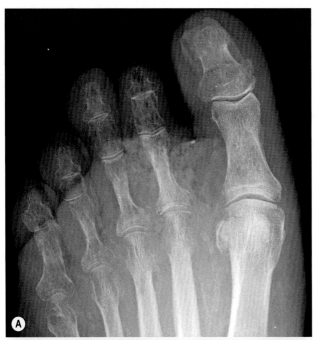

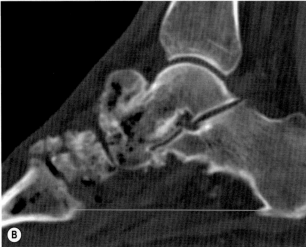

FIGURE 1-27 ■ **Soft-tissue gas.** (A) Radiograph of the forefoot in a diabetic patient with the dappled low-density appearances of gas in the soft tissues of the second toe; note vascular calcification and osteopenia. (B) Reformatted sagittal CT image shows extensive soft tissue, joint and intraosseous low-density gas due to infection in a different patient.

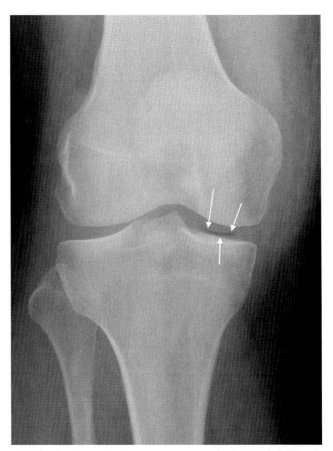

FIGURE 1-28 ■ **Radiograph of the knee shows intra-articular gas (arrows) following penetrating injury.**

recognise breach of a joint capsule following a soft-tissue laceration as joint washout is indicated to prevent septic arthritis (Fig. 1-28). Associated foreign bodies can be diagnosed on radiographs when they are radio-opaque: for example, glass. Organic foreign bodies such as wood are better assessed using ultrasound.

Periosteal Reaction

The periosteum is a dense layer of specialised connective tissue which invests the outer bony cortex except at the articulating surfaces of synovial joints. The outer periosteal stratum is a dense, innervated and vascularised fibrous sheath providing nourishment and sensory innervation. The inner layer or cambium is more loosely arranged and contains osteoblasts and osteoprogenitor cells, which are essential for bone repair and growth. Compact Sharpey's fibres anchor the periosteum to the underlying bone lamellae. Functionally, the periosteum also provides attachment for ligaments and tendons.

Direct or indirect insult to the periosteal layer causes it to elevate from the underlying bony cortex. This causes a non-specific radiological finding termed periosteal reaction. The insult can take many forms, including trauma, infection, malignancy, arthritis and drug reaction (Table 1-2). There is considerable overlap in the different appearances of periosteal reaction; although it is not possible to discriminate between malignant and benign

bacteria such as coliforms, *Bacteroides*, anaerobic *Streptococcus* species and *Aerobacter aerogenes* may also produce gas, although these tend to be less severe, causing more localised infection than *Clostridium* spp.

Soft-tissue gas is frequently seen in conjunction with trauma. Breach of the respiratory or gastrointestinal tract may occur following blunt trauma, for example, and is also seen following surgery and as a complication following interventional procedures such as central line insertion. Gas within the soft tissues of the chest or retroperitoneum is termed surgical emphysema and locules of air may be palpated deep to the skin.

Air can be introduced into the soft tissues following penetrating injury through the skin. It is important to

TABLE 1-2 Differential Diagnosis of Periosteal Reaction

Congenital	Periosteal reaction of the newborn
Genetic	Caffey disease
	Pachydermoperiostosis
Arthritides	Psoriatic arthritis
	Reactive arthritis
Infection	
Trauma	Fracture
	Stress injury
Metabolic	Hypertrophic osteoarthropathy
	Thyroid acropachy
Drugs	Prostaglandins
	Fluorosis
	Hypervitaminosis A
Tumours	Primary bone malignancy
	Leukaemia and lymphoma
	Osteoid osteoma
	Eosinophilic granuloma
	Chondroblastoma
Vascular	Venous stasis

TABLE 1-3 Types of Periosteal Reaction

Non-aggressive	Thin
	Solid
	Thick and irregular
	Septated
Aggressive	Spiculated
	Hair-on-end
	Sunburst
	Laminated
	Disorganised
	Interrupted
	Codman triangle

conditions, certain features differentiate between non-aggressive and aggressive forms (Table 1-3).

Non-aggressive Periosteal Reaction

Congenital. Physiologic periosteal reaction of the newborn is a well-recognised radiological finding of unknown aetiology causing symmetrical continuous periosteal reaction, typically of the long bones. It is seen in term and pre-term neonates and is important to differentiate from non-accidental injury.

Genetic. Also known as infantile cortical hyperostosis, Caffey's disease is a rare and benign self-limiting genetic condition of early infancy which can be either familial or sporadic in terms of transmission. Developing as a triad of rapidly evolving cortical thickening, soft-tissue swelling and hyperirritability,[29] the disorder most commonly affects the mandible but can involve any bone and often more than one site is affected. Long bone involvement is confined to the diaphysis; there is marked cortical thickening with bony expansion and abnormality may persist for months or even years. Given the features, it is vital to exclude osteomyelitis, trauma and malignancy.

Pachydermoperiostosis or primary hypertrophic osteoarthropathy occurs in older children, classically in pubertal boys. This rare familial condition characteristically causes insidious thickening of the skin of the face

and clubbing of the digits. Radiologically there is symmetrical development of often exuberant irregular periosteal reaction of the long bones. Unlike secondary hypertrophic osteoarthropathy, in pachydermoperiostosis the periosteal reaction extends to involve the epiphysis.

Arthritis. Psoriatic arthritis may develop before the dermatological manifestations are exhibited. Bone proliferation, enthesopathy and periosteal reaction, in addition to marginal erosions, are well-recognised features. The periosteal reaction can be exuberant and aggressive in appearance and is classically juxta-articular. As the periosteal reaction matures with time it progresses into solid new bone.

Reactive arthritis is a seronegative arthritis occurring as an autoimmune response to infection. There is a strong relationship to human leucocyte antigen (HLA) B27. A wide range of infectious agents have been described but the majority of cases relate to genitourinary infection, particularly *Chlamydia trachomatis* or gastrointestinal infection with *Campylobacter*, *Shigella* or *Salmonella* species. The resultant periosteal reaction is identical to that seen in psoriatic arthritis but typically affects the lower limbs.

Trauma. Subtle periosteal reaction at a site of pain may be the only radiographic feature of a stress fracture (Fig. 1-29A); it should be emphasised that up to 80% of stress fractures are radiographically occult at presentation and delayed or additional imaging may be warranted. Periosteal reaction occurring at a fracture site can have a variable appearance, ranging from smooth, solid periostitis to disorganised and aggressive periosteal reaction (Fig. 1-29).

Metabolic. Secondary hypertrophic osteoarthropathy (HOA) is a common manifestation of extraskeletal disease causing symmetric, generalised periosteal reaction of tubular bones. Unlike primary hypertrophic osteoarthopathy, there is sparing of the epiphyses. HOA is classically described related to pulmonary abnormalities when it may be termed hypertrophic pulmonary osteoarthopathy. Lung cancer, and non-small cell cancer in particular, is the most common cause but HOA is also recognised in conjunction with tumours of the pleura and mediastinum, suppurative lung disease (for example, bronchiectasis or empyema), pulmonary metastases and cystic fibrosis. Less commonly, HOA occurs due to gastrointestinal disease such as biliary cirrhosis or inflammatory bowel disease.

Developing as digital clubbing, swelling of the hands and feet and exophthalmos, thyroid acropachy is a rare complication of autoimmune thyroid disease. There is generalised and relatively symmetrical periosteal reaction which is irregular and may be spiculated that typically involves the mid-diaphyses of the metacarpals, metatarsals and phalanges.

Drugs. Several drugs are known to cause periosteal reaction. Excess intake of fluorine causes dental abnormalities when occurring in childhood. In adults excess fluorine intake results in increased bone density with reduced bone elasticity, giving an increased fracture risk. Osteosclerosis is accompanied by a thick and undulating periosteal reaction and widening of the diaphyses.

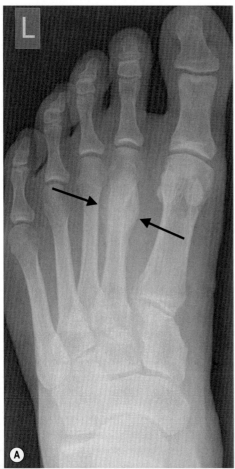

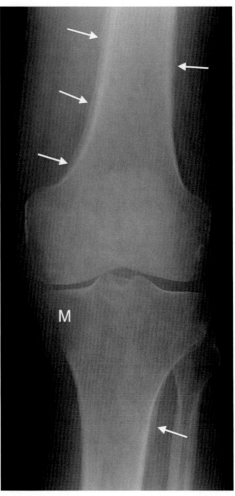

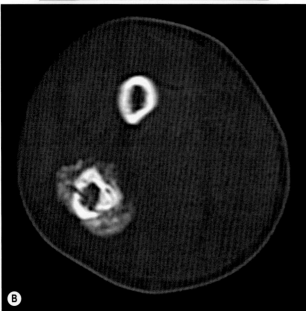

FIGURE 1-29 ■ **Different patients.** (A) Radiograph shows stress fracture of the second metatarsal with periosteal reaction (arrows). (B) Axial CT of healing ulna fracture. The fracture remains ununited with florid surrounding periosteal reaction and callus.

FIGURE 1-30 ■ **Hypertrophic osteoarthropathy in a patient with lung cancer.** Periosteal reaction of the distal femur and proximal tibia (arrows). Lytic metastasis (M) within the medial tibia with cortical destruction.

Calcification or ossification of ligaments, tendons and interosseous membranes is a distinctive feature. Fluorosis is endemic in areas such as China and India.

Prostaglandins are used in infants to maintain a patent ductus arteriosus in ductal-dependent congenital heart disease. They can produce a diffuse cortical proliferation believed to occur due to decreased osteoclast activity.[30] This is associated with limb swelling and pain which resolves following the cessation of treatment.

Chronic hypervitaminosis A may present with anorexia and dermatological symptoms in adults and children. Radiologically there is a smooth and solid periosteal reaction of the long bones, which in the immature skeleton can be associated with metaphyseal splaying, thinning of the growth plate and premature fusion. In the distal femur, in particular, the epiphysis may evolve into a conical shape invaginating into the metaphysis.

Tumours. Slow-growing bone tumours typically exhibit non-aggressive periosteal reaction. The most common example is the benign osteoid osteoma which develops as fusiform, smooth, focal and eccentric periosteal reaction with a central lucent nidus which may

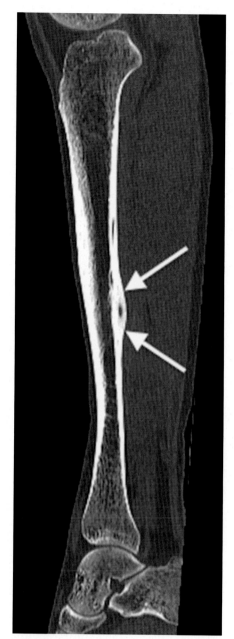

FIGURE 1-31 ■ **Osteoid osteoma of the tibia.** Reformatted sagittal CT shows smooth fusiform periosteal reaction and lucent nidus (arrows).

contain a dense calcified centre (Fig. 1-31). Occurring in the second and third decades, osteoid osteomas most often affect the femur, tibia and humerus. These tumours are chemically active, producing prostaglandins that stimulate new bone formation in the area around the lesion.

Vascular. Periosteal reaction due to chronic vascular insufficiency is commonly seen in the older population, almost exclusively affecting the tibia and fibula and occasionally the metatarsals and phalanges. Radiographs reveal a solid and undulating, non-aggressive periosteal reaction which initially is separate from the underlying cortex but blends with it over time. There may be other features of venous stasis such as phleboliths, and soft-tissue swelling is a common finding.

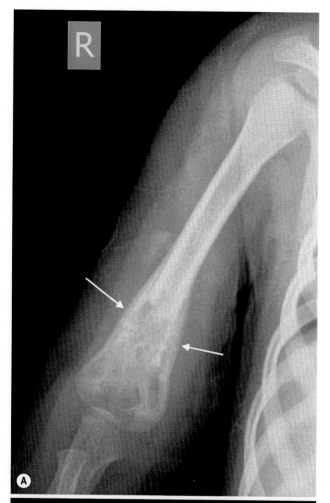

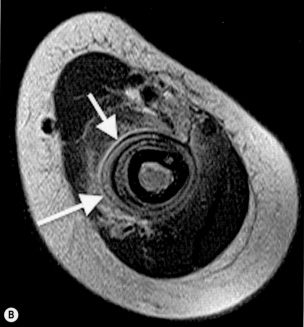

FIGURE 1-32 ■ **Aggressive periosteal reaction in Langerhans cell histiocytosis in a paediatric patient.** Bone destruction and lamellated periosteal reaction (arrows) shown on (A) AP radiograph and (B) axial T2 MRI.

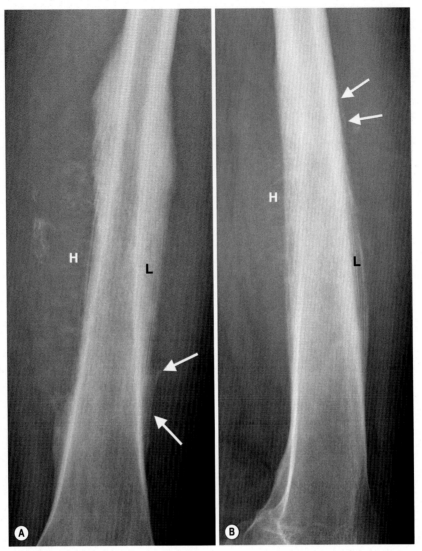

FIGURE 1-33 ■ **Ewing's sarcoma of the femur.** (A) AP and (B) lateral radiographs show lamellated (L) and hair-on-end (H) periosteal reaction with Codman triangle formation (arrows).

Aggressive Periosteal Reaction. Aggressive periosteal reaction occurs due to a rapidly progressive disease process, typically primary bone malignancy, osteomyelitis or metastatic bone disease. Some benign bone disorders such as aneurysmal bone cysts, however, are well recognised as having periosteal reaction with aggressive features. Several subtypes of aggressive periosteal reaction are described; although certain traits are more common with specific conditions, there is sizable overlap in appearance.

Lamellated periosteal reaction occurs parallel to the long axis of the bone and can be seen as multiple layers of concentric new bone formation. Sometimes referred to as 'onion-skin' periosteal reaction, this is described as a feature of Ewing's sarcoma but may also be seen in osteosarcoma, lymphoma and rarely infection (Figs. 1-32 and 1-33). Periosteal reaction with a radial orientation to the bone represents invasion of perforating vascular channels and along Sharpey's fibres. This can have the perpendicular 'hair-on-end' pattern (Fig. 1-33) seen in

Ewing's sarcoma, osteosarcoma and rarely infection, or there may be a divergent 'sunburst' arrangement more typical of osteosarcoma, osteoblastoma and osteoblastic metastases (Fig. 1-25).

A Codman triangle is a zone of periosteal elevation seen in association with a soft-tissue mass or at the border of cortical destruction or tumour extension (Fig. 1-33A). It is a feature of primary bone tumours such as osteosarcoma and Ewing's sarcoma but can also be caused by metastases, infection or trauma.

REFERENCES

1. Horsfield D, Murphy G. Stress views of the ankle joint in lateral ligament injury. Radiography 1985;51(595):7–11.
2. Ozcelik A, Gunal I, Kose N. Stress views in the radiography of scapholunate instability. Eur J Radiol 2005;56(3):358–61.
3. Dobbins JT 3rd. Tomosynthesis imaging: at a translational cross-roads. Med Phys 2009;36(6):1956–67.
4. Fahey FH, Webber RL, Chew FS, Dickerson BA. Application of TACT to the evaluation of total joint arthroplasty. Med Phys 2003;30(3):454–60.

5. Jamadar DA, Robertson BL, Jacobson JA, et al. Musculoskeletal sonography: important imaging pitfalls. Am J Roentgenol 2010;194(1):216–25.

6. Ophir J, Céspedes I, Ponnekanti H, et al. Elastography: a quantitative method for imaging the elasticity of biological tissues. Ultrason Imaging 1991;13(2):111–34.

7. Danielson P, Alfredson H, Forsgren S. Distribution of general (PGP 9.5) and sensory (substance P/CGRP) innervations in the human patellar tendon. Knee Surg Sports Traumatol Arthrosc 2006;14(2):125–32.

8. McNally EG. Ultrasound of the small joints of the hands and feet: current status. Skeletal Radiol 2008;37(2):99–113.

9. McCollough CH, Primak AN, Braun N, et al. Strategies for reducing radiation dose in CT. Radiol Clin North Am 2009;47(1):27–40.

10. Choi HK, Al-Arfaj AM, Eftekhari A, et al. Dual energy computed tomography in tophaceous gout. Ann Rheum Dis 2009;68(10):1609–12.

11. Nicolaou S, Yong-Hing CJ, Galea-Soler S, et al. Dual-energy CT as a potential new diagnostic tool in the management of gout in the acute setting. Am J Roentgenol 2010;194(4):1072–8.

12. Pache G, Krauss B, Strohm P, et al. Dual-energy CT virtual noncalcium technique: detecting posttraumatic bone marrow lesions—feasibility study. Radiology 2010;256(2):617–24.

13. Durie BG. The role of anatomic and functional staging in myeloma: description of Durie/Salmon plus staging system. Eur J Cancer 2006;42(11):1539–43.

14. Yanny S, Cahir JG, Barker T, et al. MRI of aseptic lymphocytic vasculitis-associated lesions in metal-on-metal hip replacements. Am J Roentgenol 2012;198(6):1394–402.

15. Rhee RB, Chan KK, Lieu JG, et al. MR and CT arthrography of the shoulder. Semin Musculoskelet Radiol 2012;16(1):3–14.

16. Gold GE, Chen CA, Hargreaves BA, Bangerter NK. Recent advances in MRI of articular cartilage. Am J Roentgenol 2009;193(3):628–38.

17. Ringleb SI, Bensamoun SF, Chen Q, et al. Applications of magnetic resonance elastography to healthy and pathologic skeletal muscle. J Magn Reson Imaging 2007;25(2):301–9.

18. Hiltunen J, Suortti T, Arvela S, et al. Diffusion tensor imaging and tractography of distal peripheral nerves at 3 T. Clin Neurophysiol 2005;116(10):2315–23.

19. Sarikaya I, Sarikaya A, Holder LE. The role of single photon emission computed tomography in bone imaging. Semin Nucl Med 2001;31(1):3–16.

20. Filer A, de Pablo P, Allen G, et al. Utility of ultrasound joint counts in the prediction of rheumatoid arthritis in patients with very early synovitis. Ann Rheum Dis 2011;70(3):500–7.

21. Abedin M, Tintut Y, Demer LL. Vascular calcification: mechanisms and clinical ramifications. Arterioscler Thromb Vasc Biol 2004;24(7):1161–70.

22. Simonsen LL, Sonne-Holm S, Krasheninnikoff M, Engberg AW. Symptomatic heterotopic ossification after very severe traumatic brain injury in 114 patients: incidence and risk factors. Injury 2007;38(10):1146–50.

23. Carter SR, Davies AM, Evans N, Grimer RJ. Value of bone scanning and computed tomography in fibrodysplasia ossificans progressiva. Br J Radiol 1989;62(735):269–72.

24. Trapnell DH. Calcification of nerves in leprosy. Br J Radiol 1965;38(454):796–7.

25. Airio A, Pukkala E, Isomaki H. Elevated cancer incidence in patients with dermatomyositis: a population based study. J Rheum 1995;22(7):1300–3.

26. Razzaque MS, et al. FGF-23, vitamin D and calcification: the unholy triad. Nephrol Dial Transplant 2005;20(10):2032–5.

27. Christensen WR, Liebman C, Sosman MC. Skeletal and periarticular manifestations of hypervitaminosis D. Am J Roentgenol Radium Ther 1951;65(1):27–41.

28. Lafforgue PF, Chagnaud CJ, Daver LM, et al. Intervertebral disk vacuum phenomenon secondary to vertebral collapse: prevalence and significance. Radiology 1994;193(3):853–8.

29. Caffey J. Infantile cortical hyperostosis; a review of the clinical and radiographic features. Proc R Soc Med 1957;50(5):347–54.

30. Letts M, Pang E, Simons J. Prostaglandin-induced neonatal periostitis. J Pediatr Orthop 1994;14(6):809–13.

CHAPTER 2

Internal Derangements of Joints: Upper and Lower Limbs

Robert S.D. Campbell • Andrew J. Dunn • Eugene McNally • Ahmed Daghir

---

CHAPTER OUTLINE

INTRODUCTION

THE SHOULDER

THE ACROMIOCLAVICULAR JOINT

THE STERNOCLAVICULAR JOINT

THE ELBOW

HAND AND WRIST

THE HIP

THE KNEE

THE ANKLE AND FOOT

INTRODUCTION

Magnetic resonance imaging (MRI) and ultrasound now allow the radiologist to undertake detailed examinations of the soft tissues of joints including tendons, ligaments, cartilage and fibrocartilagenous structures such as the menisci. Injuries that previously had to be inferred from patterns of bone injury shown on conventional radiographs can now be assessed in great detail allowing prognosis for conservative management and planning for surgical decision making. While common features exist in terms of the appearance of tendon and ligament abnormalities, the individual biomechanical properties of the different joints and the varying requirements of these joints strongly influence the patterns of injury seen. Broadly, soft-tissue joint injury falls into two patterns: acute injuries such as an acute ligament tear or osteochondral injury and chronic injury. Chronic injury generally occurs as a result of chronic and repetitive microtrauma to the structure concerned. Examples include tendinopathy and impingement syndromes. In this chapter we have used the term 'tendinopathy' (sometimes also known as tendinosis) to refer to chronic degenerative change in tendons. This was previously referred to as tendinitis, but this term has fallen out of use as it implies an inflammatory process which is not a feature of the chronic pattern of tendon injury being described.

THE SHOULDER

The shoulder is the most mobile joint in the human body. Movement occurs primarily through the glenohumeral joint, but with a large contribution from the scapulothoracic articulation. The upper limb and scapula articulate with the trunk through the acromioclavicular and sternoclavicular joints. The wide range of movement that can occur at the shoulder is possible because of the shallow cup provided by the glenoid and relatively large humeral head. This configuration has been likened to a golf ball on a golf tee and is inherently unstable. Stability to the glenohumeral joint is provided through the soft tissues of the rotator cuff tendons and ligaments, which are susceptible to injury.

The glenoid fossa of the scapula articulates with the head of the humerus to form the glenohumeral joint (GHJ). The glenoid is shallow, pear shaped and anteverted in both the sagittal and axial planes. The fibrocartilaginous labrum runs circumferentially around the glenoid, increasing the overall surface area and contributing to the stability of the joint.

The GHJ is surrounded by a number of synovial-lined bursae that communicate with each other and provide lubrication for the motion of the rotator cuff tendons. The subscapularis bursa (SSB) lies anteriorly between the subscapularis tendon and the anterior deltoid muscle. The subacromial bursa (SAB) lies between the supraspinatus and infraspinatus tendons and the undersurface of the acromion, ACJ and lateral end of the clavicle. The subdeltoid bursa (SDB) is continuous with the lateral aspects of the SAB and SSB and continues posteriorly beneath the posterior belly of the deltoid muscle.

The rotator cuff muscles and tendons along with the long head of biceps are the dynamic stabilisers of the GHJ. The rotator cuff muscles arise from the scapula, passing laterally, to insert on the proximal humerus. They contribute to abduction as well as internal and external rotation of the humerus. The coracoacromial arch is formed by the coracoid, the acromion and the intervening coracoacromial ligament, under which the supraspinatus tendon (SST) passes. The rotator cuff comprises:

- Subscapularis: inserts on lesser tuberosity
- Supraspinatus: inserts anterior facet of greater tuberosity
- Infraspinatus: inserts middle facet of greater tuberosity
- Teres minor: inserts posterior facet of greater tuberosity.

The long head of biceps (LHB) tendon arises from the supraglenoid tubercle and superior labrum. The intra-articular component passes between the subscapularis and supraspinatus tendons in a region known as the rotator interval, and enters the bicipital groove on the anterior aspect of the humeral head. The LHB is stabilised within the rotator interval by the biceps pulley comprised of coracohumeral and superior glenohumeral ligaments.

The static stabilisers of the GHJ are the glenohumeral (G-H) ligaments which are condensations of the joint capsule. They comprise the superior, middle and inferior glenohumeral ligaments. The IGHL is the most important of the G-H ligaments. It is divided into anterior and posterior components, which act like a hammock to support the humeral head in abduction.

The commonest types of internal derangement of the shoulder relate to:

- rotator cuff disease
- GHJ instability
- superior labral tears.

Rotator Cuff Disease

The commonest cause of rotator cuff tendon tears is external impingement occurring mostly in patients over the age of 40 years. Acute injuries are uncommon in the younger population, except in athletes. Impingement of the rotator cuff tendons occurs between the humeral head and coracoacromial arch during abduction of the upper arm. Initially there is reversible oedema and haemorrhage in the tendons, which may lead to tendinopathy and eventually failure of the tendon.[1] The subacromial space may be reduced by bony abnormalities such as AC joint osteophytes and abnormalities of the shape of the acromion. Secondary impingement may occur through abnormal coordination of the rotator cuff muscles and abnormal scapulothoracic movement.

The impingement phenomenon is associated with the development of subacromial bursitis, and acromial bone spur formation. This further limits the subacromial space and aggravates the impingement process.[1]

Tendinopathy is defined as tendon injury on a cellular level that is most commonly age related and degenerative in nature but may also occur following trauma in younger individuals. The connective tissue that binds and organises the collagen bundles of the tendon undergoes microscopic tearing that leads to activation of inflammatory mediators and disorganised tendon healing. The tendon often thickens and may show features of delamination, mucoid degeneration and eventually partial tearing

on imaging.[2] Calcific tendinopathy is characterised by intrasubstance deposition of calcium hydroxyapatite crystals of unknown aetiology. The calcific deposits may be asymptomatic but can become painful when they produce focal tendon swelling that may contribute to external impingement. Release of calcium from the tendon into the overlying SAB can produce an acute inflammatory bursal reaction.

Rotator cuff tendon tears are defined as partial or full thickness. A partial thickness tear (PTT) involves either the articular surface (commonest) or the bursal surface (less common), but does not extend all the way through the tendon.[2] A full thickness tear (FTT) extends from the articular surface to the bursal surface and creates an abnormal communication between the GHJ and SAB. The term full thickness only indicates that the tear extends through the full thickness of the tendon; it does not imply the tear extends from the anterior edge of the tendon to the posterior edge. However, as the tear size increases, the whole tendon may become torn (anterior to posterior) creating a massive tear with medial tendon retraction. The supraspinatus is most commonly affected, but tears may progress to involve both infraspinatus and subscapularis.

Tears of the LHB pulley and subscapularis tendon may lead to medial subluxation of the LHB tendon from the bicipital groove. The LHB may also show features on tendinopathy or may eventually rupture.

Radiography is useful for demonstrating bony abnormalities of the AC joint and acromion and excluding associated GHJ arthrosis (Fig. 2-1). Marked narrowing of the subacromial space is a specific but insensitive sign of a full thickness rotator cuff tear[3] (Fig. 2-2). MRI and ultrasound (US) directly visualise the rotator cuff tendons.

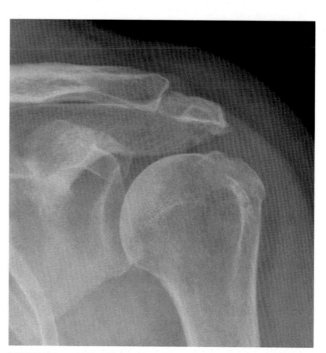

FIGURE 2-1 ■ AP radiograph of the shoulder demonstrating bony enthesophyte formation on the lateral margin of the acromion and the greater tuberosity secondary to external impingement.

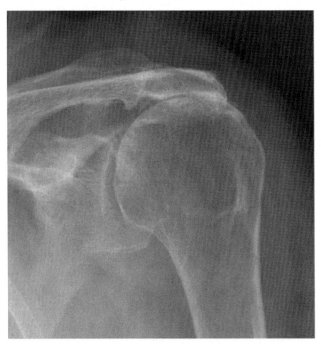

FIGURE 2-2 ■ AP radiograph of the shoulder demonstrating narrowing of the subacromial space and bony impingement of the humerus and acromion secondary to chronic rotator cuff tear.

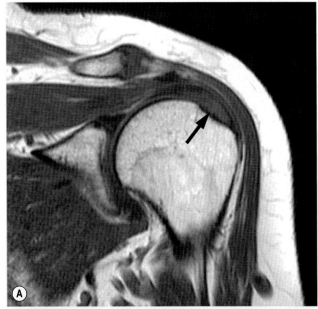

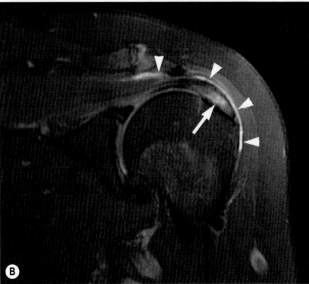

FIGURE 2-3 ■ Coronal oblique T1W (A) and T2FS (B) MR images of a patient with external impingement. High SI fluid is present in the subacromial bursa on the T2W image, indicating bursitis (arrowheads). The supraspinatus tendon is thickened with increased SI on both T1W and T2W sequences as a result of associated tendinopathy (arrows).

Both techniques are capable of diagnosing tendinopathy (Fig. 2-3), and have nearly 100% accuracy rates for FTTs of the rotator cuff.[4] MR arthrography is not usually indicated for primary rotator cuff disease. The most important features to describe that help determine management include the following:
- size of cuff tear
- location of cuff tear
- presence of associated rotator cuff muscle atrophy
- dislocation or rupture of the LHB tendon
- bony abnormalities of the coracoacromial arch
- secondary arthrosis of the GHJ.

The primary sign of a rotator cuff FTT is a focal deficiency of the tendon (Figs. 2-4 and 2-5). This nearly always occurs at the tendon insertion on the tuberosity. The margins of the tear are best delineated when there is fluid within the tendon defect. Secondary signs of an FTT include the presence of fluid in both the GHJ and SAB, and flattening or concavity of the subacromial fat plane.

PTTs are less reliably demonstrated by both MRI and US, and it may be difficult to differentiate tendinopathy from partial tears. Focal clefts, tears, or tendon thinning affecting the articular margin of the footprint of the tuberosity are most common (Figs. 2-6 and 2-7). Tendon thickening is not always present. It is important not to mistake magic angle phenomenon on short TE MR sequences or anisotropy on US as evidence of tendinopathy.[2]

Calcific tendinopathy can be visualised on radiographs as discrete amorphous deposits of calcium density. On US they are echogenic and may or may not cast acoustic shadowing (Fig. 2-8). Small deposits of calcium may be

difficult to detect on MRI as both the calcification and surrounding tendon are of low SI.

GHJ Instability

The GHJ is an inherently unstable joint. Injury or abnormality of the static stabilisers renders the joint susceptible to recurrent dislocation, and further injury. Chronic GHJ instability may lead to secondary arthrosis if untreated. Imaging is used to document the extent of internal derangement in order to determine the therapeutic options.[5]

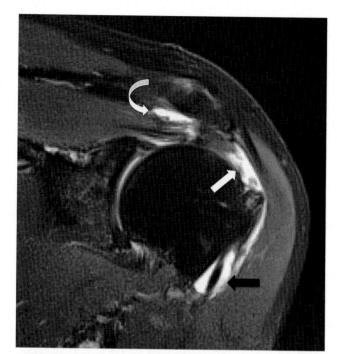

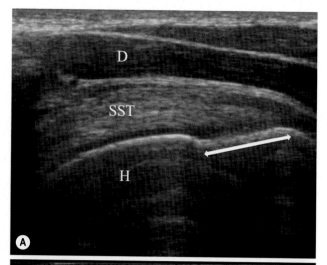

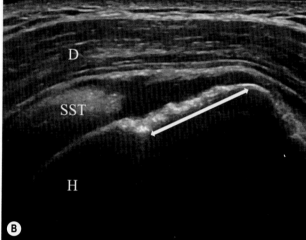

FIGURE 2-4 ■ **Coronal oblique T2FS image.** There is a partial thickness tear of the supraspinatus tendon which is filled by high SI fluid (white arrow). There is also fluid within the glenohumeral joint around the biceps tendon sheath (black arrow), and within the subacromial bursa (curved white arrow), indicating the abnormal communication between the two compartments created by the tendon tear.

FIGURE 2-5 ■ Normal longitudinal US image of the supraspinatus tendon (A). The echogenic tendon inserts across the footprint of the greater tuberosity (double arrow). A full thickness tear of supraspinatus (B) is demonstrated as a focal deficiency of the tendon which is filled by low reflective joint fluid. D, deltoid muscle; H, humeral head; SST, supraspinatus tendon.

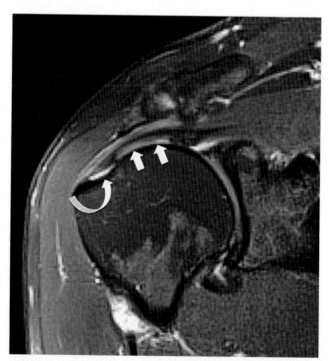

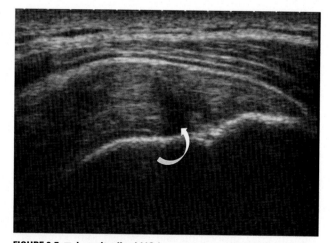

FIGURE 2-6 ■ **Coronal oblique T2FS image.** There is a partial thickness tear of the supraspinatus tendon, with a linear area of fluid SI tracking part way across the insertion point of the tendon on the footprint of the tuberosity (curved white arrow). There is also more extensive partial articular surface tearing of the proximal tendon (white arrows).

FIGURE 2-7 ■ **Longitudinal US images of a partial thickness tear of the supraspinatus tendon.** There is a focal low reflective area on the articular surface of the tendon (curved arrow). The tear does not extend across the whole of the tuberosity, and does not involve the full tendon width.

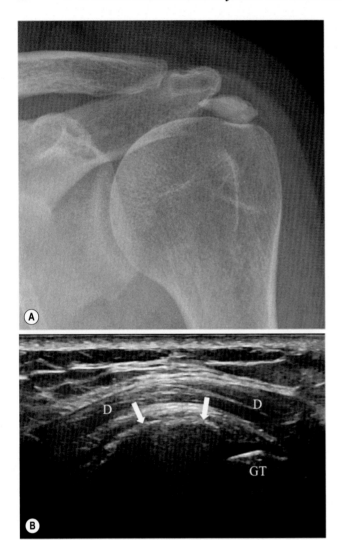

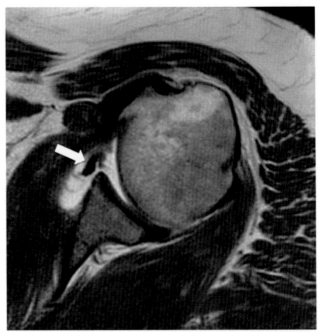

FIGURE 2-9 ■ **Axial T1W image from an MR arthrogram study acquired through the inferior glenoid below the level of the coracoid process.** There is high SI contrast medium extending deep to the low SI fibrocartilaginous labrum (white arrow) as a result of labral detachment (compare with the appearance of the posterior labrum). This is a typical Bankart lesion, with no associated bony defect of the glenoid rim.

FIGURE 2-8 ■ AP radiograph of the shoulder (A) demonstrating calcific tendonitis with an amorphous deposit of calcium density overlying the greater tuberosity. The longitudinal US image (B) shows the calcific deposit within the suprasinatus tendon as a highly reflective curvilinear area (white arrows). There is posterior acoustic shadowing which partly obscures the underlying humeral head. D, deltoid muscle; GT, greater tuberosity.

Instability of the GHJ may be dependent on three factors, referred to as the Bayley triangle:

- traumatic structural
- atraumatic structural
- habitual non-structural (abnormal muscle patterning).

A combination of these factors may be present in any one patient, but trauma is the commonest cause of instability. Anteroinferior dislocation is the commonest presentation. Posterior dislocation is frequently encountered following epileptic seizures. Inferior dislocation is rare.

Radiographs are the primary imaging technique to confirm GHJ dislocation and establish joint congruity following reduction. Anteroposterior and axial views or a modified caudal angled axial are most appropriate. MRI, MR arthrography or CT arthrography are used in the non-acute setting to assess the static stabilisers.[6]

Anterior GHJ dislocation causes tearing and detachment of the anteroinferior glenoid labrum, known as a Bankart lesion. The location of the labral tear is described according to clockface terminology: 12 o'clock represents the biceps anchor, and 3 o'clock is anterior at the equator of the glenoid. Fluid signal intensity or contrast medium extending between the glenoid and labrum is the primary sign of a labral tear (Fig. 2-9). The labrum may become displaced, and it is important to assess the position of the labrum with respect to the face of the glenoid.

More severe injury may be associated with a bony injury of the glenoid rim, usually called a bony Bankart lesion (Fig. 2-10). Non-enhanced CT may occasionally be preferred to assess the size of the bony defect of the glenoid. There is usually associated impaction injury on the posterosuperior aspect of the humeral head called a Hill–Sachs defect (Figs. 2-11 and 2-12).

In posterior dislocation the location of labral and humeral injury is opposite to anterior dislocation, and are termed reverse Bankart lesions and reverse Hill–Sachs defects.

Injury to the joint capsule and glenohumeral ligaments is common. The anterior band of IGHL is the most important joint stabiliser. It may be torn at the humeral insertion or less commonly from its origin on the glenoid. Imaging with the arm in *ab*duction and *ex*ternal *ro*tation (ABER imaging) is sometimes used to assess the integrity of the ligament, to identify the degree of labral displacement and loss of joint congruity.[5]

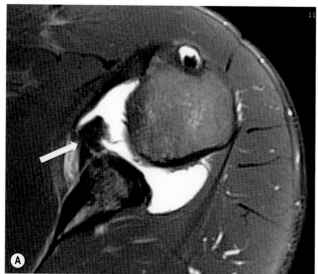

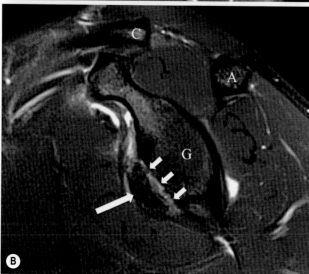

FIGURE 2-10 ■ Axial FS T1W (A) and sagittal oblique FS T1W (B) MR arthrogram images demonstrating a bony Bankart lesion resulting from anterior glenohumeral dislocation. The fibrocartilaginous anterior labrum and glenoid rim are separated from the remainder of the glenoid and displaced medially (white arrow). The fracture line is best seen on the sagittal image (small white arrows). A, acromion; C, clavicle; G, glenoid.

The most important features to describe that help determine management include:
- Location and extent of labral defect
  - use clockface terminology.
- Pattern of labral displacement.
- Presence of bony glenoid rim defects.
  - assess the cross-sectional area of involvement.
- Associated GHJ ligament deficiency.
- Glenoid version.
- Secondary arthrosis of the GHJ.
- Size and depth of the Hill–Sachs defect.

Superior Labral Tears

Tears of the superior labrum and biceps anchor are commonly encountered injuries in overhead throwing

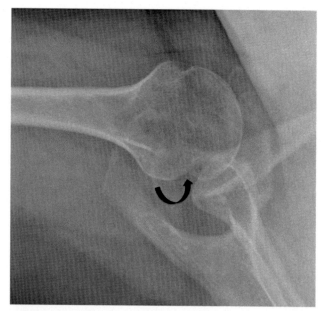

FIGURE 2-11 ■ Subaxial radiograph of the shoulder showing a Hill–Sachs deformity (curved black arrow) secondary to previous traumatic dislocation.

athletes. Abnormal traction on the biceps anchor and superior labrum results in tears that usually extend posteriorly. They are often referred to as *s*uperior *l*abral tears *a*nterior to *p*osterior (SLAP tears).[7] MRI, MR arthrography or CT arthrography may assess the glenoid labrum.

Contrast medium or fluid signal intensity extending into the substance of the labrum or through the chondrolabral junction is the primary sign of a SLAP tear (Fig. 2-13). Tears may be localised to the posterosuperior labrum, or may be more extensive. There may be tear extension into the LHB tendon. There are many grades of SLAP tears described but the extent of the tear and the structures involved are the most important features.[8]

The most important features to describe that help determine management include:
- Extent of labral tear
  - use clockface terminology.
- Involvement of biceps anchor and tendon.
- Presence of associated rotator cuff tears.

THE ACROMIOCLAVICULAR JOINT

The AC joint is a synovial plane joint. All the forces of glenohumeral and scapulothoracic movements are transmitted to the trunk through the ACJ and sternoclavicular joint. Osteoathritis (OA) of the ACJ is common and the associated capsular thickening and osteophyte formation is a contributor to external impingement of the shoulder.

The ACJ has strong capsular ligaments, and is also stabilised by the coracoclavicular (C-C) ligaments. Traumatic disruption and dislocation of the joint is described by the Rockwood classification:

Grade I: undisplaced injury with sprain of acromioclavicular ligaments.

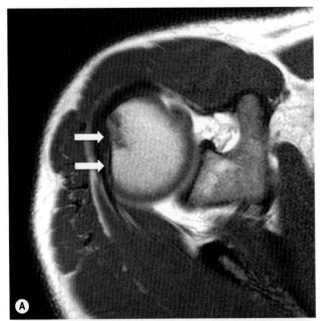

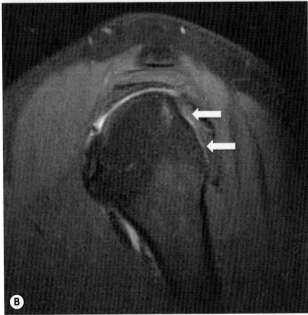

FIGURE 2-12 ■ Axial T1W image from an MR arthrogram study demonstrating a Hill–Sachs lesion (A). There is flattening of the posterolateral humeral head (white arrows), which should normally be approximately spherical at the level of the coracoid process. The same lesion is also seen on the corresponding sagittal oblique T2FS image (B).

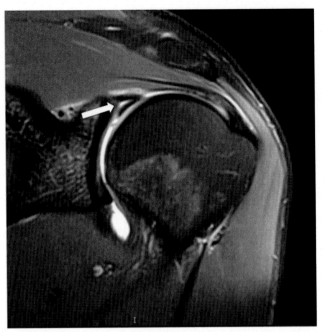

FIGURE 2-13 ■ **Coronal FS T2W MR arthrogram image.** There is high SI contrast medium extending into the substance of the superior labrum, indicating a superior labrum anterior to posterior (SLAP) tear.

may demonstrate abnormal joint widening, and the C-C ligaments can be visualised directly by MRI (Fig. 2-14).

Post-traumatic osteolysis of the lateral clavicle occurs in approximately 6% of ACJ disruptions and may also be seen with repetitive ACJ microtrauma such as weight-lifting (Fig. 2-15).

THE STERNOCLAVICULAR JOINT

The sternoclavicular joint (SCJ) is a synovial saddle joint, with a cartilaginous articular disc. It has limited movement, but like the AC joint transmits the forces of shoulder movement to the trunk. It is very prone to osteoarthritis, which may be associated with chronic anterior subluxation. Radiographic evaluation of the SC joints may be difficult but CT or MRI readily demonstrate the features of arthrosis.[10]

Traumatic subluxation and dislocation usually occurs anteriorly. Posterior dislocation is a rare but important injury, as the displaced medial clavicle may be associated with vascular injury in the superior mediastinum.[11]

THE ELBOW

The elbow is a complex synovial hinge joint. It comprises the ulnotrochlear and radiocapitellar articulations which allow flexion and extension of the elbow. The proximal radioulnar joint (in conjuction with the distal radioulnar joint) enables pronation and supination of the forearm by rotation of the radius around the ulna.[12]

The primary flexors are biceps brachii, brachialis and brachoradialis. Triceps is the main extensor. Supination

Grade II: ACJ widening with <50% superior displacement of lateral clavicle.
Grade III: >100% superior displacement of lateral clavicle.
Grade IV: posterior displacement of lateral clavicle.
Grade III and IV injuries are associated with disruption of the C-C ligaments and above are treated surgically. Grade I and II injuries usually resolve spontaneously. However, some patients may present with persistent pain and instability. Ligament reconstruction may be required in the athletic population.[9] Weight-bearing radiographs

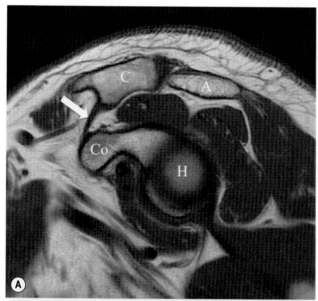

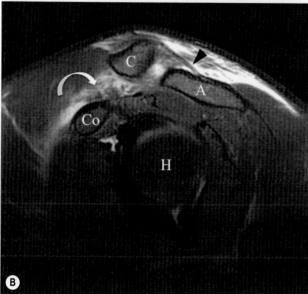

FIGURE 2-14 ■ Sagittal oblique T1W image (A) of the normal coracoclavicular (C-C) ligament. The FS T2W MR image (B) was acquired in a patient following traumatic disruption of the acromioclavicular joint. The joint is normally aligned, but there is fluid within the joint, there is stripping of the superior joint capsule (arrowhead) and there is high SI haemorrhage in the overlying soft tissues. In addition there is haemorrhage between the coracoid and clavicle secondary to C-C ligament disruption (white arrow). A, acromion; C, clavicle; Co, coracoid; H, humeral head.

of the forearm occurs through the action of biceps and supinator. Pronation is by pronator teres, and pronator quadratus (at the wrist). The common tendon for wrist and hand extension arises from the lateral humeral epicondyle, and the common flexor tendon from the medial epicondyle.

The joint is stabilised by the ulnar collateral and radial collateral ligaments. The radial collateral complex includes the annular ligament which supports the radial head.

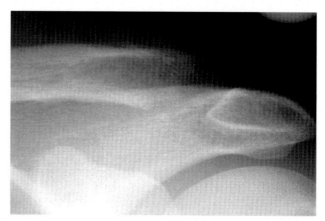

FIGURE 2-15 ■ **AP radiograph of the AC joint.** There is widening of the joint, with resorption and loss of the cortical margin of the lateral clavicle as a result of post-traumatic osteolysis.

Tendons

Insertional tendinopathy around the elbow joint most commonly affects:
- common extensor origin: tennis elbow
- common flexor origin: golfer's elbow
- distal biceps tendon.

The triceps and other tendons are rarely involved.

Tendinopathy of the common extensor and flexor tendons presents with localised pain over the distal humeral epicondyles. It is often a clinical diagnosis, although imaging may be performed in refractory cases to confirm the diagnosis and exclude a tear. Ultrasound is frequently used to guide injection therapy.

The affected tendon is thickened and hyporeflective on US, with neovascularisation on Doppler imaging (Fig. 2-16). High SI is demonstrated on fluid-sensitive MRI sequences (Fig. 2-17). Tendon tears are demonstrated as focal areas of deficiency.[13] In chronic cases, new bone formation may be seen on radiographs at the tendon enthesis. Calcific tendinopathy is much less common than in the rotator cuff of the shoulder.

The distal biceps tendon inserts on the tuberosity of the proximal radius. It does not have a tendon sheath, but surrounding connective tissue is known as a paratenon. It is surrounded near the insertion by the bicipitoradial bursa. Distal biceps tears are often clinically unrecognised, but may be amenable to surgery if diagnosed early. In the early stages the tendon is thickened and there may be an effusion in the bicipitoradial bursa (Fig. 2-18). In complete rupture the tendon retracts proximally. MRI and US may be used to confirm the diagnosis and locate the tendon end (Figs. 2-19 and 2-20).

Bone and Cartilage

The capitellum is the third most commonly affected site in osteochondritis dissecans (after the knee and ankle). It commonly affects teenagers and young adults. A focal osteochondral fragment or defect may be visualised on radiographs. Cross-sectional imaging with MRI, MR arthrography or CT arthrography is used to detect radiographically occult lesions and for grading osteochondral

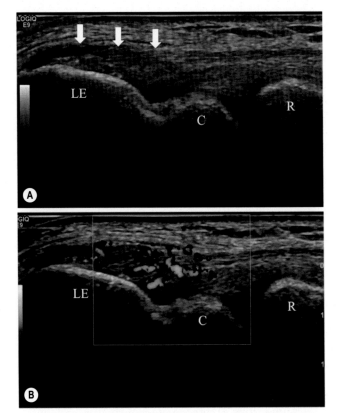

FIGURE 2-16 ■ **Longitudinal US images of tennis elbow.** The common extensor tendon is low reflective and thickened (white arrows) on the grey-scale image (A). The power Doppler image (B) demonstrates prominent neovascularisation. C, capitellum; LE, lateral epicondyle; R, radial head.

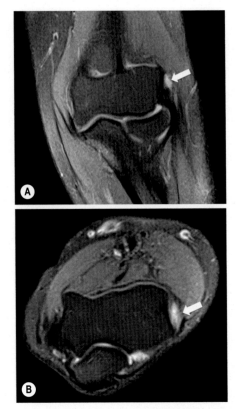

FIGURE 2-17 ■ Coronal (A) and axial (B) FS T2W MR images of the elbow. There is a focal area of high SI intensity tendinopathy in the common extensor tendon origin (white arrows) secondary to insertional tendinopathy (tennis elbow).

lesions (Fig. 2-21). The osteochondral fragment may remain in situ or lie remotely within the elbow joint. Fluid SI at the base of the osteochondral lesion on MRI, or contrast medium tracking around the fragment on arthrographic images, is a sign of an unstable lesion. Integrity of the overlying articular cartilage is a good sign of stability.

Reports should include:
- size and location of osteochondral defect;
- stability of the lesion and integrity of overlying cartilage; and
- presence of any remote intra-articular bodies.

Intra-articular bodies are also frequently encountered in OA of the elbow. They may be calcified, but non-calcified chondral bodies may also occur. CT is often utilised to assess the size and location of osteophytes before surgery, as well as identify small loose bodies. Chondral bodies are not visualised on radiographs or conventional CT. In some cases pre- and post-angiography CT may be performed (Fig. 2-22). Conventional MRI is less sensitive for detection of small intra-articular bodies.

Ligaments

The collateral ligaments of the elbow may be torn as the result of an elbow dislocation, and may require surgical repair. A coronoid process fracture is a sign of an

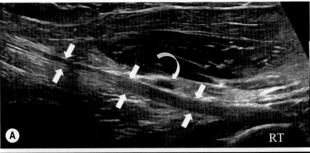
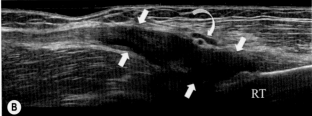

FIGURE 2-18 ■ Longitudinal US (A) of a normal distal biceps tendon (white arrows). The tendon is of uniform size and echo-texture and inserts on the radial tuberosity. In a patient with elbow pain, severe tendinopathy is present, with marked tendon thickening and low reflective change (B). Note the relationship of the tendon to the brachial vessels (curved white arrows). RT, radial tuberosity.

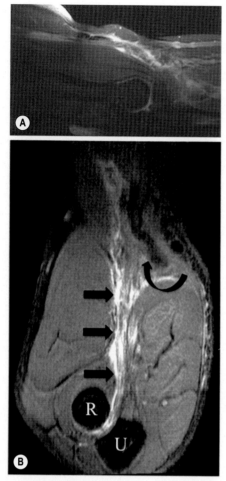

FIGURE 2-19 ■ **FS T2W MR images of a complete distal biceps tendon tear.** The sagittal image (A) demonstrates high SI haemorrhage around the poorly defined retracted tendon end (white arrows). The corresponding FABS image (B) acquired with the arm above the head with the elbow flexed demonstrates the torn tendon end (curved black arrow), and the empty fluid-filled tendon sheath extending down to the insertion on the radial tuberosity (black arrows). B, biceps muscle; R, radius; T, trochlea; U, ulna.

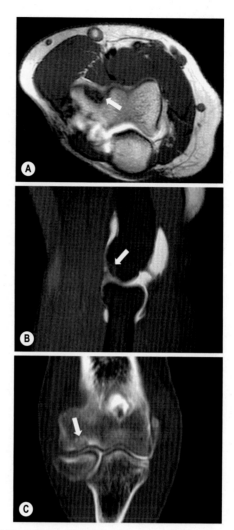

FIGURE 2-21 ■ **Osteochondritis dissecans (OCD) of the capitellum.** The OCD lesion is seen on the T1W (A) and FS T1W (B) MR arthrogram images as an area of low SI in the subchondral bone. There is no high SI contrast medium extending around of the base of the lesion, indicating the articular cartilage is intact, and the lesion is stable. The corresponding coronal CT arthrogram image (C) also confirms the integrity of the articular cartilage.

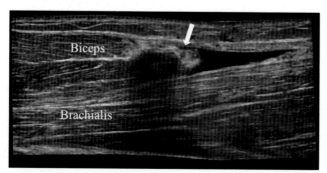

FIGURE 2-20 ■ **Longitudinal US image of a distal biceps tendon tear.** The torn retracted tendon end (white arrow) is accentuated by the presence of acoustic shadowing because of edge artefact and the low reflective fluid in the tendon sheath distally.

unrecognised elbow dislocation. Chronic tears of the ulnar collateral ligament are infrequently encountered in some throwing sports and in weightlifters.

In acute injuries MRI shows the presence of soft-tissue oedema and haemorrhage around the affected ligament. MR arthrography may be preferred for diagnosis of chronic tears. Acute ulnar collateral ligament (UCL) tears often occur at the proximal origin on the medial humeral epicondyle (Fig. 2-23). In chronic tears the defect is usually at the insertion on the sublime tubercle of the ulna.[14]

HAND AND WRIST

The wrist is a synovial joint, formed from the articulations between the radius and ulna, the eight carpal bones

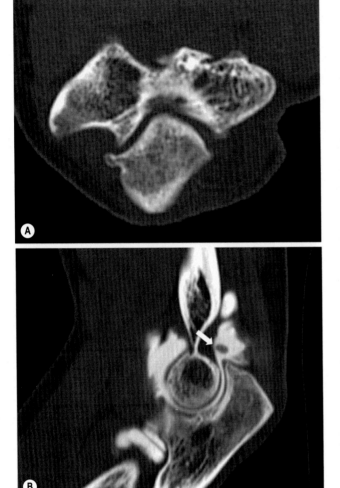

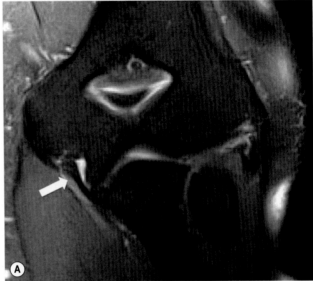

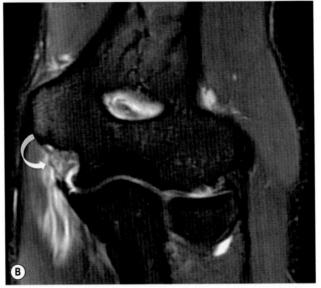

FIGURE 2-22 ■ Axial CT image (A) of early OA of the elbow. There is an osteophyte arising from the olecranon. The corresponding sagittal CT arthrogram image (B) demonstrates a non-radiopaque chondral body in the posterior joint recess (white arrow).

FIGURE 2-23 ■ Coronal FS T2W MR image (A) of a normal ulnar collateral ligament (UCL) of the elbow (white arrow). In a patient with an acute valgus strain injury (B), there is a tear of the UCL at the proximal origin on the lateral humeral epicondyle (curved white arrow), and there is surrounding soft-tissue haemorrhage.

and the metacarpal bones. The distal radioulnar joint allows supination and pronation of the forearm.

The mechanics of the wrist are complex, but movement occurs primarily through the proximal carpal row, comprising the scaphoid, lunate and triquetrum. This acts as a bridge between the forearm bones and the distal carpal row, which is relatively rigid. The proximal carpal row is referred to as the intercalated segment, and the lunate acts as the keystone. Stability between the segments of the proximal row is maintained by the intrinsic scapholunate and lunotriquetral ligaments. Stability between the radius and ulna, the proximal and distal carpal rows is maintained by multiple dorsal and volar extrinsic ligaments. Carpal alignment is assessed on PA radiographs, by identifying continuity of the articular surfaces of the carpal bones (known as the arcs of Gilula).

The first carpometacarpal joint between the trapezium and first metacarpal is more mobile than the other CMC joints to allow for the greater range of movements of the thumb. It has a separate synovial compartment.

The distal radioulnar joint and ulnocarpal joint are stabilised by the triangular fibrocartilage (TFC) complex. The TFC is a cartilaginous disc that arises from the ulnar border of the distal radius and attaches to the fovea of the ulnar styloid. Its margins blend with the dorsal and volar radioulnar ligaments, and the extensor carpi ulnaris (ECU) tendon sheath.

The flexor tendons of the fingers and thumb pass through the carpal tunnel, which is maintained superficially by the flexor retinaculum, which extends from the hook of hamate and pisiform to the scaphoid and trapezium. The median nerve passes through the carpal tunnel to enter the palm. The extensor tendons are stabilised by the extensor retinaculum on the dorsal aspect of the wrist at the level of the first carpal row.

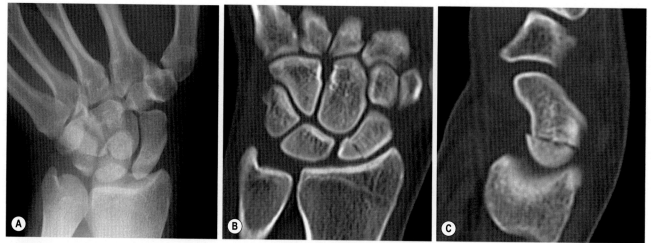

FIGURE 2-24 ■ Follow-up oblique radiograph (A) of the wrist in a patient with previous scaphoid fracture. There is an ill-defined sclerotic area in the proximal pole but there is no visible fracture line. However, the corresponding coronal (B) and sagittal oblique (C) CT MPRs clearly show fracture non-union.

Bone

Fractures around the wrist are common. Waist of scaphoid fractures may be associated with avascular necrosis of the proximal pole. The more proximal the fracture site, the higher the incidence of fracture non-union.

Radiological signs of avascular necrosis (AVN) include sclerosis of the proximal pole, which may progress to articular collapse and bone fragmentation. CT is used to assess the state of fracture union (Fig. 2-24). Signs of AVN on MRI include low SI sclerosis on T1-weighted (T1W) images and short T1 inversion recovery (STIR) images. Marrow oedema on STIR images is an indicator of persistent vascular perfusion in the proximal segment. The absence of enhancement with gadolinium contrast medium on fat-saturated T1W images in areas of sclerosis is a reliable indicator of lack of vascularity[15] (Fig. 2-25).

Spontaneous AVN of the lunate is known as Keinböck's disease. The radiographic and MRI features are the same as AVN of the scaphoid (Fig. 2-26). It may be associated with negative ulnar variance (short ulna). Advanced bony collapse in both proximal scaphoid fractures and AVN of the lunate results in late-stage secondary osteroarthritis.

Wrist Ligaments

Tears of the ligaments of the wrist can result in carpal instability. Disruption of the intrinsic ligaments results in intercalated segment instability. This is also termed dissociative carpal instability because there is dissociation between the segments of the proximal carpal row.

The scapholunate ligament is most frequently involved. Radiographs may show scapholunate diastasis (>3 mm). The lunate demonstrates dorsal rotation on lateral views and volar rotation of the scaphoid. This results in an increase in the scapholunate angle (>60°) known as dorsal intercalated segment instability (DISI) (Fig. 2-27). A DISI deformity of the carpus may also be associated with fractures of the scaphoid.

Disruption of the lunotriquetral ligament is less common. In this situation there is volar rotation of the lunate on lateral radiographs, with reduction of the scapholunate angle (<30°). On PA radiographs there may be an obvious step between the distal articular surface of the lunate and triquetrum. This is termed volar intercalated segment instability (VISI).

More subtle degrees of instability may be demonstrated by an instability series of radiographs acquired with radial and ulnar deviation and with a clenched fist view. Video fluoroscopy is also useful for assessing dynamic wrist instability.

Abnormal communication between the radiocarpal and midcarpal joints may be seen on arthrography (Fig. 2-28), which is usually combined with MRI or CT[16] (Figs. 2-29 and 2-30). However, direct visualisation of the ligaments is possible with conventional MRI. The most important features to describe that help determine management include the following:
- Carpal alignment
  - scapholunate angle
  - scapholunate diastasis
  - disruption of the arcs of Gilula.
- Integrity of the intrinsic ligaments.
- Presence of associated arthrosis.

Injuries to the extrinsic ligaments result in a variety of complex radiocarpal and midcarpal non-dissociative instabilities.

Lunate and perilunate dislocations are important injuries. In lunate dislocation, the lunate dislocates in a volar direction with loss of the articulation of the radius and other carpal bones. In perilunate dislocation, the lunate retains the articulation with the radius and the remainder of the carpus dislocates in a dorsal or volar direction. PA radiographs show an abnormal triangular appearance of the lunate. Differentiation of lunate versus perilunate dislocation is best made on a lateral radiograph. Both injuries may be associated with scaphoid (or other carpal) fractures, which indicates a greater degree of wrist instability.

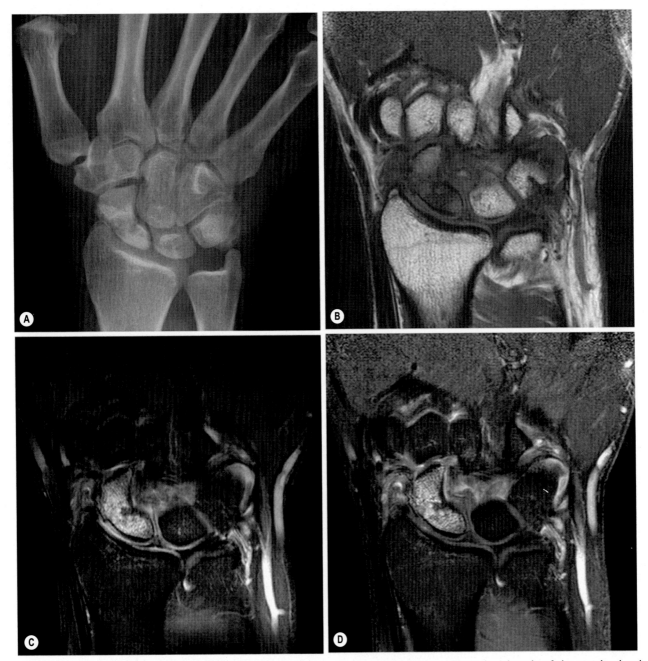

FIGURE 2-25 ■ PA radiograph of the wrist (A) showing non-union of a scaphoid fracture. There is sclerosis of the proximal pole segment indicating possible avascular necrosis (AVN). The corresponding coronal T1W MR image (B) demonstrates low SI within the marrow cavity, which is also consistent with AVN. However, there is high SI oedema on the T2FS image (C), and the post-contrast medium T1FS image (D) shows marked enhancement, indicating persistent vascularity of the scaphoid.

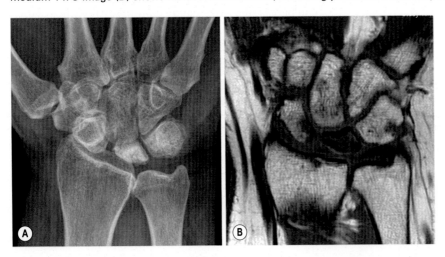

FIGURE 2-26 ■ AP radiograph (A) of the wrist with avascular necrosis of the lunate (Keinböck's disease). The lunate is small and sclerotic with features of early subchondral fragmentation. The coronal T1W image (B) shows the same features with low SI marrow indicating bone sclerosis. No marrow oedema was present on the T2FS images (not shown).

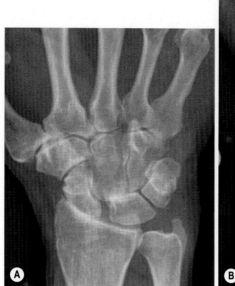
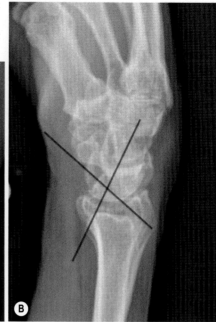

FIGURE 2-27 ■ AP (A) and lateral (B) radiographs of the wrist in a patient with scapholunate ligament rupture, dorsal intercalated segment instability (DISI), and secondary OA. There is scapholunate diastasis on the AP view, with widening of the joint space. The scapholunate angle (black lines) is increased above 60° on the lateral view with dorsal tilt of the lunate (normal scapholunate angle = 30–60°).

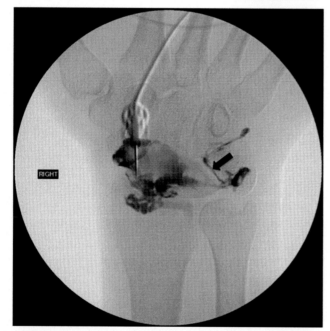

FIGURE 2-28 ■ **Fluoroscopic image acquired during digital subtraction arthrography of the wrist.** The radiocarpal joint has been injected and contrast medium fills the joint space. There is leak of contrast medium through the lunotriquetral joint into the midcarpal joint (black arrow), indicating ligament rupture.

Triangular Fibrocartilage

The TFC is composed of fibrocartilage and is normally low SI on all MRI pulse sequences (Fig. 2-31). Tears of the TFC complex may present as ulnar-sided wrist pain. They occur as either a degenerative phenomenon or as an acute injury. Degenerative tears frequently result in central perforation of the TFC (Fig. 2-32), and are associated with positive ulnar variance (long ulna). This in turn may lead to ulnar abutment on the triquetrum, which is another cause of ulnar-sided wrist pain.

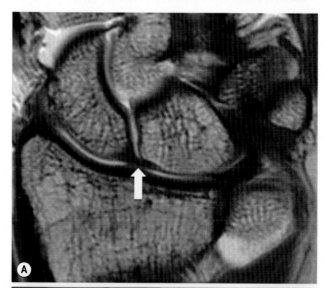
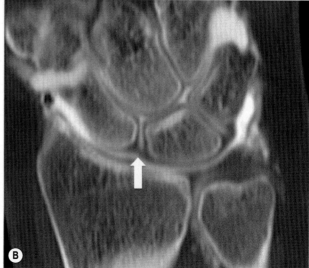

FIGURE 2-29 ■ Normal scapholunate ligament on coronal T1W MR arthrogram (A) and CT arthrogram (B) images (white arrows).

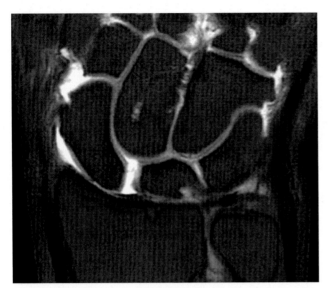

FIGURE 2-30 ■ **Scapholunate ligament disruption on an FS T1W MR arthrogram image.** The ligament is absent, and there is scapholunate diastasis. There are features of early secondary OA change with loss of articular cartilage on the scaphoid and lunate with a subchondral cyst in the lunate.

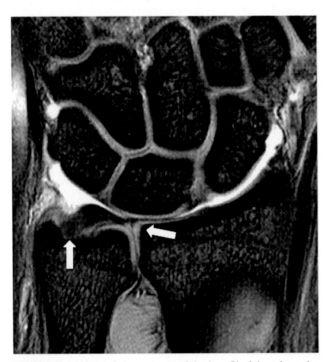

FIGURE 2-31 ■ Normal appearance of the low SI of the triangular fibrocartilage (TFC) on a coronal T2W gradient-echo MR arthrogram. The radial and ulnar attachments are well demonstrated (white arrows).

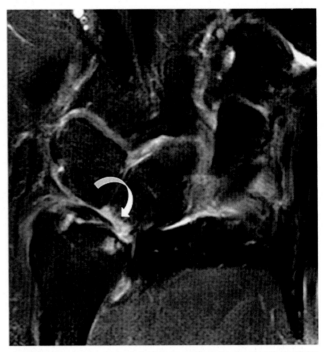

FIGURE 2-32 ■ **Degenerative TFC perforation on a coronal FS T1W MR arthrogram.** There is a large central defect of the TFC (curved white arrow), outlined by the high SI intra-articular contrast medium. There are associated OA changes in the wrist and DRUJ, with loss of articular cartilage and a subchondral cyst in the distal ulna.

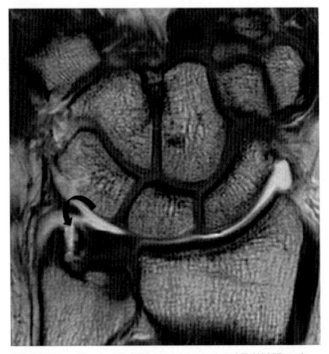

FIGURE 2-33 ■ **Traumatic TFC tear on a coronal T1W MR arthrogram.** There is avulsion of the ulnar styloid attachment of the TFC, with contrast medium extending between the TFC and styloid process (curved black arrow).

Traumatic TFC tears often affect the ulnar attachments and are associated with ulnar styloid fractures (Fig. 2-33). These injuries may also involve the dorsal and volar radioulnar ligaments and can lead to DRUJ instability.

Wrist Tendons

The tendons of the wrist are divided into extensor and flexor tendons. The extensor tendons form six groups with separate synovial sheaths, numbered from a radial to ulnar direction at the level of the radiocarpal joint.

Extensor tendinopathy is commonly seen in the extensor carpi ulnaris (ECU) tendon as it passes over the ulnar

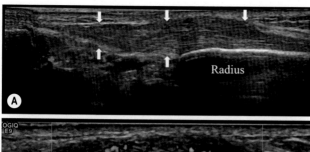

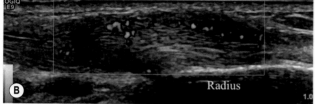

FIGURE 2-34 ■ Longitudinal grey-scale US image of the extensor group I tendons of the wrist (A). There is thickening of the tendon with echogenic thickening of the tendon sheath (white arrows) representing stenosing tenosynovitis (De Quervain's disease). There is associated tendon neovascularisation on the corresponding power Doppler image (B).

styloid. This is a common site for tenosynovitis in the setting of inflammatory arthropathy that may produce erosion of the ulnar styloid. Another commonly encountered extensor tendinopathy affects the extensor group I tendons of abductor pollicis longus and extensor pollicis brevis.[17] This is frequently associated with a stenosing tendosynovitis known as De Quervain's tenosynovitis (Fig. 2-34).

The flexor tendons are grouped within the carpal tunnel, with the exception of the flexor carpi ulnaris and radialis tendons. Isolated flexor tendinopathy is uncommon, though generalised flexor tenosynovitis may occur with rheumatoid arthritis. This increases the pressure within the carpal tunnel and may cause a secondary carpal tunnel syndrome by compression of the median nerve.

Median Nerve

Carpal tunnel syndrome is a neuropathy of the median nerve. It is usually idiopathic, or associated with pregnancy. Direct nerve compression may occur within the carpal tunnel in patients with synovitis of the wrist or flexor tendons. Lesions with mass effect arising from the tendon sheath or peripheral nerve sheath tumours are occasionally encountered.

Diagnosis is often made by a combination of clinical findings and nerve conduction studies. US or MRI may be required in cases with atypical features. Imaging is used to visualise abnormalities of the nerve, and to exclude secondary causes of carpal tunnel syndrome. The changes in the nerve are variable and include flattening of the nerve within the carpal tunnel, and proximal thickening. A cross-sectional area of > 10 mm^2 is suggestive of carpal tunnel syndrome. Qualitative changes within the nerve such as loss of normal fascicular pattern on US or increased SI on MRI are unreliable signs in isolation.[18]

UCL of Thumb

Tears of the ulnar collateral ligament of the thumb are common. They are often referred to as gamekeeper's thumb or skier's thumb. Undisplaced ligament tears can be treated conservatively, but displaced tears will not heal and require surgical repair.

In a displaced tear the ligament is torn from the distal insertion and retracts proximally around the aponeurosis of the adductor pollicis. This is known as a Stener lesion.[19] The displaced ligament can be demonstrated on both MRI and US (Fig. 2-35).

THE HIP

The hip is a large ball-and-socket joint which allows a wide range of movement while maintaining strong stability such that dislocation is much less frequent than in the shoulder. The cup-shaped acetabulum is formed at the junction of the ilial, ischial and pubic bones. The depth of the acetabulum is increased by the fibrocartilaginous labrum. Stability is further increased by the iliofemoral, ischiofemoral and pubofemoral ligaments which reinforce the joint capsule. The acetabulum and femoral head are lined by hyaline cartilage. The ligamentum teres is a weak ligament attaching to the fovea of the femoral head. It transmits the foveal artery, though in adults most of the blood supply of the femoral head is provided by the circumflex femoral arteries.

Labrum and Cartilage

The fibrocartilaginous labrum forms a ring at the margin of the acetabulum, increasing the stability of the joint by deepening the acetabular fossa. Lesions of the acetabular labrum constitute one of the most common internal derangements of the hip. Tears of the labrum may be traumatic or degenerative and are a cause of pain and mechanical symptoms. The gold standard imaging technique is MRI following injection of gadolinium contrast medium into the joint (MR arthrography). However, with modern high field strength systems some centres make use of conventional MRI without arthrographic contrast medium. The torn labrum may appear small, irregular, absent or may demonstrate linear penetration of contrast agent into the tear (Fig. 2-36). The anterosuperior and superior portions of the labrum are most frequently affected. Fluid tracking through the tear may form a paralabral cyst which is a useful indication of an underlying labral tear. Occasionally intra-articular contrast material can be seen communicating with the cyst on MR arthrographic images. Labral tears are often associated with adjacent articular cartilage damage and it is proposed that a labral tear is a precursor to the development of osteoarthritis. However, it is also important to recognise that labral degenerative tears are seen in association with osteoarthritis and the precise relationship between the two entities is as yet unclear.

Traumatic tears may arise from impingement between the femoral head and neck and the acetabular rim. This condition is known as femoroacetabular impingement.

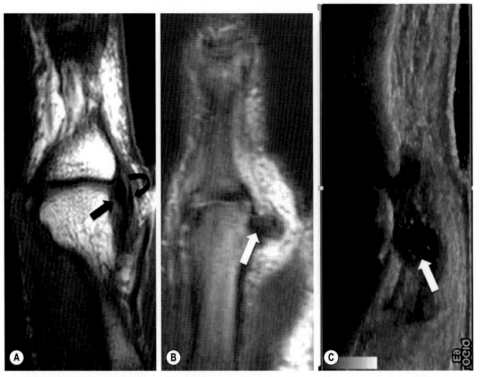

FIGURE 2-35 ■ Coronal T1W image (A) demonstrating the normal low SI ulnar collateral ligament (UCL) of the metacarpal joint of the thumb (black arrow), and the overlying adductor aponeurosis (curved black arrow). The coronal FS T2W MR image (B) and corresponding longitudinal US image (C) show a retracted UCL tear (Stener lesion) in a patient following a valgus strain injury (white arrows).

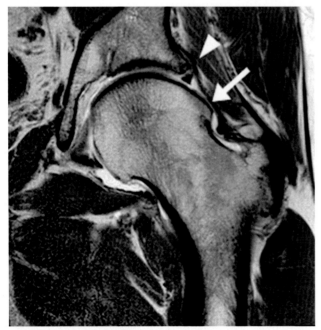

FIGURE 2-36 ■ **Cam deformity and labral tear.** Coronal T1-weighted MR arthrographic image. High signal intra-articular contrast medium is shown penetrating between the labrum and acetabulum (arrowhead) indicating a labral tear. There is an osseous bump, or cam deformity of the lateral femoral head (arrow).

Two kinds of femoroacetabular impingement are described, cam type and pincer type, though these often coexist.[20] Cam impingement is caused by the presence of an abnormal osseous 'bump' found on the anterior or lateral aspect of the femoral head–neck junction (Fig. 2-36). This produces abnormal contact between femur and acetabular rim in certain positions and typically presents in young athletic men. The α angle can be used to identify this loss of sphericity on a cross-table lateral radiograph or axial oblique MRI (Fig. 2-37). An α angle measuring greater than 50° may be taken as abnormal.[21] Repeated contact between the osseous bump and the anterior acetabulum during hip flexion results in a labral tear and/or cartilage damage. CT is an excellent technique for demonstrating the bone morphology in this condition, although MR arthrography is able to show the cartilage and labral damage. Acetabular cartilage delamination (separation of the cartilage from the underlying bone), sometimes termed a 'carpet lesion', is common in cam-type impingement and may be detected on MR arthrography.[22] The information provided by arthrographic MRI is important, as joint-sparing treatment (such as cam re-contouring) is unlikely to give effective symptom relief if there is established severe cartilage damage.

Pincer-type impingement, more common in middle-aged women, results from overcoverage of the femoral head by the acetabulum. This can be due to a deep acetabulum, bone hypertrophy at the acetabular rim or abnormal acetabular retroversion, the latter leading to an

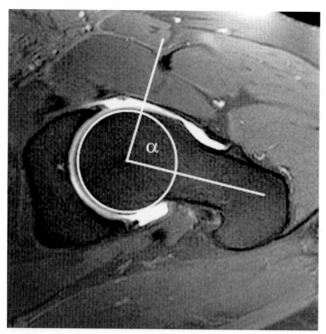

FIGURE 2-37 ■ The α angle measured on an axial oblique T1-weighted fat-saturated MR arthrographic image shows loss of sphericity of the femoral head (cam deformity). A circle of best fit is drawn around the femoral head. A line is drawn along the femoral neck axis. A second line is drawn from the centre of the femoral head to the point on the circle where the femoral head begins to protrude from it. The α angle is measured between the two lines.

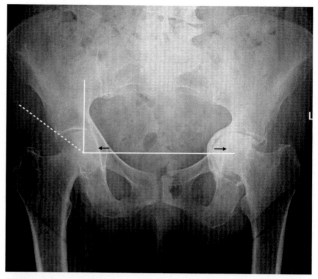

FIGURE 2-38 ■ **AP pelvic radiograph.** At both hips the femoral head is seen to overlap the ilioischial line (arrows) indicating bilateral protrusio acetabuli, which in this female patient was idiopathic. Note severe secondary degeneration in the left hip joint. The centre-edge angle detects overcoverage of the femoral head. A line is drawn perpendicular to an axis through both femoral head centres. A second line is drawn from the femoral head centre to the most lateral point of the acetabular roof. The centre-edge angle lies between the two lines.

effective overcoverage of the femoral head anteriorly. On hip flexion the abnormal morphology results in impingement between the acetabular rim and the femoral neck, leading to labral and cartilage damage. The centre-edge angle is a method to identify acetabular overcoverage on an AP radiograph of the pelvis (Fig. 2-38). A centre-edge angle greater than 40° may be considered abnormal.[23] Coxa profunda and protusio acetabuli are two types of deformity that predispose to pincer-type impingement. Coxa profunda is identified on an AP radiograph when the floor of the acetabular fossa overlaps the ilioischial line. Protrusio acetabuli, more severe, is present when the femoral head itself overlaps the ilioischial line (Fig. 2-38).

Muscle and Tendon

Muscle and tendon injury around the hip is common. This may result from acute trauma such as may be sustained in sporting activities or, particularly in the case of tendon injury, from chronic repetitive microtrauma. The hamstring and adductor origins are commonly affected in young athletes while gluteus medius tendon degeneration (tendinopathy) and tears are more common in the elderly. On MRI and ultrasound, the appearances vary depending on the severity of the injury. In the case of muscle injury, findings may range from minor muscle oedema to discontinuity of fibres and muscle retraction. In chronic cases there may be fatty atrophy or muscle ossification. Tendon disease in the form of tears or tendinopathic change may also be demonstrated; the latter is

seen as loss of the normal tendon low signal on T1- and T2-weighted MR images along with thickening of the tendon. Ultrasound will also show tendon discontinuities and tendinopathy.

Avulsion of an unfused apophysis at a muscle attachment may occur in children undertaking athletic activities. The anterior superior iliac spine (sartorius muscle), the anterior inferior iliac spine (rectus femoris) and ischial tuberosity (hamstring) are common sites of involvement (Fig. 2-39). Because avulsed apophyses continue to form bone, this can lead to bizarre mass-like appearances on imaging when presentation is delayed. The location of the bone 'mass' and the age of the patient are key to making the correct diagnosis.

While mechanical snaps and clicks can arise from within the joint, for instance in the presence of a labral tear or loose body, such mechanical symptoms may also arise from extra-articular causes. The snapping hip describes a snap or clunk felt by the patient when undertaking a particular movement. It may be associated with pain and the snap may be audible. Two of the most common extra-articular varieties are the snapping iliotibial band (external type) and the snapping iliopsoas tendon (internal type). Both can be imaged using ultrasound, which allows continuous visualisation of the relevant structures while the patient reproduces the snapping. In the external type the gluteus maximus muscle can be shown initially lying over the greater trochanter before abruptly moving posteriorly to bring the iliotibial band into contact with the greater trochanter.[24] In the internal type the iliopsoas tendon rotates abnormally before abruptly reversing and forcefully striking the superior pubic ramus.[25]

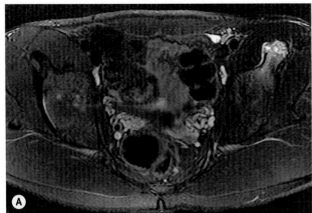

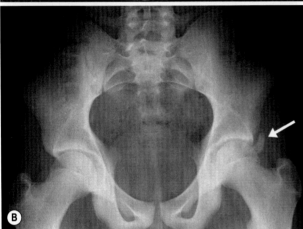

FIGURE 2-39 ■ **Avulsion of the straight head of rectus femoris from the anterior inferior iliac spine (AIIS).** (A) Axial T2-weighted fat-saturated image of the pelvis demonstrates oedema at the left AIIS and irregularity of the apophysis. (B) Plain radiograph taken 5 months later shows displacement of the apophysis from the AIIS.

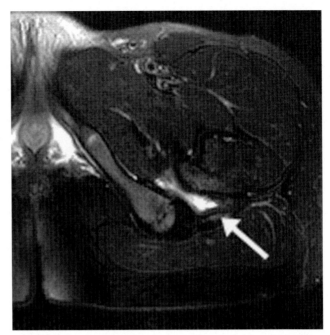

FIGURE 2-40 ■ **Ischiofemoral impingement.** Axial T2-weighted fat-saturated image shows bursa formation in a narrowed ischiofemoral space.

TABLE 2-1   **Potential Causes of Hip AVN**
• Idiopathic
• Trauma and vascular
• Fracture (including complication of fracture fixation)
• Radiotherapy
• Dysbaric osteonecrosis (caisson disease)
• Arteritis
• Inflammatory
• Pancreatitis
• Connective tissue disease
• Rheumatoid arthritis
• Metabolic and endocrine
• Pregnancy
• Diabetes
• Cushing's syndrome
• Gaucher's disease
• Toxic
• Steroids
• Alcohol
• Immunosuppressives
• Haematological disorders
• Sickle cell anaemia
• Polycythemia rubra vera
• Haemophilia

Ischiofemoral impingement is a recently described condition predominantly affecting women associated with narrowing of the space between the ischial tuberosity and lesser trochanter of the femur. It is thought that the quadratus femoris muscle which passes through this space may be impinged during repetitive hip movement, giving rise to pain. MRI reveals narrowing of the space associated with oedema of the quadratus femoris muscle belly and adjacent free fluid (Fig. 2-40).[26] However, similar appearances may be found in asymptomatic individuals and the clinical significance of this has not yet been established.

Bone

Avascular necrosis of the femoral head has many potential underlying causes (Table 2-1). MRI is the preferred technique, allowing early detection of signal change in the subchondral region of the femoral head. The 'double line' sign on fluid-sensitive sequences, characteristic of AVN, describes a low signal sclerotic line next to a high signal hypervascular line which demarcates the extent of the lesion (Fig. 2-41). There may be accompanying bone marrow oedema in the femoral head and neck. The extent of involvement on MRI has prognostic value in determining the outcome after decompressive surgery.[27] Conventional radiographs are much less sensitive in the early stages of AVN, but as the process progresses they will typically show a linear subchondral lucency that progresses to articular collapse and sclerosis. Both hips should be imaged together, as bilateral involvement is common.

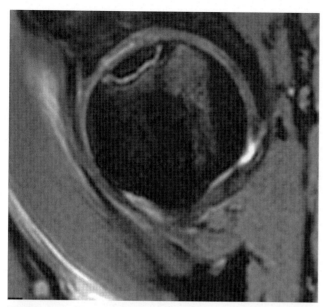

FIGURE 2-41 ■ **Avascular necrosis (AVN) in the femoral head.** Sagittal oblique T2-weighted fat-saturated image demonstrates a region of subchondral AVN demarcated by the characteristic 'double line' sign.

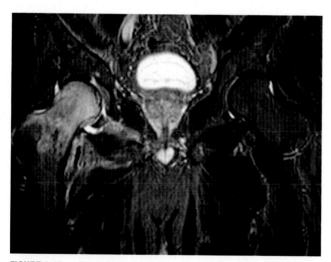

FIGURE 2-42 ■ **Transient osteoporosis of the right hip.** Coronal T2-weighted fat-saturated image shows extensive bone marrow oedema in the right femoral head and neck. See text for the differential diagnosis.

Transient osteoporosis of the hip (TOP), also known as bone marrow oedema syndrome, is a self-limiting painful condition of uncertain aetiology.[28] On MRI this appears as extensive bone marrow oedema signal involving the femoral head and/or neck (Fig. 2-42). Conventional radiographs may show reduced bone density but MRI is the most important tool in diagnosis. Following resolution in the hip, the condition may go on to involve other parts of the skeleton, in which case the condition is called regional migratory osteoporosis. Bone marrow high signal (oedema) seen in the femoral head and/or neck raises several possible diagnoses, including transient osteoporosis, that should also be considered (Table 2-2).

TABLE 2-2	Causes of Femoral Head/Neck Bone Marrow Oedema

- Transient osteoporosis
- Avascular necrosis
- Fracture
  - Including fatigue and insufficiency fractures
- Arthropathy (including joint sepsis)
  - Will normally involve both sides of the joint
- Osteoid osteoma
- Osteomyelitis
- Myeloma and metastases

Bursae

Bursae are synovial-lined structures found in many sites around the musculoskeletal system, and it is their normal function to facilitate the movement between muscles and adjacent structures. Bursal inflammation, or bursitis, may result from overuse injury or from involvement by systemic inflammatory conditions such as inflammatory arthritis. On imaging, a normal bursa will often be unseen, or appear as a thin layer of fluid between tissues. When inflamed (bursitis), imaging will show the bursa as a more substantial fluid-containing structure. There may be thickening of the bursal walls and adjacent soft-tissue oedema. Several bursae are recognised around the hip, but the most common to be associated with symptoms are the iliopsoas and the greater trochanteric bursae. The trochanteric bursae are a group of bursae found deep to the gluteus maximus, gluteus medius and gluteus minimus muscles.[29] 'Trochanteric bursitis' is a relatively common condition which may involve one or more of the bursae and typically occurs in middle-aged women. Trochanteric bursitis presents with lateral hip pain and may be associated with tendinopathy of gluteus medius (Fig. 2-43). The iliopsoas bursa is the largest bursa in the body and communicates with the hip joint in approximately 15% of individuals. It lies deep to the iliopsoas muscle and passes directly over the anterior hip joint capsule. Iliopsoas bursitis typically presents with anterior hip pain related to movement or with an anterior groin mass if large.

THE KNEE

The knee is the largest joint in the body and comprises three compartments, the medial and lateral femorotibial compartments and the patellofemoral compartment. The femoral condyles articulate with the tibial condyles, and the patella articulates with the femoral trochlea. The joint capsule encloses the articular surfaces, menisci and cruciate ligaments. The collateral ligaments and tendons are extra-articular, apart from the popliteus tendon, which has an intra-articular portion. The bony articular surfaces alone are inherently unstable, so these soft-tissue supporting structures are vital to the joint stability and are prone to injury. MRI remains the imaging technique of choice for evaluating most internal knee derangements. It is well suited for demonstrating the menisci,

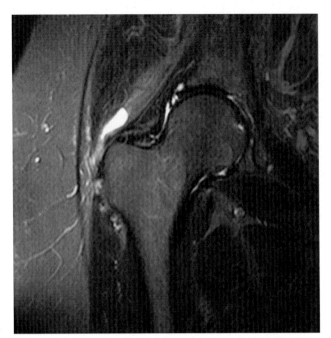

FIGURE 2-43 ■ **Trochanteric bursitis.** Coronal T2-weighted fat-saturated image shows fluid distension of the subgluteus medius bursa. There is associated thickening and oedema of the gluteus medius tendon insertion.

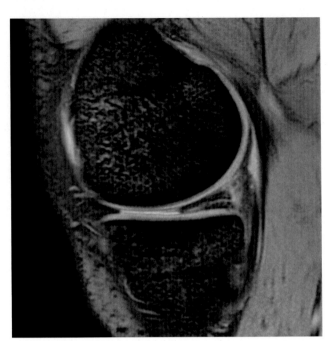

FIGURE 2-44 ■ **Horizontal tear of the medial meniscus.** Sagittal gradient-echo image shows linear high signal in the posterior meniscus extending to the free edge.

tendons and ligaments. However, ultrasound can be used to demonstrate the peripheral joint structures, showing the medial and lateral collateral ligaments and soft tissues of the extensor mechanism well.

Menisci

The menisci are two semilunar fibrocartilaginous structures located between the articular cartilage of the femoral and tibial condyles. They each have a crescent shape with an anterior and posterior horn and a body. The tips of the horns are attached to the tibial plateau adjacent to the intercondylar eminence. These attachments are known as the meniscal roots. The medial meniscus is larger than the lateral and has a larger posterior horn than anterior horn. In the case of the lateral meniscus, the horns are of similar size, but in approximately 5% of individuals the lateral meniscus has a discoid morphology. A discoid meniscus is associated with increased incidence of pathology from a young age. Sagittal MRI sequences of the normal meniscus show a bow-tie configuration at the periphery. On progressive images toward the intercondylar fossa the meniscus appears as two triangles representing the anterior and posterior horns. The normal menisci exhibit uniform low signal on all MRI sequences, although in children some increased signal is frequently identified in the posterior third. Degeneration may lead to intrameniscal high signal, or 'myxoid change', particularly in the posterior medial meniscus. A tear is diagnosed on MRI when high signal is demonstrated extending to the articular surface of the meniscus. Tears may be horizontal or vertical depending on whether they reach one meniscal surface or two. A complex tear is diagnosed when two or more tear configurations are present. The configuration

of a meniscal tear has important implications for management. Horizontal tears are frequently degenerative in nature and may be asymptomatic (Fig. 2-44). Joint fluid may escape through a horizontal tear, forming a parameniscal cyst. Two types of vertical tear are recognised. Longitudinal tears lie within the substance of the meniscus, tracking circumferentially. They often involve the periphery of the meniscus where the blood supply is better and may therefore heal spontaneously. As the name suggests, radial tears extend radially into the meniscus from the free edge; they take several forms. A small oblique slit is a common form and is called a parrot beak tear (Fig. 2-45). If it traverses the full width, a radial tear may split the meniscus, leading to separation of the two parts. A 'ghost meniscus' describes the MRI appearance of a complete radial tear where the image section passes through the split (Fig. 2-46). This sign is most often found in tears involving the posterior root of the medial meniscus. Some tears have a fragment which may displace and cause locking; this is particularly common with longitudinal tears, which, in particular, can give rise to a 'bucket handle' tear. Here the meniscal fragment remaining attached at both ends flips into the intercondylar notch (Fig. 2-47). The 'double PCL sign' describes a sagittal view showing the posterior cruciate ligament (PCL) and a second parallel low signal structure representing the displaced bucket handle fragment of a torn meniscus (Fig. 2-48).

Anterior Cruciate Ligament

The anterior cruciate ligament (ACL) attaches proximally at the posteromedial margin of the lateral femoral condyle in the intercondylar fossa and distally at the anterior aspect of the tibial intercondylar eminence. The

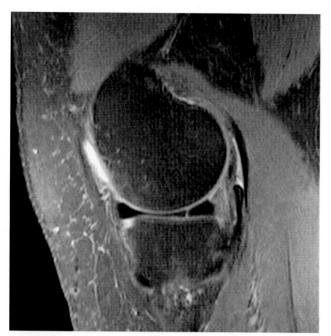

FIGURE 2-45 ■ Radial tear of the medial meniscus on a sagittal proton density fat-saturated image.

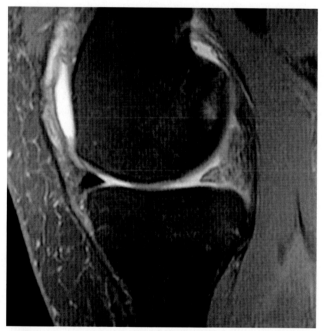

FIGURE 2-46 ■ 'Ghost meniscus'. Sagittal proton density fat-saturated image shows abnormal high signal of the posterior medial meniscus due to a complete radial tear.

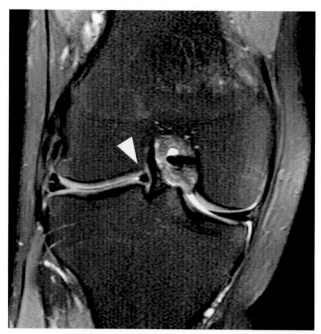

FIGURE 2-47 ■ 'Bucket handle' tear of the lateral meniscus. Coronal proton density fat-saturated image demonstrates a flipped fragment of the lateral meniscus (arrowhead) in the intercondylar fossa.

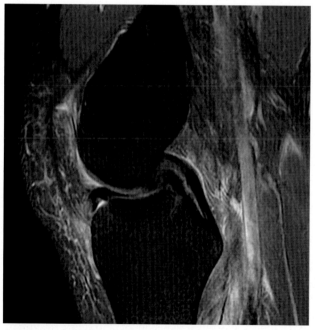

FIGURE 2-48 ■ Double PCL sign. Sagittal proton density fat-saturated image shows a flipped fragment of a 'bucket handle' meniscal tear that lies in the intercondylar fossa deep to the PCL.

ACL acts to restrain anterior translation and, to a lesser extent, internal rotation of the tibia relative to the femur. On MRI, the ligament is best visualised on sagittal images, appearing normally as fan-shaped bundles of taut fibres. Two bundles, the anteromedial and posterolateral, may be differentiated on the coronal and axial sequences. As fluid and loose connective tissue may be interspaced between the bundles, the ACL often appears larger and of more mixed signal intensity than the PCL.

ACL tears are common sporting injuries. On MRI, complete tears appear as discontinuity of the fibres, increased signal and/or laxity (Fig. 2-49). The

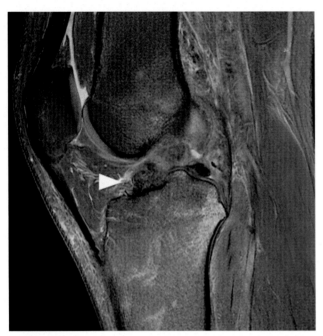

FIGURE 2-49 ▪ Complete intrasubstance ACL tear. Sagittal proton density fat-saturated image reveals retracted ACL fibres (arrowhead) at the distal attachment and no intact proximal fibres. Note bone marrow oedema in a typical location in the posterior tibia.

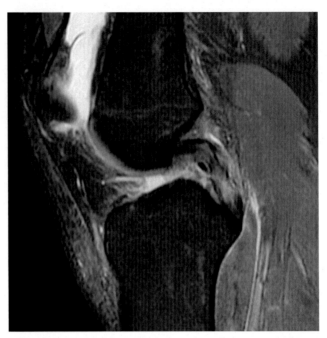

FIGURE 2-50 ▪ PCL tear. Sagittal proton density fat-saturated image shows abnormal signal and thickening of the distal PCL.

mid-substance of the ligament is injured more frequently than the proximal or distal portions. Partial tears or sprains of the ACL are recognised on MRI by altered signal and/or laxity in the presence of continuity of some fibres. There are several secondary imaging signs associated with ACL injury. Typically there is microfracture in the posterior aspect of the lateral tibial plateau and the subarticular lateral femoral condyle, reflecting impaction between these sites during subluxation of the knee at the time of the injury (pivot shift injury). ACL tears may be accompanied by anterior translation of the tibia relative to the femur. This can be detected on sagittal images as it will cause buckling of the PCL. The lateral notch sign, which is specific but not very sensitive for ACL injury, describes abnormally deep indentation of the condylopatellar sulcus of the lateral femoral condyle on a lateral conventional radiograph.[30] ACL injuries are commonly associated with injury to other structures. O'Donaghue's triad describes tears of the ACL, MCL and medial meniscus. A Segond fracture, which has a high association with ACL injury, describes avulsion of a fracture fragment from the lateral margin of the lateral tibial condyle at the attachment of the joint capsule.

Posterior Cruciate Ligament

The posterior cruciate ligament (PCL) extends from the anterolateral margin of the medial femoral condyle to the posterior aspect of the tibial intercondylar eminence. It normally appears as a thick low signal bundle that is visualised well in all planes on MRI. Tears of the PCL, e.g. from a sporting or dashboard-type injury, may result in

instability characterised by posterior translation of the tibia relative to the femur. Partial intrasubstance ruptures of the PCL are more common than complete tears and avulsions. Intrasubstance tears exhibit thickening and altered signal on MRI while usually maintaining the appearance of a continuous structure (Fig. 2-50).[31] Microfracture of the anterior aspect of the tibial plateau is typical. Associated soft-tissue injury is common, including tears of the ACL, medial collateral ligament and posterolateral corner.

Medial Collateral Ligament

The medial collateral ligament (MCL) has superficial and deep components; the former are more important for maintaining knee stability in the presence of valgus forces. The posterior oblique ligament is found more posteriorly and is formed by contributions from the superficial and deep MCL. Together with the semimembranosus tendon, it is an important stabiliser of the knee posteromedially. Coronal MRI sequences clearly identify the MCL as a thin low signal band, differentiating the superficial portion from the much shorter deep portion which has attachments to the middle third of the lateral meniscus. Injury to the MCL may be classified according to severity.[32] A Grade 1 sprain is a periligamentous injury characterised by oedema around the ligament which maintains low signal. A Grade 2 injury represents a partial tear with focal intraligamentous thickening and altered signal intensity as a result of oedema and/or haemorrhage. A Grade 3, or complete, tear shows complete discontinuity across the ligament. Chronic ossification of the proximal MCL following injury is known as a Pellegrini–Stieda lesion.

Lateral Collateral Ligament Complex and Posterolateral Corner

Lateral joint stability is provided by a number of structures including anteriorly, the iliotibial band, which attaches onto the proximal tibia. The lateral collateral ligament (LCL), or fibular collateral ligament, passes between the lateral femoral condyle and the fibular head. The biceps femoris tendon has a common attachment with the LCL to the fibular head known as the conjoint tendon. LCL tears may arise within the ligamentous substance or from avulsion at the fibular head.

The LCL is a component of the posterolateral corner complex of supporting structures which also includes the popliteus tendon, biceps tendon, arcuate ligament, popliteofibular ligament and posterior joint capsule. Injury to the posterolateral corner is often associated with damage to other ligamentous structures, most commonly tears of the ACL. Posterolateral corner injuries may lead to posterolateral instability which has implications for surgical management, particularly when associated with ACL injuries. While the LCL, biceps tendon and popliteus are seen well on MRI, it is often difficult to reliably evaluate the smaller components of the posterolateral corner individually because of their small size and orientation.

The Extensor Mechanism and Patellofemoral Joint

The patella is a sesamoid bone (the largest in the body) that lies between the quadriceps tendon proximally and the patellar tendon distally. The medial and lateral patellar retinacula also form part of the extensor mechanism. The patella articulates with the trochlea groove, or sulcus, of the femur. This groove is an important component in providing stability to the patella. Trochlea dysplasia describes a shallow sulcus (this can be measured on imaging) that predisposes to patellar dislocation. An abnormally high position of the patella (patella alta) may contribute to patellar maltracking and/or cartilage damage. The Insall–Salvati ratio assesses relative patella height and is given by the ratio of patellar tendon length to the length of the patella itself. It can be calculated from conventional radiographs or sagittal MRI images.[33,34] Axial MRI or CT images may be used to measure the tibial tubercle–trochlea groove distance (TTD) which identifies lateralisation of the patellar tendon insertion (which predisposes to lateral dislocation).[35] The patella is prone to dislocate laterally due to the valgus force of the quadriceps muscle group, although in the majority of cases this dislocation is transient and by the time of presentation to hospital the patella has reduced. Nevertheless there are characteristic MRI findings in acute patellar dislocation–relocation (Fig. 2-51). These include subcortical bone marrow oedema of the medial patella and lateral femoral condyle reflecting 'kissing contusions'. There is usually an associated tear of the medial patellar retinaculum and/or an osteochondral fracture of the patella.

Cartilage degeneration in the knee is common as a feature of osteoarthritis. Chondromalacia patellae

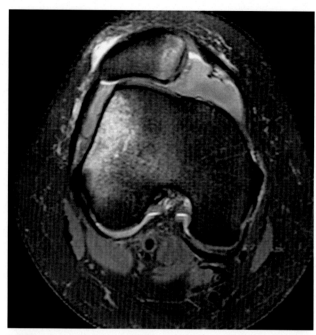

FIGURE 2-51 ■ **Acute patellar dislocation–relocation.** Axial proton density fat-saturated image shows typical bone marrow oedema reflecting 'kissing contusions' of the medial patella and lateral femoral condyle. Note the shallow trochlea sulcus and lateral patella tilt which predispose to dislocation.

describes cartilage damage occurring in adolescents and young adults which primarily involves the patellofemoral compartment. This may be associated with patellar misalignment or trauma. Cartilage damage can be graded according to severity. Early damage is demonstrated on MRI as signal abnormality and thinning. Progressive damage appears as full-thickness fissuring or a defect. The presence of subchondral oedema or cyst formation indicates the most severe damage.

Patellar tendinopathy involving the proximal tendon attachment is commonly referred to as 'jumper's knee' because of its association with athletic activities that involve jumping. It can be demonstrated on MRI and ultrasound where it typically appears as focal thickening of the central deep portion of the proximal tendon with increased Doppler vascularity (Fig. 2-52). On ultrasound the tendinopathic tendon shows low reflectivity and on MRI increased intrasubstance signal. Patellar tendinopathy may also involve the more distal tendon. Osgood–Schlatter disease is a common condition in children aged between 8 and 13 years and is characterised by distal patellar tendinopathy, tibial tubercle enlargement or fragmentation and thickening of the overlying soft tissues. The condition is thought to result from repetitive traction injury related to sporting activity. Tears of the patella or quadriceps tendons may occur, typically on the background of tendinopathy. They are readily evaluated with ultrasound or MRI.

Bone and Cartilage

Osteochondritis dissecans is a common condition of uncertain aetiology affecting children and adolescents. It is characterised by focal cartilage and subchondral bone

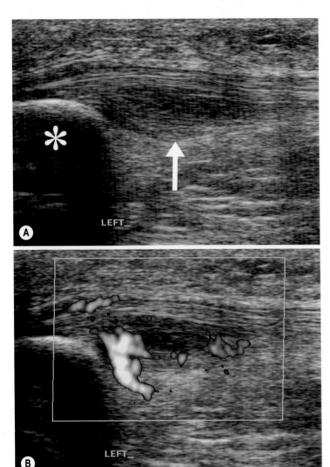

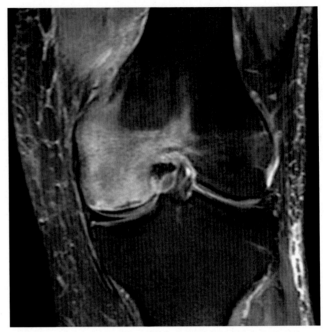

FIGURE 2-53 ■ **Transient osteoporosis of the knee.** Coronal proton density fat-saturated image shows extensive bone marrow oedema in the medial femoral condyle. Note there is subchondral linear low signal indicating associated insufficiency fracture.

FIGURE 2-52 ■ **Jumper's knee.** Longitudinal ultrasound images of proximal patellar tendinopathy. (A) Note thickening and hypoechogenicity of the deep part of the proximal tendon (arrow); * indicates the patella. (B) Doppler interrogation reveals marked neovascularity of the proximal tendon (in orange).

abnormality, and most commonly involves the lateral aspect of the medial femoral condyle. Conventional radiographs may reveal linear subarticular lucency with adjacent sclerosis but they are not sensitive. MRI clearly demonstrates these lesions, allowing measurement and localisation. A rim of fluid signal which undercuts the involved bone implies the lesion has become detached and may go on to displace into the joint space.

Repeated mechanical trauma to the articular surfaces of the knee may lead to subchondral fractures. Often occult on conventional radiographs, these lesions are demonstrated on fluid-sensitive MRI sequences as focal linear subchondral low signal (indicating the fracture line) with intense surrounding oedema-like signal in the bone marrow. Cartilage and meniscal damage may predispose to such injuries. Normal forces in the absence of predisposing abnormality may cause subchondral fracture if the underlying bone is weak (insufficiency fracture). Subchondral insufficiency fracture was sometimes previously referred to as 'spontaneous osteonecrosis of the knee', a term that is incorrect and becoming archaic. Recent interest has focused on a condition called 'bone marrow oedema syndrome' or 'transient osteoporosis' which is believed to predispose to insufficiency fracture in the knee and elsewhere (Fig. 2-53).[28]

Bursae

There are numerous anatomical bursae around the knee. Inflammation of a bursa, or bursitis, is commonly caused by friction from repetitive movement, though bursae may also be involved in systemic inflammatory conditions such as rheumatoid arthritis. Around the patellar tendon there are the superficial infrapatellar, deep infrapatellar and prepatellar bursae. Bursitis may affect any of these, and involvement of the last is called 'housemaid's knee'. Friction between the distal iliotibial band and lateral femoral condyle may give rise to bursitis known as 'runner's knee'. Inflammation of the pes anserine bursa gives rise to pain over the anteromedial aspect of the proximal tibia. The most commonly involved bursa in the popliteal region lies between the medial head of gastrocnemius and the semimembranosus tendon, the popliteal bursa. This communicates with the joint and distension of this bursa is called a popliteal or baker's cyst.

THE ANKLE AND FOOT

The ankle allows a wide range of movement, but also has to transmit considerable forces. It is the most commonly injured joint, with ligamentous injury in the form of sprains and tears particularly common. Patients typically present with pain and/or instability following such injury. The talar dome articulates with the tibial plafond and small facets on the medial and lateral malleoli. The malleoli contribute to the joint stability and provide attachments for the collateral ligaments, which are themselves important stabilisers of the ankle. The distal tibiofibular joint is a fibrous joint that contains a synovial recess extending from the ankle joint. Several tendons crossing the ankle joint are also prone to injury.

Ligaments

Injuries sustained to the ankle usually result from inversion or eversion. Inversion injuries are significantly more common than eversion injuries, with the result that the lateral ankle ligaments are torn more frequently than the medial. Three components of the lateral collateral ligament complex are recognised: the anterior and posterior talofibular ligaments and the calcaneofibular ligament. The anterior talofibular ligament is the most vulnerable to injury, followed by the calcaneofibular ligament. The posterior talofibular ligament is rarely injured except in the most severe cases. MRI or ultrasound may be used for assessment of these structures. On imaging, ligament damage may appear as altered signal/echogenicity, thickening, thinning, or absence (indicating a complete tear) (Fig. 2-54).[36] Damage to the lateral ligaments may lead to chronic anterolateral impingement in the absence of frank instability. Anterolateral impingement describes repetitive soft-tissue injury in the anterolateral gutter, causing synovitis and haemorrhage, which may be identified on MRI.[37]

The most important medial ankle ligaments include the anterior and posterior tibiotalar (also known as deltoid), tibio-spring and spring ligaments. The spring ligament extends from the calcaneus to the navicular and functions as an important stabiliser of the foot arch together with the posterior tibial tendon. The distal tibiotalar syndesmosis comprises anterior, interosseous and posterior tibiofibular ligaments. Strong forces are usually required to disrupt the syndesmotic ligaments such as those resulting in an ankle fracture. However, syndesmotic ligament injuries do occur, typically as a sports injury.

Tendons

Tendon abnormalities are common about the ankle. The tendons crossing the ankle anteriorly, medially and laterally do so in tendon sheaths and symptoms may relate to tenosynovitis as well as to tendinopathy if there is symptomatic intrinsic degeneration, tear, or subluxation/dislocation of the tendon itself. The last of these may occur if there is retinacular injury. The Achilles tendon is the largest tendon in the body. It is also vulnerable to tendinopathy and tears. Like the patellar tendon, the Achilles does not have a tendon sheath, but its surrounding tissues may still become inflamed. This is known as paratenonitis. Ultrasound and MRI are both excellent techniques for assessing the tendons. Ultrasound has the advantage of greater spatial resolution, Doppler flow to show inflammatory hyperaemia and dynamic imaging with ankle movement.

The posteromedial ankle tendons comprise the tibialis posterior (TP), flexor digitorum longus (FDL) and flexor hallucis longus (FHL) tendons. TP is the strongest of these, with approximately twice the cross-sectional area of FDL. It is also the most frequently affected by pathology. TP function is important in maintaining the medial arch of the foot (with the spring ligament) and tears of TP may lead to flat foot deformity. An os naviculare is a sesamoid bone located at the insertion of TP. Tenosynovitis appears as increased fluid in the tendon sheath, sometimes with altered appearance of the tendon itself. Ultrasound can help confirm the diagnosis by demonstrating hyperaemia on Doppler interrogation of the tendon or its sheath (Fig. 2-55). On MRI, a greater cross-sectional area of fluid than tendon is suggestive of tenosynovitis. The FHL and very occasionally the FDL tendon sheaths communicate with the ankle joint in a minority of individuals. Therefore fluid in these tendon sheaths may relate to an ankle joint effusion.

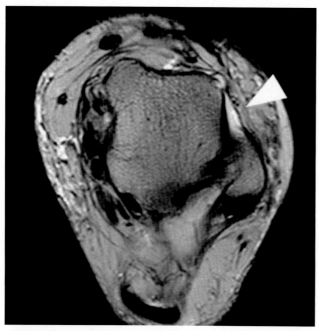

FIGURE 2-54 ■ **Anterior talofibular ligament tear.** Axial oblique T2-weighted image shows absence of ligament fibres in the usual position (arrowhead), indicating a chronic tear.

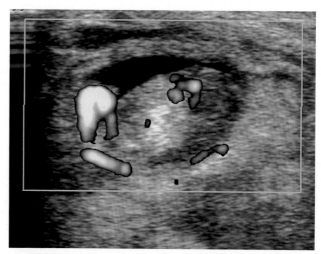

FIGURE 2-55 ■ **Tibialis posterior tenosynovitis.** Transverse ultrasound image reveals anechoic fluid in the tendon sheath and marked neovascularity of the tendon sheath (orange) on Doppler interrogation.

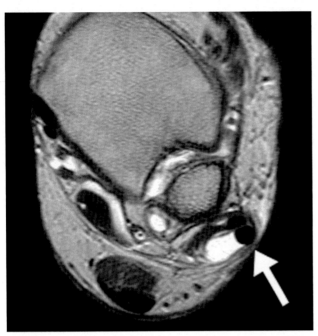

FIGURE 2-56 ■ Peroneal tendon dislocation. Axial oblique T2-weighted image shows anterolateral dislocation of the peroneal tendons (arrow). Note abnormal fluid in the tendon sheath.

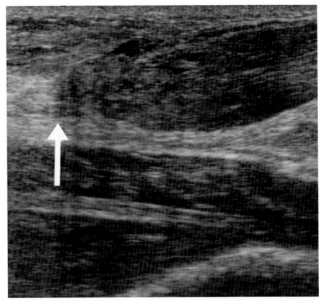

FIGURE 2-57 ■ Complete tear of Achilles tendon. Longitudinal ultrasound image reveals the position of the retracted proximal tendon end (arrow).

The peroneal tendons pass posterior to the lateral malleolus, where the peroneus brevis (PB) tendon is normally located between the peroneus longus (PL) tendon and the malleolus in the fibular groove. Both tendons are retained by the superior peroneal retinaculum (SPR). The SPR extends from the posterolateral fibular periostium to the Achilles tendon aponeurosis. The PB tendon is prone to longitudinal tears or 'splits'. In the early stages the PB tendon adopts a semilunar or boomerang shape which progresses to a split with inter-positioning of the PL tendon between the split fibres of PB. Tears of the SPR may lead to peroneal tendon dislocation (Fig. 2-56). Dynamic imaging with ultrasound shows lateral dislocation of the peroneal tendons from the fibular groove with provocative movements.[38] A sesamoid os peroneum within the PL tendon is present in a minority of individuals. The os peroneum may be associated with PL tendinopathy or may itself be fractured or inflamed, giving rise to pain. Tears of PL tend to occur at the level of the cuboid tunnel or just distal to an os perineum, if present. Pathology of the anterior ankle tendons, comprising the tibialis anterior, extensor hallucis longus and extensor digitorum longus tendons, is infrequent. Tears of tibialis anterior occur more commonly in older age groups particularly close to the insertion of the medial cuneiform.

Achilles tendinopathy is common and may be related to athletic activities in young adults. However, more typically it occurs in the middle aged. It results from chronic microtrauma to the tendon, leading to tendon degeneration. Typically there is focal fusiform thickening of the tendon involving the mid-portion, with increased signal on short and long TE MRI and low reflectivity and loss of normal tendon echotexture on US. The insertion is less often involved, although this can be affected by enthesopathy or by mechanical impingement from a prominent posterior calcaneal process (Haglund's bump). Ultrasound also demonstrates hyperaemia on Doppler

interrogation of the tendon or deep fat pad (Kager's fat pad). The Achilles tendon lacks a tendon sheath. However, inflammation of the surrounding tissues or paratenon, (paratenonitis) may be seen, particularly in runners. The paratenon is found on the superficial, medial and lateral aspects of the tendon and when inflamed appears on MRI as a rim of ill-defined increased signal on these aspects of the tendon. On ultrasound the paratenon appears as a hyporeflective rim. Acute tears of the Achilles tendon may be partial or complete. Complete tears (which are much more common) exhibit no continuity of fibres and may show retraction (Fig. 2-57). Dynamic ultrasound imaging is useful for measuring the separation of the tendon ends for surgical planning.[39] The retrocalcaneal bursa is located deep to the insertion of the Achilles tendon. Inflammation of this bursa may be found in association with Achilles tendinopathy and usually results from chronic and repetitive microtrauma, frequently described as overuse injury. Systemic inflammatory disorders including rheumatoid and seronegative arthritis may also cause inflammation of the Achilles tendon insertion or retrocalcaneal bursa. Retro-Achilles bursitis involves the bursa superficial to the Achilles tendon.

Bone

Osteochondral lesion (OCL) of the talar dome is a common cause of persisting deep ankle pain. Most talar OCL occur following trauma, though some medial lesions arise without a history of injury.[40] OCL is easily missed on conventional radiographs of the ankle. MRI is very sensitive for OCL, allowing assessment of location and size (Fig. 2-58). The presence of fluid signal around the lesion helps to determine whether the lesion is partially detached, detached or displaced.

Impingement may occur in various locations around the ankle, the commonest types being anterolateral (see

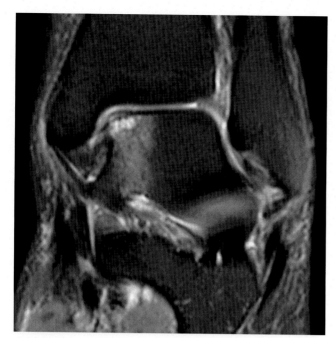

FIGURE 2-58 ■ **Osteochondral lesion of the talar dome.** Coronal T2-weighted fat-saturated image shows subchondral cyst formation in the medial talar dome and surrounding bone marrow oedema.

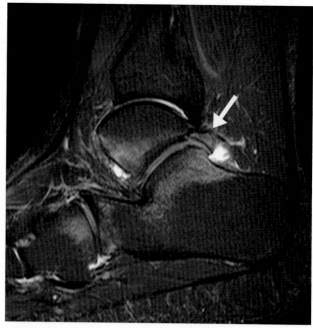

FIGURE 2-59 ■ **Posterior ankle impingement.** Sagittal T2-weighted fat-saturated image shows bone marrow oedema within a prominent os trigonum (arrow) and the posterior calcaneus.

above), anterior and posterior. Anterior impingement occurs between bony spurs on the dorsal talar neck and anterior tibial plafond, a condition associated with kicking activities like soccer. These spurs can be readily identified on lateral radiographs. MRI may additionally reveal synovitis and lateral ankle ligament damage.[41] Posterior impingement is most frequently associated with a large os trigonum or Stieda process of the talus (Fig. 2-59). These give rise to chronic compression of soft tissues against the posterior tibia in activities that involve repetitive forced plantar flexion as in ballet dancing.[42]

Tarsal Coalition

Tarsal coalition refers to developmental fusion of two (rarely three) bones in the hind-foot. Coalition may be osseous or non-osseous (the latter may be fibrous or cartilaginous). The most common type is calcaneonavicular followed by subtalar, other types being much less common. In calcaneonavicular coalition the navicular is fused to the calcaneus through an elongated anterior calcaneal process (Fig. 2-60). In subtalar coalition there is fusion between the talus and calcaneus at or adjacent to the middle subtalar joint. This results in a characteristic 'C-sign' on a lateral radiograph reflecting continuation of the bone contour through the coalition. MRI and CT are much more sensitive than plain radiographs for tarsal coalition. Stress changes may also be demonstrated at the site of coalition or in nearby structures.

Other Soft-Tissue Abnormalities

Plantar fasciitis is a common cause of heel pain thought to result from chronic microtrauma of the plantar fascia from biomechanical stress. The central band is most

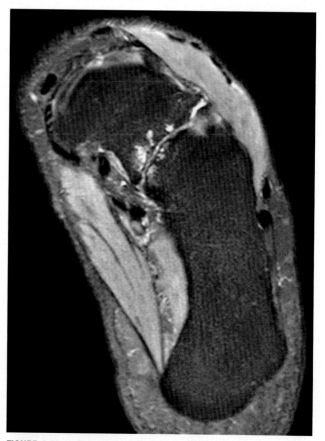

FIGURE 2-60 ■ **Calcaneonavicular coalition.** Axial T2-weighted fat-saturated image reveals abnormal articulation between the calcaneus and navicular without marrow continuity, indicating non-osseous coalition. Note there is subcortical cyst formation resulting from abnormal stresses.

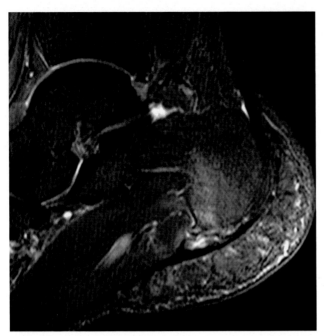

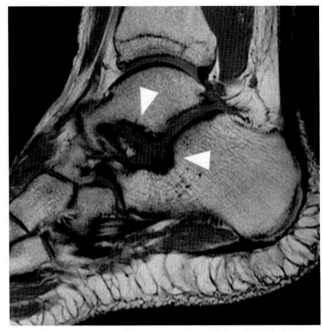

FIGURE 2-61 ■ **Plantar fasciitis.** Sagittal T2-weighted fat-saturated image demonstrates oedema and thickening of the origin of the plantar fascia. Note the presence of bone marrow oedema in the adjacent part of the calcaneus.

FIGURE 2-62 ■ **Sinus tarsi syndrome.** Sagittal T1-weighted image reveals replacement of the normal high signal of the fat in the sinus tarsi with intermediate signal (arrowheads), indicating inflammation.

frequently involved near its calcaneal origin. The diagnosis is made on ultrasound when there is thickening of the fascia (normally measuring up to 5 mm[43]) and loss of normal echogenic fibrillar texture. MRI reveals thickening and increased signal on fluid-sensitive sequences, indicating inflammation (Fig. 2-61). A calcaneal spur may be present but this is often found in the absence of plantar fasciitis and there is no role for conventional radiographs in the diagnosis of plantar fasciitis. Other less common causes of plantar fascia thickening to consider include seronegative arthropathy, plantar fibroma and hyperlipidaemia.

The sinus tarsi is a cone-shaped space between the anterior and posterior subtalar joints containing fat surrounding ligaments, small vessels and nerve endings. Sinus tarsi syndrome describes pain arising from this structure, typically occurring with a history of an ankle sprain. The exact aetiology is unclear and it may be that this syndrome has a number of different causes. The condition is identified on MRI as loss of the normal high T1 fat signal in the sinus tarsi (Fig. 2-62).[44]

Tarsal tunnel syndrome is an entrapment neuropathy of the posterior tibial nerve giving rise to pain/paraesthesia on the plantar aspect of the foot and a positive Tinel's sign. Muscle weakness is less common. The posterior tibial nerve is compressed within the tarsal tunnel, a compartment in the posteromedial ankle which is bounded by the flexor retinaculum. The tunnel transmits the posterior tibial nerve as part of a neurovascular bundle and the tendons of TP, FDL and FHL. MRI or ultrasound may be used to identify a lesion compressing the nerve such as a ganglion, bone fracture, nerve sheath tumour or accessory FDL. MRI may additionally reveal oedema in denervated muscles supplied by the nerve.

The plantar plate is a fibrocartilaginous structure extending from the metatarsal neck to the base of the proximal phalanx of each toe. Its function is to resist hyperextension of the MTP joint. Plantar plate rupture most commonly affects the great toe. It may be diagnosed with ultrasound or MRI. MRI with injection of contrast medium into the MTP joint dorsally demonstrates escape of the contrast agent through the torn plantar plate, leading to opacification of the flexor tendon sheath.

Morton neuroma is another cause of metatarsalgia, most commonly arising in the third web space. It is thought to result from repetitive compression of the plantar common digital nerve, leading to perineural fibrosis. On ultrasound a Morton's neuroma typically appears as a rounded hypoechoic mass. On MRI it appears as a low-to-intermediate signal intensity mass in a characteristic position. The advantage of ultrasound in this setting is to guide injection therapy after the diagnosis has been confirmed.

REFERENCES

1. Campbell RS, Dunn A. External impingement of the shoulder. Semin Musculoskelet Radiol 2008;12(2):107–26.
2. Opsha O, Malik A, Baltazar R, et al. MRI of the rotator cuff and internal derangement. Eur J Radiol 2008;68(1):36–56.
3. Sanders TG, Jersey SL. Conventional radiography of the shoulder. Semin Roentgenol 2005;40(3):207–22.
4. Smith TO, Back T, Toms AP, Hing CB. Diagnostic accuracy of ultrasound for rotator cuff tears in adults: a systematic review and meta-analysis. Clin Radiol 2011;66(11):1036–48.
5. Macmahon PJ, Palmer WE. Magnetic resonance imaging in glenohumeral instability. Magn Reson Imaging Clin N Am 2012;20(2): 295–312, xi.
6. Sanders TG, Zlatkin M, Montgomery J. Imaging of glenohumeral instability. Semin Roentgenol 2010;45(3):160–79.

7. Modarresi S, Motamedi D, Jude CM. Superior labral anteroposterior lesions of the shoulder: part 1, anatomy and anatomic variants. Am J Roentgenol 2011;197(3):596–603.

8. Modarresi S, Motamedi D, Jude CM. Superior labral anteroposterior lesions of the shoulder: part 2, mechanisms and classification. Am J Roentgenol 2011;197(3):604–11.

9. Melenevsky Y, Yablon CM, Ramappa A, Hochman MG. Clavicle and acromioclavicular joint injuries: a review of imaging, treatment, and complications. Skeletal Radiol 2011;40(7):831–42.

10. Johnson MC, Jacobson JA, Fessell DP, et al. The sternoclavicular joint: can imaging differentiate infection from degenerative change? Skeletal Radiol 2010;39(6):551–8.

11. Restrepo CS, Martinez S, Lemos DF, et al. Imaging appearances of the sternum and sternoclavicular joints. Radiographics 2009; 29(3):839–59.

12. Tomsick SD, Petersen BD. Normal anatomy and anatomical variants of the elbow. Semin Musculoskelet Radiol 2010;14(4): 379–93.

13. Hayter CL, Adler RS. Injuries of the elbow and the current treatment of tendon disease. Am J Roentgenol 2012;199(3):546–57.

14. Delport AG, Zoga AC. MR and CT arthrography of the elbow. Semin Musculoskelet Radiol 2012;16(1):15–26.

15. Taljanovic MS, Karantanas A, Griffith JF, et al. Imaging and treatment of scaphoid fractures and their complications. Semin Musculoskelet Radiol 2012;16(2):159–73.

16. Cerezal L, de Dios Berna-Mestre J, Canga A, et al. MR and CT arthrography of the wrist. Semin Musculoskelet Radiol 2012;16(1): 27–41.

17. Jacob D, Cohen M, Bianchi S. Ultrasound imaging of non-traumatic lesions of wrist and hand tendons. Eur Radiol 2007; 17(9):2237–47.

18. Wilson D, Allen GM. Imaging of the carpal tunnel. Semin Musculoskelet Radiol 2012;16(2):137–45.

19. Ebrahim FS, De Maeseneer M, Jager T, et al. US diagnosis of UCL tears of the thumb and Stener lesions: technique, pattern-based approach, and differential diagnosis. Radiographics 2006;26(4): 1007–20.

20. Beck M, Kalhor M, Leunig M, Ganz R. Hip morphology influences the pattern of damage to the acetabular cartilage: femoroacetabular impingement as a cause of early osteoarthritis of the hip. J Bone Joint Surg Br 2005;87(7):1012–18.

21. Tannast M, Siebenrock KA, Anderson SE. Femoroacetabular impingement: radiographic diagnosis—what the radiologist should know. Am J Roentgenol 2007;188(6):1540–52.

22. Pfirrmann CW, Duc SR, Zanetti M, et al. MR arthrography of acetabular cartilage delamination in femoroacetabular cam impingement. Radiology 2008;249(1):236–41.

23. Kutty S, Schneider P, Faris P, et al. Reliability and predictability of the centre-edge angle in the assessment of pincer femoroacetabular impingement. Int Orthop 2012;36(3):505–10.

24. Choi YS, Lee SM, Song BY, et al. Dynamic sonography of external snapping hip syndrome. J Ultrasound Med 2002;21(7):753–8.

25. Deslandes M, Guillin R, Cardinal E, et al. The snapping iliopsoas tendon: new mechanisms using dynamic sonography. Am J Roentgenol 2008;190(3):576–81.

26. Torriani M, Souto SC, Thomas BJ, et al. Ischiofemoral impingement syndrome: an entity with hip pain and abnormalities of the quadratus femoris muscle. Am J Roentgenol 2009;193(1):186–90.

27. Lafforgue P, Dahan E, Chagnaud C, et al. Early-stage avascular necrosis of the femoral head: MR imaging for prognosis in 31 cases with at least 2 years of follow-up. Radiology 1993;187(1):199–204.

28. Korompilias AV, Karantanas AH, Lykissas MG, Beris AE. Bone marrow edema syndrome. Skeletal Radiol 2009;38(5):425–36.

29. Woodley SJ, Mercer SR, Nicholson HD. Morphology of the bursae associated with the greater trochanter of the femur. J Bone Joint Surg Am 2008;90(2):284–94.

30. Cobby MJ, Schweitzer ME, Resnick D. The deep lateral femoral notch: an indirect sign of a torn anterior cruciate ligament. Radiology 1992;184(3):855–8.

31. Rodriguez W Jr, Vinson EN, Helms CA, Toth AP. MRI appearance of posterior cruciate ligament tears. Am J Roentgenol 2008; 191(4):1031.

32. Schweitzer ME, Tran D, Deely DM, Hume EL. Medial collateral ligament injuries: evaluation of multiple signs, prevalence and location of associated bone bruises, and assessment with MR imaging. Radiology 1995;194(3):825–9.

33. Insall J, Salvati E. Patella position in the normal knee joint. Radiology 1971;101(1):101–4.

34. Miller TT, Staron RB, Feldman F. Patellar height on sagittal MR imaging of the knee. Am J Roentgenol 1996;167(2):339–41.

35. Dejour H, Walch G, Nove-Josserand L, Guier C. Factors of patellar instability: an anatomic radiographic study. Knee Surg Sports Traumatol Arthrosc 1994;2(1):19–26.

36. Perrich KD, Goodwin DW, Hecht PJ, Cheung Y. Ankle ligaments on MRI: appearance of normal and injured ligaments. Am J Roentgenol 2009;193(3):687–95.

37. Ferkel RD, Tyorkin M, Applegate GR, Heinen GT. MRI evaluation of anterolateral soft tissue impingement of the ankle. Foot Ankle Int 2010;31(8):655–61.

38. Neustadter J, Raikin SM, Nazarian LN. Dynamic sonographic evaluation of peroneal tendon subluxation. Am J Roentgenol 2004;183(4):985–8.

39. Kotnis R, David S, Handley R, et al. Dynamic ultrasound as a selection tool for reducing achilles tendon reruptures. Am J Sports Med 2006;34(9):1395–400.

40. Anderson IF, Crichton KJ, Grattan-Smith T, et al. Osteochondral fractures of the dome of the talus. J Bone Joint Surg Am 1989; 71(8):1143–52.

41. Haller J, Bernt R, Seeger T, et al. MR-imaging of anterior tibiotalar impingement syndrome: agreement, sensitivity and specificity of MR-imaging and indirect MR-arthrography. Eur J Radiol 2006; 58(3):450–60.

42. Russell JA, Kruse DW, Koutedakis Y, et al. Pathoanatomy of posterior ankle impingement in ballet dancers. Clin Anat 2010;23(6):613–21.

43. Schmidt WA, Schmidt H, Schicke B, Gromnica-Ihle E. Standard reference values for musculoskeletal ultrasonography. Ann Rheum Dis 2004;63(8):988–94.

44. Klein MA, Spreitzer AM. MR imaging of the tarsal sinus and canal: normal anatomy, pathologic findings, and features of the sinus tarsi syndrome. Radiology 1993;186(1):233–40.

BONE TUMOURS (1): BENIGN TUMOURS AND TUMOUR-LIKE LESIONS OF BONE

Asif Saifuddin

CHAPTER OUTLINE

GENERAL CHARACTERISTICS OF BONE TUMOURS
Radiological Assessment of Bone Tumours
BENIGN BONE TUMOURS
Cartilage Tumours
Osteogenic Tumours
Fibrogenic Tumours
Fibrohistiocytic Tumours

Giant Cell Tumour
Vascular Tumours
Smooth Muscle Tumours
Lipogenic Tumours
Neural Tumours
Miscellaneous Lesions

GENERAL CHARACTERISTICS OF BONE TUMOURS

Bone tumours may be benign or malignant, and are currently classified according to the World Health Organisation Classification of 2002.[1] The pre-biopsy diagnosis of a bone tumour depends upon several features, including patient age, lesion location and finally the radiological characteristics. The latter allows an assessment of rate of growth (generally indicative of benignity or malignancy) and underlying histological subtype, based predominantly upon patterns of matrix mineralisation (Table 3-1).

Age at Presentation

Patient age is of huge importance in suggesting a differential diagnosis of a focal bone lesion. Primary bone tumours are rare below the age of 5 years and over the age of 40 years, with the exception of myeloma and chondrosarcoma. Metastases are the commonest lesions over the age of 40 years.

RADIOLOGICAL ASSESSMENT OF BONE TUMOURS[1]

Location

The location of the lesion within the skeleton (appendicular, axial) and within the individual bone (epiphysis, metaphysis, diaphysis; intramedullary, intracortical, surface) must be considered in detail when discussing individual tumours, since it has a considerable influence on differential diagnosis.

Rate of Growth

When considering rate of growth, the most important feature is the lesion margin. In benign and low-grade malignant neoplasms, this margin is sharp (geographical; Type 1). Type 1A has a rim of sclerosis between the lesion and the host bone (Fig. 3-1A), Type 1B is a very well defined lytic lesion but with no marginal sclerosis (Fig. 3-1B), while Type 1C has a slightly less sharp, non-sclerotic margin (Fig. 3-1C). Type 2 is moth-eaten destruction, which represents the next most aggressive pattern and is characterised by multiple lucent areas measuring 2–5 mm in diameter separated by bone which has yet to be destroyed (Fig. 3-2). Type 3 is permeative destruction, which is the most aggressive pattern and is composed of multiple coalescing small ill-defined lesions 1 mm or less in diameter with a zone of transition of several centimetres (Fig. 3-3). Radiographs inevitably underestimate the extent of medullary involvement, which is more clearly shown on magnetic resonance imaging (MRI).

Regions with apparently intact cortex may show extra-cortical tumour masses. This phenomenon often leads, in highly malignant tumours such as Ewing's sarcoma, to 'cortical saucerisation' as the tumour, temporarily restrained by the periosteum, erodes back through the cortical bone.

Benign or low-grade malignant neoplasms tend to remain within the medullary cavity until late in their development. Typically, the cortex is not destroyed, but slow erosion of its endosteal surface (endosteal scalloping) together with periosteal new bone formation results

TABLE 3-1   Classification of Primary Benign Bone Tumours

Cartilage tumours	Osteochondroma
	Chondroma
	• Enchondroma
	• Periosteal chondromas
	• Multiple chondromatosis
	Chondroblastoma
	Chondromyxoid fibroma
Osteogenic tumours	Osteoid osteoma
	Osteoblastoma
Fibrogenic tumours	Desmoplastic fibroma
Fibrohistiocytic tumours	Benign fibrous hystiocytoma
	• Fibrous cortical defect
	• Non-ossifying fibroma
Giant cell tumour	Giant cell tumour
Vascular tumours	Haemangioma
Smooth muscle tumours	Leiomyoma
Lipogenic tumours	Lipoma
Neural tumours	Neurilemmoma
Miscellaneous lesions	Aneurysmal bone cyst
	Solitary bone cyst
	Fibrous dysplasia
	Osteofibrous dysplasia
	Langerhans cell histiocytosis (eosinophilic granuloma)
	Erdheim–Chester disease
	Chest wall hamartoma

Modified from WHO 2002 Classification.[1]

in expansion of bone (Fig. 3-1A). Conversely, high-grade malignant tumours commonly extend through the cortex by the time of presentation, resulting in cortical destruction and an adjacent extraosseous mass (Fig. 3-3).

Periosteal Reaction[2]

Periosteal reaction is of various types with none being pathognomonic of any particular tumour: rather, the type helps to indicate the aggressiveness of the lesion. A thick, well-formed (solid) periosteal reaction (Fig. 3-4A) indicates a slow rate of growth but not necessarily a benign tumour, since it may be seen with chondrosarcoma. Laminated periosteal reaction (Fig. 3-4B) indicates subperiosteal extension of tumour, infection or haematoma. Lesions demonstrating periodic growth may show a multi-laminated pattern (Fig. 3-4C). A Codman's triangle indicates the limit of subperiosteal tumour in a longitudinal direction (Fig. 3-4B). Vertical (sunburst spiculation or 'hair-on-end') types of periosteal reaction are seen with the most aggressive tumours such as osteosarcoma (Fig. 3-4D) and Ewing's sarcoma. However, the most rapidly growing lesions may not be associated with any radiographically visible periosteal response, since mineralisation of the deep layer of periosteum can take 2 weeks.

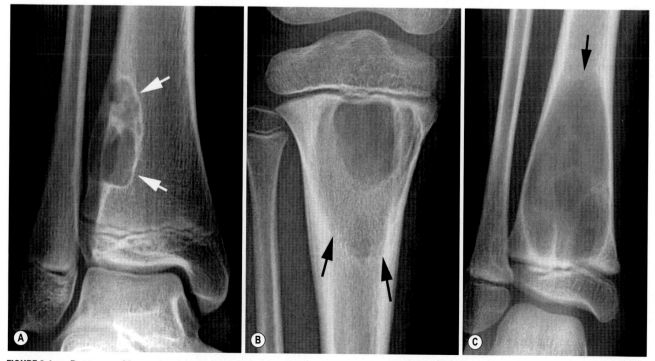

FIGURE 3-1 ■ **Patterns of bone destruction. Geographic.** (A) Type 1A AP radiograph of the distal tibia in a patient with non-ossifying fibroma (NOF), demonstrating the sharp, thin sclerotic margin (arrows). (B) Type 1B AP radiograph of the proximal tibia in a patient with an aneurysmal bone cyst (ABC) showing a well-defined, non-sclerotic margin (arrows). (C) Type 1C AP radiograph of the distal tibia in a patient with an ABC showing a slightly less well-defined, non-sclerotic margin (arrows).

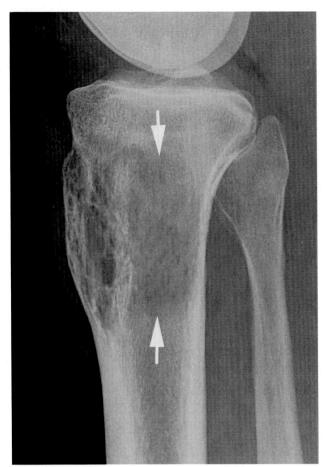

FIGURE 3-2 ■ Patterns of bone destruction. Moth-eaten. Lateral radiograph of the proximal tibia showing a 'moth-eaten' appearance (arrows) caused by the coalescence of multiple small lytic areas.

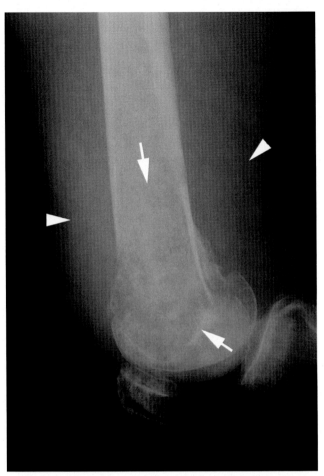

FIGURE 3-3 ■ Patterns of bone destruction. Permeative. Lateral radiograph of the distal femur showing a 'permeative' pattern of bone destruction (arrows). Note also the large circumferential extraosseous mass (arrowheads).

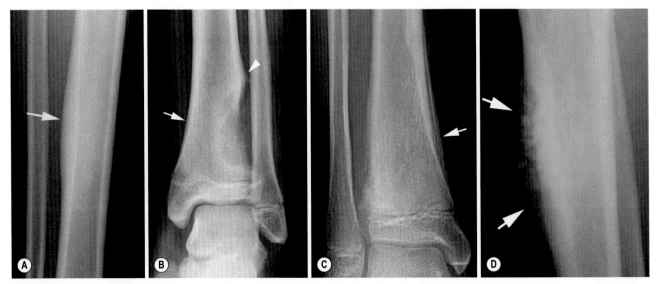

FIGURE 3-4 ■ Patterns of periosteal reaction. (A) Coned AP radiograph of the tibial diaphysis showing solid periosteal reaction (arrow) due to an occult osteoid osteoma. (B) AP radiograph of the distal tibia showing a single, laminated periosteal reaction (arrow) associated with an ABC. Note also the Codman's triangle (arrowhead). (C) AP radiograph of the distal tibia showing a multi-laminated periosteal reaction (arrow) associated with acute osteomyelitis. (D) Coned lateral radiograph of the proximal tibia showing a coarse 'sunburst'-type vertical periosteal reaction associated with osteosarcoma.

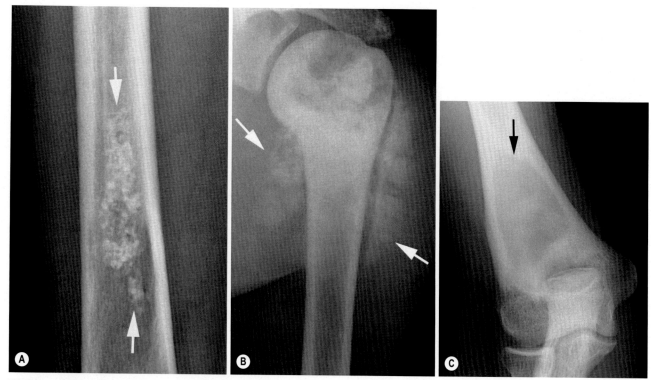

FIGURE 3-5 ■ Patterns of matrix mineralisation. (A) Coned AP radiograph of the femoral diaphysis in a patient with grade 2 chondrosarcoma, showing typical punctate chondral calcification. (B) AP radiograph of the proximal humerus in a patient with osteoblastic osteosarcoma showing typical 'cloud-like' osseous mineralisation (arrows). (C) AP radiograph of the distal humerus femur in a patient with fibrous dysplasia showing typical 'ground-glass' mineralisation (arrow).

Matrix Mineralisation

The matrix of a tumour represents the extracellular material produced by the tumour cells within which the cells lie. Certain tumours produce characteristic radiographically visible matrix mineralisation, which allows the histological cell type to be predicted. Chondral calcifications are typically linear, curvilinear, ring-like, punctate or nodular (Fig. 3-5A). Osseous mineralisation is cloud-like and poorly defined (Fig. 3-5B), whereas diffuse matrix mineralisation in benign fibrous tumours produces the characteristic 'ground-glass' appearance (Fig. 3-5C), seen most commonly in fibrous dysplasia. Some neoplasms, such as adenocarcinoma metastases, can provoke reactive mineralisation, whereas calcifications within an intraosseous lipoma are due to associated fat necrosis. Also, some bone sarcomas may develop on underlying calcified bone infarcts.

CT and MRI in Diagnosis and Staging

CT is excellent for demonstrating the presence of radiographically occult matrix mineralisation and the persistence of a thin cortical shell, indicating that the tumour still lies deep to the periosteum. CT also plays a major role in the investigation of cortical thickening, allowing the demonstration of the cause, such as the nidus of an osteoid osteoma or a stress fracture.

The major role of MRI is in local staging, particularly for high-grade malignant tumours such as osteosarcoma, where the intraosseous extent, identification of 'skip' lesions and relationship to the neurovascular bundle and adjacent joint can all be assessed with great accuracy.[3] Such information is vital for planning surgical management, be it limb salvage or amputation. Dynamic contrast-enhanced MRI has been advocated for determining chemotherapeutic response, but its role in routine patient management is unclear.

In the presence of a purely lytic lesion, several MRI features may help in further lesion characterisation.[4] The presence of profound low signal intensity (SI) on T2*-weighted gradient-echo images indicates chronic haemorrhage and may be seen with giant cell tumour. MRI is very sensitive to the presence of fluid–fluid levels (FFLs) and the degree of FFL change is related to histological diagnosis.[5] Lesions that are completely filled with FFLs are almost always aneurysmal bone cysts (ABCs). MRI can also demonstrate a fatty matrix, as seen with haemangioma and intraosseous lipoma. The vascular nature of renal metastases has been demonstrated by the presence of the 'flow-void' sign.[6] MRI is very sensitive to reactive medullary and soft-tissue oedema, which characterises certain lesions such as osteoid osteoma, osteoblastoma, chondroblastoma and Brodie's abscess.[7]

Bone scintigraphy plays little role in the diagnostic work-up of a suspected primary bone tumour, with the possible exception of osteoid osteoma or osteoblastoma, particularly in the spine. However, scintigraphy is still useful for the identification of skeletal metastases, although this role has recently been challenged by whole-body MRI.[8]

The position of techniques such as MR spectroscopy, positron emission tomography (PET) and computed tomography PET (CT-PET) in the management of suspected bone tumours is as yet unclear, while whole-body diffusion-weighted MRI (WBDWI) is highly sensitive for the identification of skeletal metastases.[9] Finally, the use of ultrasound[10] and CT[11] for image-guided needle biopsy is well established, while MR-guided biopsy has also been developed for targeting subtle marrow lesions.[12]

BENIGN BONE TUMOURS

Benign bone tumours are currently classified according to the 2002 World Health Organisation system based on their cell of origin[1] (Table 3-1).

CARTILAGE TUMOURS

Osteochondroma[13]

Recent genetic studies indicate that osteochondroma is a true neoplasm, which may also arise following radiotherapy and accounts for 20–50% of benign bone tumours. Osteochondromas present from 2 to 60 years, but the highest incidence is in the second decade, with a male-to-female ratio of 1.4–3.6:1.

Long bones are commonly affected, especially around the knee (~40%), the commonest locations being the distal femur, proximal humerus, proximal tibia and proximal femur. The commonest flat bones affected are the ilium and scapula. Lesions may be classified as either pedunculated, when they have a thin stalk that typically points away from the adjacent joint, or sessile when they arise from a broad base. They are typically metaphyseal in location.

Diaphyseal aclasis (hereditary multiple exostoses, HME) constitutes an uncommon autosomal dominant disorder in which the exostoses may be larger than the solitary variety and may lead to shortening or deformity of the affected limbs. The metaphyses in this condition are also typically widened and dysplastic (Fig. 3-6).

Osteochondromas present with mechanical problems such as an enlarging mass, pressure on adjoining structures (muscles, nerves, vessels), or rarely with fracture of the bony stem. Mechanical irritation of overlying soft tissues may result in adventitial bursa formation, which can mimic sarcomatous degeneration. MRI is highly accurate in the assessment of symptomatic osteochondromas.[14] The incidence of chondrosarcomatous change in the cartilage cap is very small in a solitary osteochondroma (probably <1%), while malignant degeneration in diaphyseal aclasis is approximated at 3–5%.

Radiological Features

The lesion appears as an outgrowth from the normal cortex, with which it is continuous. Pedunculated lesions have a long slim neck (Fig. 3-7A), whereas sessile lesions have a broad base from the bone of origin (Fig. 3-7B). Continuity between the medullary cavity of the lesion and that of the underlying bone is essential for the diagnosis and is best demonstrated on either CT or MRI (Fig. 3-8A). The cartilage cap is optimally demonstrated on axial proton density-weighted (PDW) or T2W fast spin-echo (FSE) MRI, when the hyperintense cartilage contrasts well against the adjacent iso-/hypointense muscle (Fig. 3-8A) and it should not exceed 2-cm thickness in adults. The cartilage cap can also be visualised and measured on ultrasound where it appears hypoechoic in contrast to the brightly reflective bone surfaces. Complications associated with OC include bursa formation

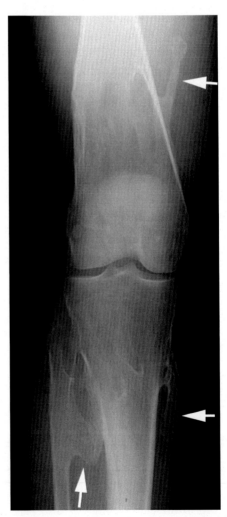

FIGURE 3-6 ■ **Diaphyseal aclasis.** AP radiograph of the right knee showing multiple osteochondromas (arrows) and associated widening of the distal femoral and proximal tibial metaphyses.

(Fig. 3-8B), neurovascular compromise and, rarely, pseudoaneurysm (Fig. 3-8C).

(En)Chondroma[13]

(En)Chondroma is an intramedullary neoplasm comprising lobules of benign hyaline cartilage and is the second

commonest benign chondral lesion after osteochondroma, accounting for approximately 8% of all primary bone tumours and tumour-like lesion in a large biopsy series. However, the true prevalence of enchondromas is unknown since the majority are asymptomatic. Incidental enchondromas have been identified in approximately 3% of routine knee MRI studies. Enchondromas affect the tubular bones of the hands and feet in 40–65% of cases and present either when they become symptomatic due to increasing size, as pathological fracture (in 60% of cases) or as incidental findings. The majority arise in the proximal phalanges (40–50%), followed by the metacarpals (15–30%) and middle phalanges (20–30%). The small bones of the feet are involved in 7% of cases. Approximately 25% are found in the femur, tibia and humerus, while other sites are very rare. The age range is 10–80 years, with most presenting in the second to fourth decades. There is equal prevalence among both genders.

Radiological Features

Most enchondromas arise centrally in the phalanges and metacarpals. Lesions are typically metaphyseal or diaphyseal, with epiphyseal location accounting for approximately 8%. Enchondromas are often eccentric and 75% are solitary. They are typically well-circumscribed, lobular or oval lytic lesions, which may expand the cortex (Fig. 3-9A). Size at presentation ranges from 10 to 50 mm. Chondral-type mineralisation may be identified within the matrix.

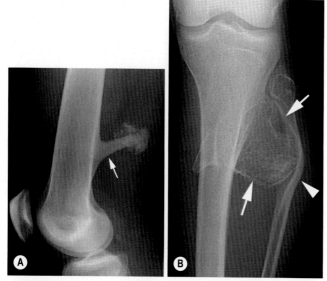

FIGURE 3-7 ■ **Osteochondroma.** (A) Lateral radiograph of the distal femur showing a typical pedunculated osteochondroma (arrow). (B) AP radiograph of the proximal tibia showing a sessile osteochondroma (arrows) with associated pressure deformity of the adjacent fibula (arrowhead).

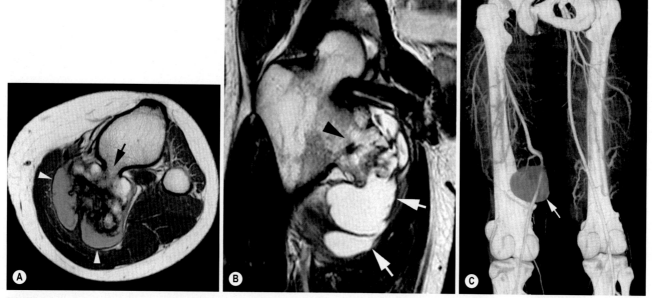

FIGURE 3-8 ■ **Osteochondroma. MRI features.** (A) Axial PDW FSE MRI through the proximal tibia showing medullary continuity (arrow) between the osteochondroma and host bone. The cartilage cap is mildly hyperintense and surrounded by a thin, hypointense perichondrium (arrowheads). (B) Coronal T2W FSE MRI of the hip showing a bursa (arrows) complicating a sessile osteochondroma (arrowhead) of the proximal femur. (C) Posterior view 3D CT maximum intensity projection (MIP) of the femora in a patient with diaphyseal aclasis showing a popliteal artery pseudoaneurysm (arrow).

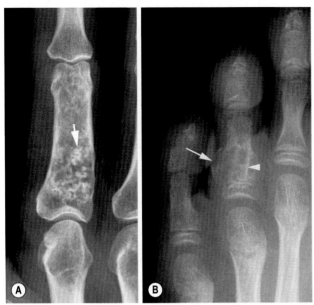

FIGURE 3-9 ■ **Enchondroma.** (A) AP radiograph of the index finger showing a lobular, mildly expansile lesion with typical chondral matrix mineralisation (arrow). (B) DP radiograph of the forefoot showing an eccentrically placed enchondroma of the fourth toe proximal phalanx (arrowhead) with an associated extraosseous component covered by a thin cortical shell (arrow).

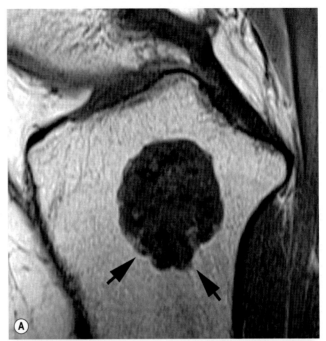

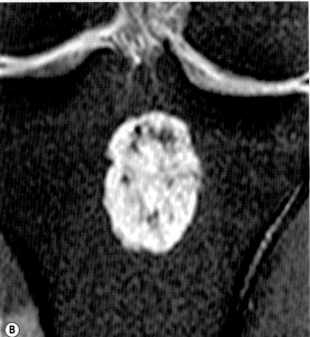

FIGURE 3-10 ■ **Enchondroma. MRI features.** (A) Sagittal T1W SE MRI showing classical appearances of a chondroma, with a lobular inferior margin (arrows). (B) Coronal fat-suppressed T2W FSE MRI showing the hyperintense lesion with matrix mineralisation manifest as punctate areas of signal void. Note the absence of surrounding reactive oedema-like SI.

The term 'enchondroma protuberans' has been used to describe an eccentrically placed enchondroma with an associated extraosseous component which is usually covered by a thin shell of intact cortical bone (Fig. 3-9B). Most cases arise in the fingers or toes and they may be difficult to distinguish from periosteal chondroma, although this may not be clinically relevant since both lesions have the same management.

The differentiation between a relatively large enchondroma and a grade 1 chondrosarcoma can be difficult. Lesion size above 5–6 cm and deep endosteal scalloping are suggestive of chondrosarcoma,[15] but prominent scalloping can also be seen with an eccentrically placed chondroma, which has been termed an 'endosteal chondroma'. However, this differentiation may not be of clinical relevance, since both can be treated in the same way, with either careful clinical and imaging follow-up, or curettage with cementation. Low-grade chondral tumours have characteristic MRI features, showing a lobular margin with intermediate T1-weighted signal intensity (T1W SI) (Fig. 3-10A) and T2-weighted/short tau inversion recovery (T2W/STIR) hyperintensity without surrounding reactive oedema (Fig. 3-10B). Matrix mineralisation manifests as punctate areas of signal void. A hypointense rim and septations may also be seen, the latter showing enhancement following IV gadolinium contrast medium.[13]

Less Common Varieties of Chondroma

Periosteal Chondroma.[16] These are rare lesions affecting children and young adults and are located in the metaphyses of tubular bones, most commonly the proximal humerus followed by the femur and tibia. They are also seen in the small bones of the hands and feet, in which

case some extension into the underlying medullary cavity is commonly seen. Radiologically, each appears as a well-defined area of cortical erosion typically measuring 1–3 cm with mature periosteal reaction and sometimes a thin external shell of bone. Cartilaginous matrix mineralisation is observed in half the cases (Fig. 3-11A). MRI shows the features of a chondral lesion with a lobular hyperintense mass on T2-weighted images adjacent to the

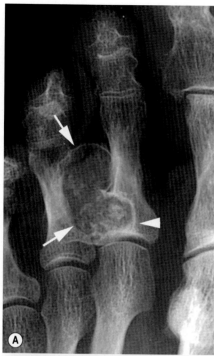

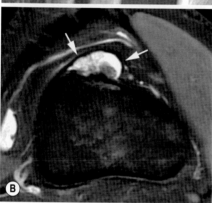

FIGURE 3-11 ■ **Periosteal chondroma.** (A) DP radiograph of the second toe showing a surface lesion with a thin surrounding calcified rim (arrows) and extension into the adjacent medullary cavity (arrowhead). (B) Axial fat-suppressed T2W FSE MRI showing a hyperintense lobular lesion (arrows) based on the anterior distal femoral cortex, without medullary infiltration.

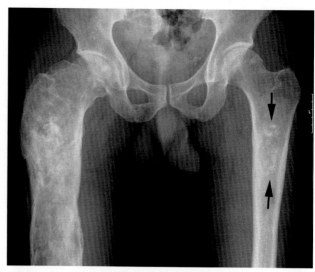

FIGURE 3-12 ■ **Enchondromatosis.** AP radiograph of the hips and proximal femora showing multiple enchondromas, with expansion of the proximal right femur and deformity consistent with Ollier's disease. A lesion is also seen on the left side (arrows).

cortex (Fig. 3-11B). The differential diagnosis includes periosteal chondrosarcoma and periosteal osteosarcoma. Malignant transformation has not been reported.

Enchondromatosis (Ollier's Disease). Rare disease. Prevalence is estimated at around 1 in 100,000. In addition to multiple enchondromas, flame-like rests of cartilage in the metaphyses impede bone growth and may result in bowing, angulation and bone enlargement (Fig. 3-12). Malignant change is reported in 5–30% of cases.

Enchondromatosis with Haemangiomas (Maffucci's Syndrome). This rare disorder combines multiple enchondromas and soft-tissue haemangiomas (occasionally lymphangiomas). The condition is unilateral in 50% of cases. Radiographically, the presence of phleboliths differentiates the disorder from Ollier's disease, while the

haemangiomas are well demonstrated by MRI. The true incidence of chondrosarcomatous change is uncertain because of the rarity of the disease, but is reported in approximately 20% of cases, usually in patients over the age of 40 years.

Chondroblastoma[13,17]

Chondroblastoma accounts for approximately 1% of all bone neoplasms, with 80–90% occurring between the ages of 5 and 25 years (mean age ~20 years). However, lesions of the flat bones such as the talus commonly present later. The male:female ratio is almost 2.7:1. Chondroblastoma has rarely been associated with metastases (especially to the lung) and a rare variant termed 'aggressive' (atypical) chondroblastoma, associated with cortical destruction and soft-tissue extension, has also been described.

Chondroblastoma commonly presents as monoarthropathy, since it is typically located in the epiphysis of a long bone, and may promote a synovial reaction. Fifty per cent arise around the knee, while the proximal femur and humeral head are also commonly affected (~20% each). Chondroblastoma is classically located eccentrically in the epiphysis (40%), but with partial closure of the growth plate it usually extends into the metaphysis (55%). The apophyses and sesamoid bones can also be involved, accounting for involvement of the greater trochanter of the femur and the greater tuberosity of the humerus. Approximately 2% are located purely within the metaphysis or diaphysis.[18] In the feet, the calcaneus and talus are most commonly involved, while chondroblastoma is the commonest tumour of the patella.

Radiological Features

The lesion is usually spherical or lobular with a fine sclerotic margin, measuring 1–4 cm in size (Fig. 3-13A).

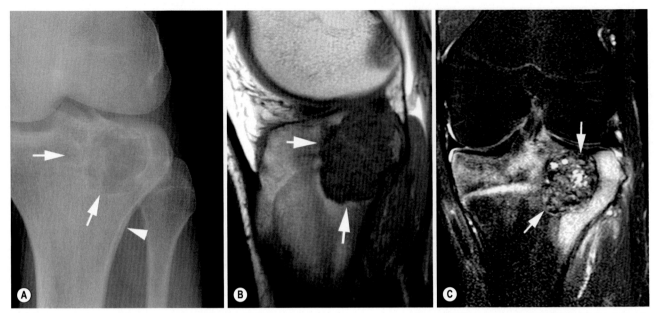

FIGURE 3-13 ■ Chondroblastoma. (A) AP radiograph of the knee showing a lobular, lytic lesion (arrows) in the proximal tibial epiphysis with extension into the metaphysis. A solid periosteal response (arrowhead) is also noted. (B) Sagittal T1W SE MRI showing an intermediate SI lesion (arrows). (C) Coronal STIR MRI demonstrates heterogeneous low SI (arrows) with prominent surrounding reactive marrow oedema-like SI.

Matrix mineralisation is demonstrated in ~30% radiographically. Linear metaphyseal periosteal reaction is present in almost 60% of long bone cases (Fig. 3-13A). MRI shows intermediate T1W SI (Fig. 3-13B) with variable SI on T2W images (Fig. 3-13C), including hypointensity and FFLs due to secondary aneurysmal bone cyst (ABC) change (~15% of cases). Associated marrow and soft-tissue oedema and reactive joint effusion are almost invariable (Fig. 3-13C). The differential diagnosis of lytic epiphyseal lesions in children includes Brodie's abscess. In adults, subchondral cysts and clear cell chondrosarcoma need to be considered.

Chondromyxoid Fibroma[13,19]

Chondromyxoid fibroma accounts for less than 0.5% of biopsied primary bone tumours, with 75% of cases occurring between 10 and 30 years of age (mean age 25 years). Most lesions are metaphyseal and eccentric within the medulla, resulting in thinning and expansion of the cortex. The long bones account for 60% of cases, with 40% arising in the flat bones (ilium 10%) or small tubular bones of the hands and feet (17%). The upper third of the tibia accounts for approximately 25% of all chondromyxoid fibromas. Juxtacortical lesions have also been reported.

Radiological Features

In the proximal tibia, chondromyxoid fibroma appears as an eccentric, lobular lesion with a sclerotic margin (Fig. 3-14). Periosteal reaction and soft-tissue extension are uncommon and matrix calcification is seen in only 12.5% of lesions. MRI shows no particular diagnostic features. Outside its classical location, it has no characteristic imaging appearances.

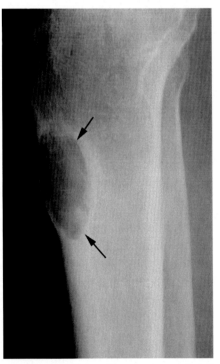

FIGURE 3-14 ■ Chondromyxoid fibroma. Lateral radiograph of the proximal tibia showing an eccentric lytic lesion with a sclerotic margin (arrows) and expansion of the anterior cortex.

OSTEOGENIC TUMOURS[20]

Osteoid Osteoma (OO)[21]

This small benign, vascular, osteoblastic tumour is often associated with a characteristic clinical picture of night pain relieved by aspirin and accounts for approximately

10% of all biopsied benign tumours. Most patients present in the second and third decades of life and the male:female ratio is 2–3:1.

OO is most common in the appendicular skeleton, with over 50% located in the diaphysis or metaphysis of the tibia or femur. However, almost no skeletal site is exempt. There are two classification systems describing the location of the lesion within bone, the first based on radiography where the nidus is either intracortical, medullary (cancellous) or subperiosteal. The second, based on CT findings, describes the nidus as being subperiosteal, intracortical, endosteal or intramedullary.[21] Approximately 13% of cases are intra-articular, causing synovitis and presenting as monoarthropathy.[22]

Radiological Features

The characteristic feature of OO is the nidus, which may appear lytic, sclerotic or most commonly of mixed density depending upon the degree of central mineralisation. The nidus measures up to15 mm in diameter and is commonly surrounded by a region of reactive medullary sclerosis and solid periosteal reaction (Fig. 3-15), the degree of which depends upon the age of the patient and the location within the bone (subperiosteal lesions and those in younger patients being more reactive than medullary or intra-articular lesions). Dense bony reactive changes may obscure a small nidus on plain radiographs (Fig. 3-4A). Rarely, a multifocal nidus is found.[23]

Bone scintigraphy now plays little role in the diagnosis or management of the lesion, while CT demonstrates the classical features of a round or oval soft-tissue density nidus, which commonly shows central dense mineralisation (Fig. 3-16A).[24] The associated reactive bone changes are also well demonstrated. A recently described finding is the 'vascular groove sign', which is manifest by the presence of thin, serpentine channels in the thickened bone surrounding the nidus (Fig. 3-16A) and has sensitivity and specificity of approximately 75 and 95%, respectively, for the diagnosis of OO.[25]

With improvements in MR technology, the nidus of an OO is now commonly visualised (Fig. 3-16B), appearing as heterogenously low–intermediate SI on both T1W and T2W images and enhancing strongly following administration of intravenous contrast medium. In addition to the reactive bony changes, oedema-like marrow and soft-tissue SI is almost invariably seen adjacent to the nidus (Fig. 3-16C). High-resolution imaging and the use of dynamic contrast-enhanced gradient-echo techniques can further improve identification of the nidus.[26] However, a very small nidus may still be occult on MRI.

Periosteal reaction is typically absent with intra-articular lesions, lesions in the terminal phalanges and those deep in medullary bone or at tendinous or ligamentous insertions. Intra-articular lesions are most commonly seen in the hip and may present with local osteopenia due to disuse (Fig. 3-17A), while MRI will show reactive bone and soft-tissue oedema-like changes and a joint effusion (Fig. 3-17B). The nidus is usually demonstrated on CT (Fig. 3-17C).

OO in the ankle and foot region may be difficult to diagnose. The subperiosteal region of the talar neck is a classical site (Fig. 3-18), but cancellous lesions of the hindfoot bones are commonly radiologically occult. MRI will show the reactive oedema-like changes, which are usually limited to a single bone, but CT is usually required to demonstrate the nidus.[27]

The natural history of OO is one of spontaneous resolution, which may be promoted with the use of non-steroidal anti-inflammatory drugs.[28] However, the current treatment of choice is CT-guided radiofrequency ablation, which is minimally invasive and has a high success rate.[24] CT in successfully treated cases commonly shows complete ossification of the nidus (Fig. 3-19) or a minimal nidus rest, while MRI may continue to show reactive bone and soft-tissue changes even after clinically successful treatment.[29]

The differential diagnosis of OO includes small areas of chronic osteomyelitis, chondroblastoma, Langerhans cell histiocytosis (LCH) and fibrous dysplasia. However, these lesions, when small enough, can also be successfully treated by CT-guided radiofrequency ablation.[24]

Osteoblastoma[30]

Osteoblastoma (OB) possesses histological similarities to OO and is differentiated primarily by its size, being

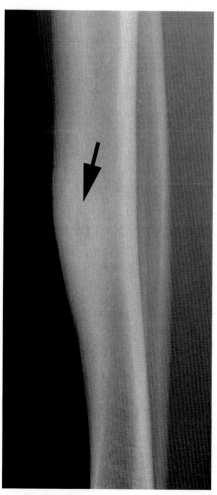

FIGURE 3-15 ■ **Osteoid osteoma.** Lateral radiograph of the tibial diaphysis shows solid thickening of the cortex, within which is a small calcified nidus (arrow).

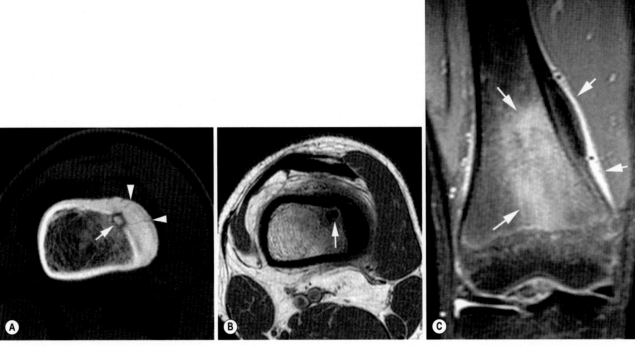

FIGURE 3-16 ■ **Osteoid osteoma.** (A) Axial CT shows a densely mineralised intracortical nidus (arrow), with solid adjacent periosteal thickening containing multiple vascular channels (arrowheads). (B) Axial T1W SE MRI clearly demonstrates the hypointense nidus (arrow) and the cortical thickening. (C) Coronal STIR MRI shows the reactive oedema-like SI changes (arrows).

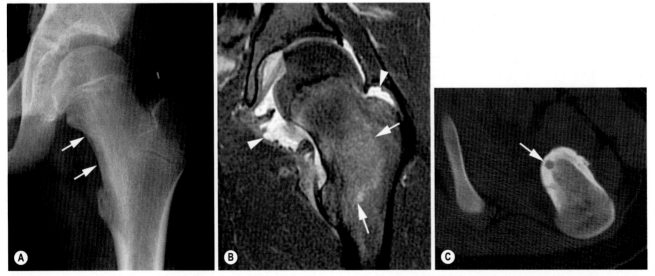

FIGURE 3-17 ■ **Intra-articular osteoid osteoma.** (A) AP radiograph of the left hip shows mild disuse osteopenia and some thickening of the calcar (arrows). (B) Coronal STIR MRI demonstrates reactive oedema-like marrow SI changes in the femoral neck (arrows) and a joint effusion (arrowheads). (C) Axial CT shows the small nidus (arrow) in the thickened calcar.

typically greater than 1.5 cm in diameter. It also shows a more aggressive growth pattern with potential for extra-osseous extension, and does not resolve spontaneously. OB is a rare tumour accounting for less than 1% of all primary bone neoplasms. Over 80% of patients are under the age of 30 years and the male:female ratio is 2–3:1.

The presentation differs from OO in that pain is not usually acute or severe and is rarely relieved by aspirin. The humerus is the commonest location in the appendicular skeleton and the lesion arises in the medullary cavity, although a periosteal location has also been described.[31]

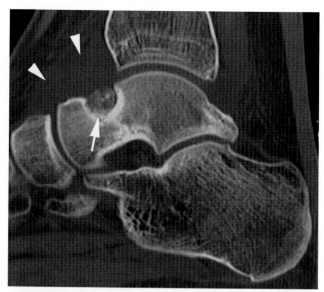

FIGURE 3-18 ■ **Osteoid osteoma of the foot.** Sagittal CT multiplanar reconstruction (MPR) showing a subperiosteal OO nidus (arrow) in the talar neck with associated reactive synovitis in the anterior recess of the joint (arrowheads).

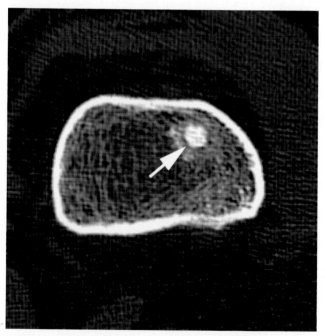

FIGURE 3-19 ■ **Radiofrequency ablation of osteoid osteoma.** Same case as described in the legend to Fig. 3-16. Axial CT shows complete ossification of the nidus (arrow) following successful CT-guided RF ablation.

Radiological Features

The lesion is predominantly lytic, measuring over 2 cm in diameter, with larger lesions showing a greater degree of matrix mineralisation (Fig. 3-20A). CT often reveals occult calcification, which can be punctate, nodular or generalised (Fig. 3-20B). Larger lesions may result in bone expansion with or without a surrounding shell of reactive bone. OB can also produce an extracortical mass, which may be reactive or due to tumour extension. As

with OO, scintigraphy is always positive and MRI shows a low–intermediate SI lesion with associated reactive changes as seen with OO, but of a lesser intensity (Fig. 3-20C). Secondary ABC change may also be seen, manifest by the development of FFLs.

In the long bones, the differential diagnosis includes Brodie's abscess and Langerhans cell histiocytosis.

FIBROGENIC TUMOURS

Desmoplastic Fibroma[32]

Desmoplastic fibroma is a rare, locally aggressive benign neoplasm with similar histological features to soft-tissue fibromatosis. It accounts for 0.06% of all bone tumours and 0.3% of benign bone neoplasms. Seventy per cent of cases present between 10 and 30 years of age (mean age 21 years) with no particular predilection for men or women. Desmoplastic fibroma usually arises in the metaphyseal region of long bones (femur, humerus, tibia and radius constitute 56% of cases), the mandible (26%) and ilium (14%). It is rarely associated with fibrous dysplasia.

Radiological Features

Most lesions are metadiaphyseal and arise as either subperiosteal or intraosseous tumours. Many are large at presentation (over 5 cm in diameter) and two patterns are seen: an ill-defined moth-eaten or permeative lesion and an expanding, trabeculated lesion (Fig. 3-21).

The MRI features are non-specific, showing heterogeneous intermediate SI on T1W images and hyperintensity on T2W images with irregular enhancement following gadolinium.[33] When the soft tissues are invaded, it may be difficult to distinguish from bony invasion by soft-tissue fibromatosis. Although desmoplastic fibroma is considered a benign lesion, metastasis has been reported following local recurrence.

FIBROHISTIOCYTIC TUMOURS[34,35]

Fibrous cortical defect, non-ossifying fibroma and benign fibrous histiocytoma all share identical histological appearances but are differentiated by their clinical and radiological features.

Fibrous Cortical Defect

Fibrous cortical defect (FCD) is most commonly identified in the distal femoral and proximal tibial metaphyses as an incidental finding, appearing as a cortically based lytic lesion commonly with a thin sclerotic margin (Fig. 3-22). The lesion typically consolidates/fades with time.

Non-Ossifying Fibroma

Non-ossifying fibroma (NOF) is a benign neoplasm, which is commonly identified incidentally, or may present with pathological fracture when large enough. The lesion may also be painful when associated with a stress fracture,

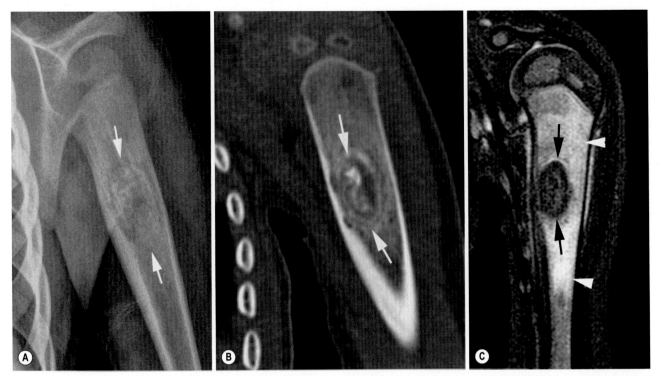

FIGURE 3-20 ■ **Osteoblastoma.** (A) AP radiograph of the left proximal humerus showing a large mixed lytic-sclerotic lesion (arrows) in the medullary cavity with associated periosteal thickening. (B) Coronal CT MPR shows the oval, mineralised lesion (arrows). (C) Coronal STIR MRI demonstrates a hypointense tumour (arrows) with extensive reactive oedema-like marrow changes (arrowheads).

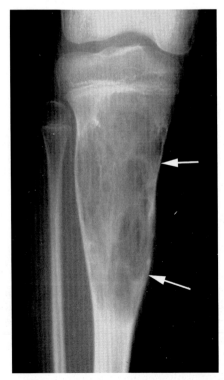

FIGURE 3-21 ■ **Desmoplastic fibroma.** AP radiograph of the proximal tibia showing an expansile aggressive metaphyseal lesion (arrows).

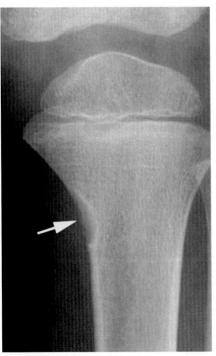

FIGURE 3-22 ■ **Fibrous cortical defect.** AP radiograph of the proximal tibia showing a small, elongated lytic lesion (arrow) in the medial proximal tibial metaphysis.

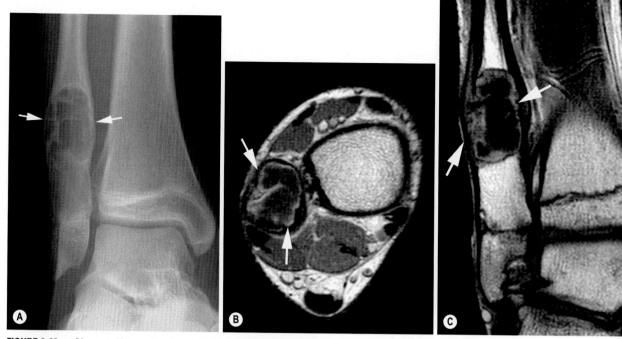

FIGURE 3-23 ■ **Non-ossifying fibroma.** (A) AP radiograph of the ankle showing a lobular lesion (arrows) expanding the distal fibular metadiaphysis. (B) Axial PDW FSE and (C) coronal T2W FSE MR images showing a lobular lesion (arrows) containing prominent areas of hypointensity due to its fibrous nature.

typically with proximal tibial lesions.[36] Patients usually present in the second decade of life and a slight male preponderance is recorded. The majority (~90%) involve the lower limbs, particularly the tibia and distal end of the femur. Multiple lesions are found and occasionally a familial incidence is reported, in which case an association with neurofibromatosis (5%) may be present. The Jaffe–Campanacci syndrome consists of multiple (usually unilateral) NOFs with café-au-lait spots but no other stigmata of neurofibromatosis. NOF can usually be diagnosed radiologically, in which case biopsy is unnecessary.

Radiological Features

The lesions are metaphyseal or diametaphyseal and essentially intracortical. A lobular appearance is classical, with the lesion usually enlarging into the medullary cavity. The tumour is oval with its long axis in the line of the bone (Fig. 3-1A). When NOF arises in a slim bone such as the fibula, it crosses the shaft readily and its characteristic intracortical origin is less obvious (Fig. 3-23A). It may then resemble other entities, such as ABC. Periosteal reaction is typically seen only after fracture.

On MRI, NOF shows low–intermediate SI on T1W and PDW images (Fig. 3-23B) and enhances following administration of intravenous gadolinium contrast medium. On T2W images, approximately 80% are hypointense (Fig. 3-23C), but with marginal or septal hyperintensity and the remainder are hyperintense. Marginal sclerosis appears as a hypointense rim.[37] Reactive marrow oedema may also be seen, particularly if the

lesion is complicated by a stress or pathological fracture, while secondary ABC change manifests as the presence of FFLs.

Benign Fibrous Histiocytoma[38]

Benign fibrous histiocytoma (BFH) is an uncommon lesion occurring in an older age group and in a different location to NOF. BFH typically presents between 20 and 50 years, with a mean age in the third decade; the male:female ratio is equal.

Radiological Features

Most frequently the lesion resembles a giant cell tumour, occurring in an eccentric subarticular location, but with a well-defined sclerotic margin indicating slower growth. About one-third occur on either side of the knee. The MRI features are also similar to GCT.

GIANT CELL TUMOUR

Giant Cell Tumour[39,40]

Giant cell tumour (GCT) is an aggressive benign neoplasm accounting for approximately 20% of benign bone tumours. However, malignant change in GCT is recognised, being either primary or secondary,[41] and benign lesions may rarely metastasise to the lungs.[42] Multifocal, metachronous GCT has also been reported,[43] which is associated with hyperparathyroidism. Hyperparathyroidism should therefore be assessed for. GCT rarely complicates familial polyostotic Paget's disease of bone.[66]

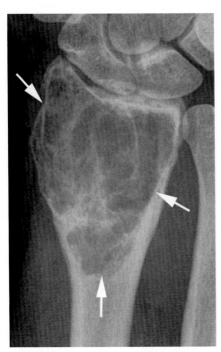

FIGURE 3-24 ■ **Giant cell tumour.** AP radiograph of the wrist showing a distal radial subarticular lytic lesion (arrows) with internal trabeculation.

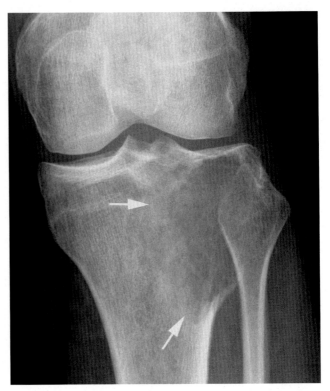

FIGURE 3-25 ■ **Giant cell tumour.** AP radiograph of the knee showing an eccentric, subarticular lytic lesion of the proximal tibia with a poorly defined margin (arrows) and destruction of the lateral cortex.

Approximately 80% occur between 18 and 45 years of age, with a male : female ratio of 2 : 3. The tumour nearly always occurs in a subarticular or subcortical region (adjacent to a fused apophysis) of a long bone, with the knee (distal femur/proximal tibia—55%), distal radius (10%) and proximal humerus (6%) being the commonest sites.

Radiological Features

GCT is classically a subarticular, eccentric, lytic lesion with a geographic, non-sclerotic margin (Fig. 3-24). However, a poorly defined margin indicative of a more aggressive lesion may be identified in 10–15% of cases (Fig. 3-25). Involvement of the subchondral or apophyseal bone is seen in 95–99% of GCTs at presentation, although lesions arising in the immature skeleton involve the metaphysis adjacent to the growth plate. The tumour usually measures 5–7 cm in size. Apparent trabeculation and cortical expansion are common features and periosteal reaction is seen in 10–15% of cases, indicating healing of a pathological fracture. Cortical destruction with extraosseous extension may occur in up to 50% of cases.

On MRI, the tumour is iso- or hypointense on T1W images (Fig. 3-26A) and shows heterogeneous hyperintensity on STIR. Areas of hyperintensity on T1W indicate the presence of subacute haemorrhage. Profound hypointensity on T2W images in solid areas of the tumour is seen in the majority of cases, being due to the deposition of haemosiderin from chronic recurrent haemorrhage (Fig. 3-26B). Marrow oedema is also demonstrated, while FFLs indicate the presence of secondary

ABC change, which is reported in approximately 15% of cases. Malignant GCT has no characteristic distinguishing features.

The most important differential diagnostic considerations are lytic osteosarcoma and, in older patients, malignant fibrous histiocytoma or a subarticular lytic metastasis, particularly from a primary renal tumour.

VASCULAR TUMOURS[44]

Haemangioma[45]

Both single and multiple haemangiomas occur in bone and may be regarded as congenital vascular malformations. However, many present as isolated bone lesions and are therefore included in the differential diagnosis of a bone tumour. Haemangiomas are classified histologically as capillary, cavernous, arteriovenous or venous. Osseous capillary haemangiomas most commonly affect the vertebral body, whereas osseous cavernous haemangiomas affect the skull vault. Involvement of the appendicular skeleton is relatively rare.

Radiological Features

As in vertebral lesions, fine or coarse vertical trabeculation is seen with haemangioma involving the epiphyses and metaphyses of long bones, with the direction of the linear striations running along the axis of the bone.

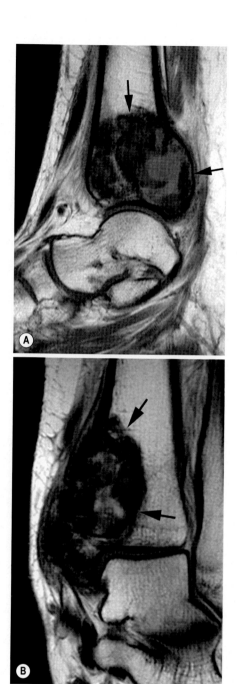

FIGURE 3-26 ■ Giant cell tumour. (A) Sagittal T1W and (B) coronal T2W FSE MRI of the ankle showing a distal tibial GCT (arrows), which demonstrates profound heterogeneous low SI due to the presence of haemosiderin from chronic haemorrhage.

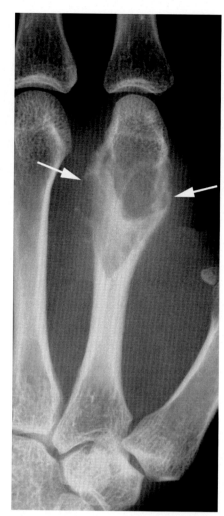

FIGURE 3-27 ■ Haemangioma. AP radiograph of the ring finger metacarpal showing an expansile lytic lesion (arrows) containing coarse trabeculation.

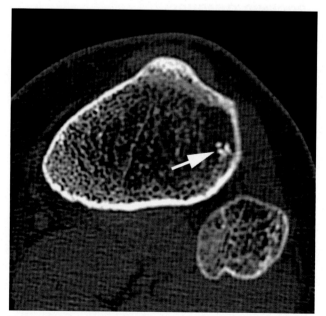

FIGURE 3-28 ■ Haemangioma. Axial CT through the proximal tibia showing a poorly defined lytic lesion containing multiple, dense thickened trabeculae (arrow).

Occasionally, well-defined vascular channels may be evident. Bone expansion and extraosseous extension are also recognised features (Fig. 3-27). Scintigraphy typically shows triple-phase uptake due to the vascular nature of the lesion, while CT demonstrates the thickened trabeculae as dense 'dots' within a fatty matrix (Fig. 3-28). On MRI, long and flat bone haemangiomas are typically of intermediate SI on T1W and hyperintense on T2W, only occasionally having a predominantly fatty matrix. The thickened trabeculae may be evident as linear areas of signal void.

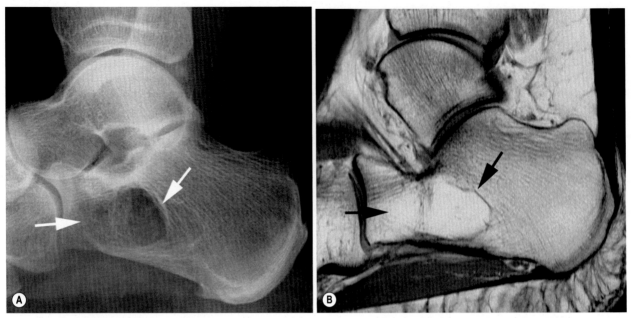

FIGURE 3-29 ■ **Intraosseous lipoma.** (A) Lateral radiograph of the calcaneus showing a well-defined lytic lesion (arrows) in the calcaneal body. (B) Sagittal T1W SE MRI shows the lesion to be hyperintense (arrows) consistent with a fatty matrix.

SMOOTH MUSCLE TUMOURS

Leiomyoma[46]

Intraosseous leiomyoma is an exceedingly rare tumour with less than 20 reported cases. It may present with non-specific pain and appears as a unilocular or multilocular lytic lesion with a sclerotic rim, mimicking a NOF. The CT and MRI features are non-specific.

LIPOGENIC TUMOURS[47]

Intraosseous Lipoma

Intraosseous lipoma[48] arises in the medulla and produces expansion, sometimes with endosteal scalloping and trabeculation, resembling a cyst or even fibrous dysplasia. Calcification is also seen. Most affect the lower limb, with a predilection for the calcaneus (Fig. 3-29A) and femur. CT and MRI (Fig. 3-29B) establish the diagnosis by demonstrating the fatty nature of the matrix. Calcification and cystic degeneration due to fat necrosis can also be identified.

Parosteal Lipoma

Parosteal lipoma is a rare lesion which is most frequently encountered around the proximal radius, where it may cause posterior interosseous nerve palsy. It may result in pressure erosion of the bone and the formation of circumferential juxtacortical new bone. The combination of such peripheral ossification with a tumour of otherwise fatty matrix, demonstrated either by CT (Fig. 3-30) or MRI,[49] establishes the radiological diagnosis.

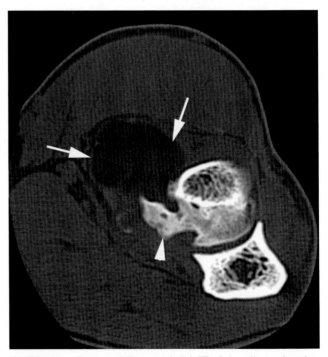

FIGURE 3-30 ■ **Parosteal lipoma.** Axial CT of the elbow showing a fatty mass (arrows) arising in association with a parosteal bony lesion (arrowhead) from the proximal radius.

NEURAL TUMOURS

Schwannoma of Bone[50]

Primary schwannomas of bone are defined as arising within the medullary cavity and are extremely rare lesions, which are usually sporadic but may be associated with the Carney complex (myxomas of the heart and skin, hyperpigmentation of the skin and endocrine overactivity). Most occur in the long bones and present with pain. The radiological features are non-specific, being those of a benign lytic bone lesion and the tumour is successfully treated by local excision.

MISCELLANEOUS LESIONS

Aneurysmal Bone Cyst[51,52]

Primary Aneurysmal bone cyst (ABC) accounts for 1–2% of all primary bone lesions and usually presents in the second decade, with 70–80% occurring between 5 and 20 years of age; the male:female ratio is equal. ABC can involve many sites, but the long bones (>50% of cases) and spine (20% of cases) are most common. Involvement of flat bones is most common in the pelvis.

Secondary ABC change can develop in a variety of benign or malignant lesions, including non-ossifying fibroma, chondroblastoma, giant cell tumour, fibrous dysplasia, osteoblastoma and osteosarcoma.

Radiological Features[53]

The classical lesion (accounting for 75–80%) is a purely lytic, expansile intramedullary lesion in the metaphysis of a long bone extending to the growth plate, which may be centrally (Fig. 3-1B, C) or, more commonly eccentrically (Figs. 3-4B, 3-31A) placed. Twenty per cent of long bone ABCs involve the diaphysis. A thin 'egg-shell' covering of expanded cortex is often identified, particularly with CT, which may also demonstrate fine septal ossification. Apparent trabeculation due to ridging of the endosteal cortex is also a feature, as is marginal periosteal reaction. Intracortical or subperiosteal ABC (Fig. 3-31B) is also observed.[54]

The lesion shows heterogeneous intermediate SI on T1W images (Fig. 3-31C) and a thin sclerotic margin with internal hypointense internal septa may be seen, which may enhance following administration of gadolinium contrast medium. T2 or PDW images almost invariably demonstrate multiple FFLs (Fig. 3-31D), which commonly fill the whole of the lesion. Reactive medullary oedema is also a frequent feature. The absence of fluid levels may indicate a 'solid' variant of ABC, which is most commonly reported in the long bones.[55]

The most important differential diagnosis of ABC is telangiectatic osteosarcoma.

Simple Bone Cyst[51,56]

Simple bone cyst (SBC) or unicameral bone cyst usually presents between the ages of 5 and 15 years, with less than 15% reported over the age of 20 years. The male:female ratio is 2.5:1 and presentation with pathological fracture is classical, especially with humeral lesions.

The proximal humerus is by far the commonest site (>60% of cases), followed by the proximal femur

(approximately 30% of cases). Other sites tend to affect adults and include the calcaneus and the posterior iliac blade.

Radiological Features

Initially, SBCs are located in the proximal metaphysis of the humerus or femur and progress toward the diaphysis with skeletal growth, eventually reaching the mid-diaphysis, by which time they are usually healed. Occasionally, the cyst adheres to the growth plate and extension into the epiphysis/apophysis is reported in 2% of lesions. SBC usually lies centrally in the shaft, expanding the bone symmetrically and thinning the cortex. The lesion is typically 6–8 cm in size. Apparent trabeculation is common, but periosteal reaction is not seen without fracture, which may result in a fragment of cortex penetrating the cyst lining, resulting in the fallen fragment sign (Fig. 3-32).

MRI demonstrates the fluid content of the lesion, homogeneous low-to-intermediate SI on T1W images and marked hyperintensity on T2W or STIR images. These appearances are altered by the presence of fracture, in which case haemorrhage may result in the presence of FFLs and pericystic oedema.[57] Following administration of intravenous contrast medium, rim enhancement is observed.

The major differential diagnosis includes ABC and fibrous dysplasia.

Fibrous Dysplasia[58]

Fibrous dysplasia (FD) accounts for approximately 7% of benign bone tumours and may either be monostotic (70–85%) or polyostotic. FD is usually painless unless a fracture has occurred. Seventy-five per cent of cases present before the age of 30 years and there is no gender predilection. The commonest sites of monostotic FD are the ribs (28%), proximal femur (23%) and craniofacial bones (20%).

Polyostotic FD may range from the involvement of two bones to more than 75% of the skeleton. Approximately 30–50% of patients with polyostotic disease have café au lait spots. FD may be associated with a variety of syndromes. McCune–Albright's *syndrome* consists of polyostotic FD (typically unilateral), ipsilateral café au lait spots and endocrine disturbance, most commonly precocious puberty in girls. Mazabraud's *syndrome* consists of FD (most commonly polyostotic) and soft-tissue myxomata.[59]

Radiological Features

Radiologically, FD presents as a geographic lesion that may cause bone expansion and deformity with diffuse ground-glass matrix mineralisation (Fig. 3-33). A thick sclerotic margin ('rind' sign) is characteristic (Fig. 3-34). Purely lytic lesions are also seen, indicating extensive cystic degeneration. The metadiaphyseal region is typically affected in long bones. Periosteal reaction is not a

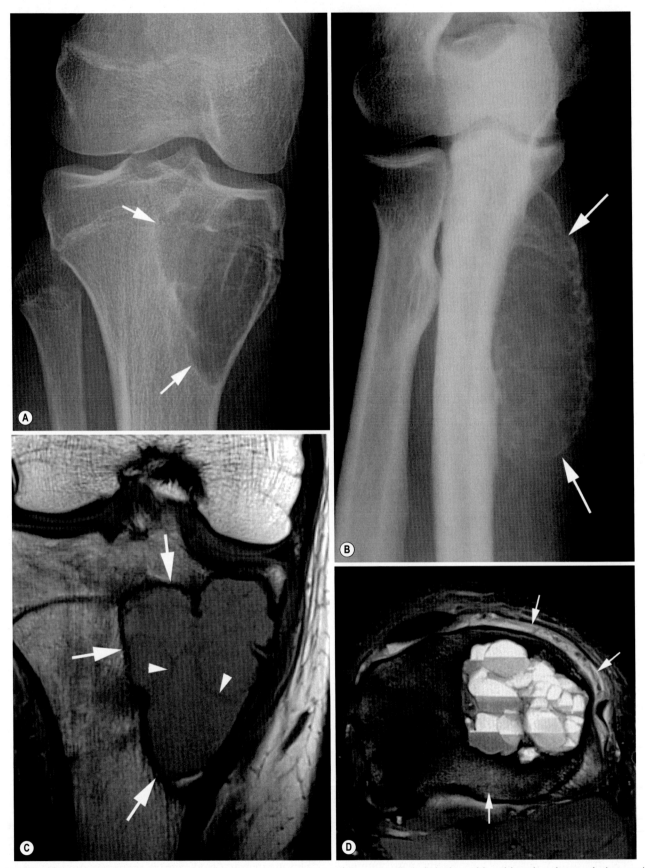

FIGURE 3-31 ■ **Aneurysmal bone cyst.** (A) AP radiograph showing a mildly expansile lytic lesion with a thin sclerotic margin (arrows) located eccentrically within the proximal tibial metaphysis. (B) AP radiograph of the proximal forearm showing an expansile lesion with a thin sclerotic margin (arrows) arising from the surface of the proximal ulna. (C) Coronal T1W SE MRI showing an intermediate SI lesion (arrows) with thin internal septae (arrowheads). (D) Axial fat-suppressed T2W FSE MRI demonstrates multiple fluid–fluid levels filling the lesion with mild surrounding reactive medullary and soft-tissue oedema (arrows).

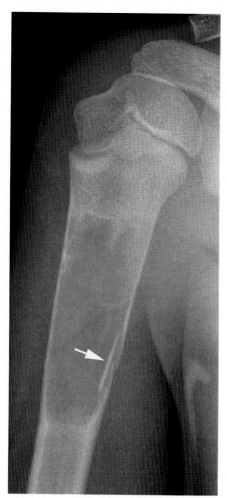

FIGURE 3-32 ■ **Simple bone cyst.** AP radiograph of the right proximal humerus showing a fractured simple bone cyst with a 'fallen fragment' (arrow).

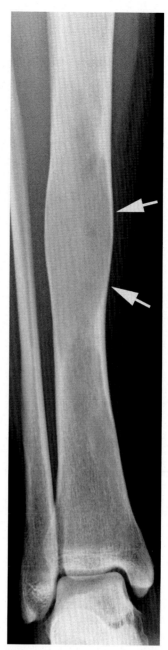

FIGURE 3-33 ■ **Fibrous dysplasia.** AP radiograph of the tibia showing a mildly expansile lesion (arrows) with diffuse 'ground-glass' matrix mineralisation.

feature in the absence of fracture. Varus deformity of the proximal femur ('shepherd's crook' deformity) is a characteristic late finding.

Skeletal scintigraphy is the best technique for identifying polyostotic disease (Fig. 3-35), although whole-body MRI may also be used. CT beautifully demonstrates the ground-glass matrix (Fig. 3-36), which may not be evident radiologically, helping to establish the diagnosis without the need for biopsy. On MRI,[60] lesions are usually isointense on T1W but may show areas of mild hyperintensity due to haemorrhage (Fig. 3-37A). Lesions may be of intermediate SI or hyperintense on T2W, depending upon whether the tumour is mainly fibrous or has undergone cystic change. Internal septa and FFLs may also be seen (Fig. 3-37B). Following administration of intravenous contrast medium, either uniform or septal enhancement is described.

The identification of associated chondroid calcification indicates a diagnosis of fibrocartilaginous dysplasia. Malignant change in fibrous dysplasia is rare, being reported in 0.5% of cases. It is more common in polyostotic disease and may follow prior radiotherapy.

Osteofibrous Dysplasia[61]

Osteofibrous dysplasia (OFD) is a rare lesion that histologically resembles fibrous dysplasia and the stroma of adamantinoma. However, it has a specific clinical and radiological picture. Presentation is from birth to 40 years, with almost 50% occurring under the age of 10 years; the male:female ratio is equal. The tibia is affected in over 90% of cases and in two-thirds of these the anterior mid-diaphyseal cortex is involved. Multiple lesions may occur in the same bone, but the ipsilateral fibula is also affected in 20% of cases. Bilateral involvement may occur.

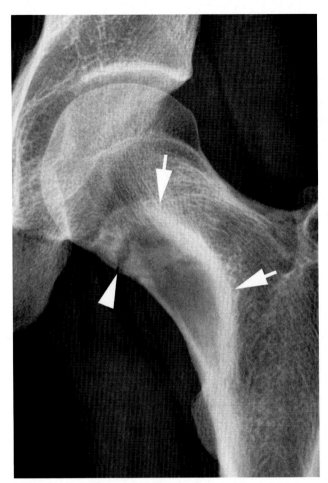

FIGURE 3-34 ■ Fibrous dysplasia. AP radiograph of the hip showing a lesion in the medial femoral neck with a thick sclerotic border (arrows) and a complicating insufficiency fracture (arrowhead).

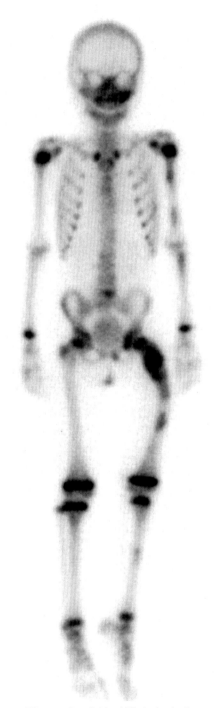

FIGURE 3-35 ■ Fibrous dysplasia. Whole-body bone scintigram showing polyostotic disease involving the left side of the body.

Radiological Features

In early infancy the lesion expands and bows the tibia with a sclerotic rim. After 3 months of age, the lesion is eccentric, multilocular and may be purely lytic (Fig. 3-38) or show ground-glass matrix mineralisation similar to that of FD. Cross-sectional imaging confirms its intracortical origin, but otherwise it shows no characteristic features, although MRI may be of value in the differentiation from osteofibous dysplasia-like adamantinoma and adamantinoma.[62]

Langerhans Cell Histiocytosis (LCH)[63]

LCH represents a spectrum of disorders characterised by the idiopathic proliferation of histiocytes (Langerhans cells), which can involve virtually any organ and present either as focal/multifocal lesions or as a multi-organ systemic disease. Three forms of the disease were classically described: eosinophilic granuloma, Letterer–Siwe disease and Hand–Schüller–Christian disease, these having different clinical and radiological manifestations. Currently, the disorder is classified as being localised (single-system

disease) or disseminated (multi-system disease), the latter cases further categorised as being either 'low risk' or 'risk'.[64]

Localised skeletal disease accounts for approximately 70% of cases of LCH and is classically seen in children between the ages of 5 and 15 years who present with focal bone pain, but lesions may also be asymptomatic. LCH can involve any bone, but most lesions involve the skull, pelvis, spine, mandible and ribs. The long bones are involved in 25–35% of cases of monostotic disease, with

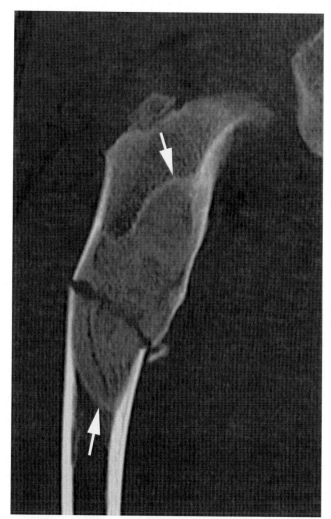

FIGURE 3-36 ■ **Fibrous dysplasia.** Coronal CT MPR of the proximal femur showing a well-defined lesion with a 'ground-glass' matrix (arrows), through which there has been a pathological fracture.

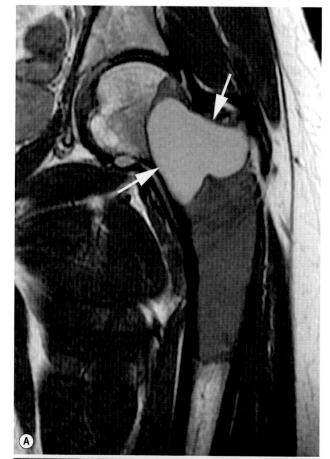

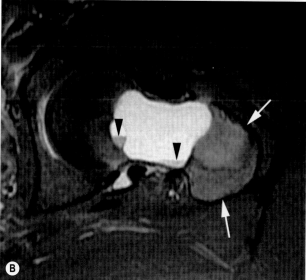

FIGURE 3-37 ■ **Fibrous dysplasia.** (A) Coronal T1W SE MRI showing a lesion in the left femoral neck with combined intermediate and increased SI (arrows), the latter due to haemorrhage. (B) Axial fat-suppressed T2W FSE MRI shows the fibrous component of the tumour to have intermediate SI (arrows), while the haemorrhagic component is hyperintense. Note also the FFLs (arrowheads).

the femur, tibia and humerus being the most common locations. Multiple lesions are seen in 10% of cases at presentation.

Radiological Features

Long bone lesions are usually located centrally within the diaphysis (~60%), followed by the metaphysis/metadiaphysis. Epiphyseal involvement is rare (~2%). The lesions are lytic, showing a fairly aggressive pattern of bone destruction (Fig. 3-39A) with occasional reactive medullary sclerosis. A multi-laminated periosteal response is commonly seen, while endosteal scalloping and mild bone expansion are also features.

MRI shows a poorly defined lesion with intermediate signal intensity. Active lesions are almost invariably associated with reactive marrow and soft-tissue oedema and periostitis (Fig. 3-39B). Cortical destruction and soft-tissue masses have rarely been described in adults with

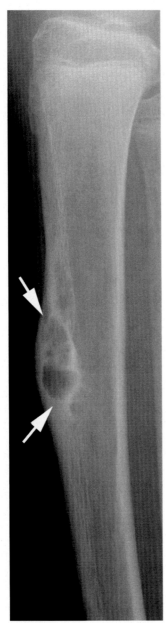

FIGURE 3-38 ■ Osteofibrous dysplasia. Lateral radiograph of the proximal tibia showing a lobular lesion (arrows) within the anterior cortex.

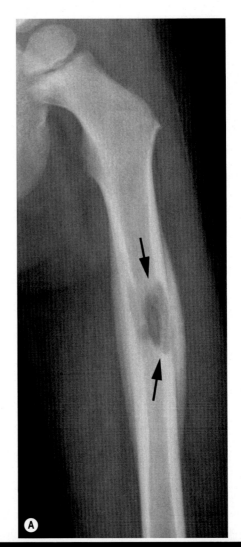

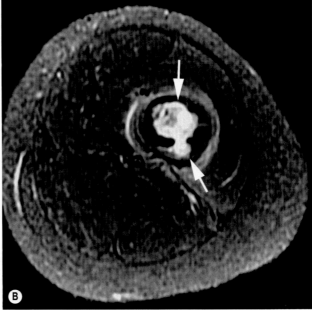

FIGURE 3-39 ■ LCH. (A) AP radiograph of the left proximal femur showing an irregular lytic lesion (arrows) with a multi-laminated periosteal response. (B) Axial fat-suppressed T2W FSE MRI showing an irregular hyperintense lesion (arrows) with associated periosteal response and soft-tissue oedema.

LCH.[64] Whole-body MRI may replace scintigraphy for the assessment of multifocal disease.

Erdheim–Chester's Disease[65]

Erdheim–Chester's disease is a rare form of histiocytosis characterised by the medullary infiltration of foamy, lipid-laden histiocytes. It usually presents in adults over the age of 40 years with bone pain most commonly related to the knees and ankles. Radiographs classically demonstrate bilateral, symmetrical metaphyseal and diaphyseal medullary sclerosis with sparing of the epiphyses.

REFERENCES

1. Fletcher DM, Unni KK, Mertens F, editors. World Health Organization Classification of Tumours. Pathology and Genetics of Tumours of Soft Tissue and Bone. Lyon: IARC Press; 2002.
2. Wenaden AE, Szyszko TA, Saifuddin A. Imaging of periosteal reactions associated with focal lesions of bone. Clin Radiol 2005;60: 439–56.
3. Saifuddin A. The accuracy of imaging in the local staging of appendicular osteosarcoma. Skeletal Radiol 2002;31:191–201.
4. Alyas F, James SL, Davies AM, Saifuddin A. The role of MR imaging in the diagnostic characterisation of appendicular bone tumours and tumour-like conditions. Eur Radiol 2007;17:2675–86.
5. O'Donnell P, Saifuddin A. The prevalence and diagnostic significance of fluid–fluid levels in focal lesions of bone. Skeletal Radiol 2004;33:330–6.
6. Choi JA, Lee KH, Jun WS, et al. Osseous metastasis from renal cell carcinoma: 'flow-void' sign at MR imaging. Radiology 2003;228:629–34.
7. James SL, Panicek DM, Davies AM. Bone marrow oedema associated with benign and malignant bone tumours. Eur J Radiol 2008;67:11–21.
8. Schmidt GP, Reiser MF, Baur-Melnyk A. Whole-body MRI for the staging and follow-up of patients with metastasis. Eur J Radiol 2009;70:393–400.
9. Khoo MM, Tyler PA, Saifuddin A, Padhani AR. Diffusion-weighted imaging (DWI) in musculoskeletal MRI: a critical review. Skeletal Radiol 2011;40:665–81.
10. Saifuddin A, Mitchell R, Burnett SJ, et al. Ultrasound-guided needle biopsy of primary bone tumours. J Bone Joint Surg Br 2000;82:50–4.
11. Jelinek JS, Murphey MD, Welker JA. Diagnosis of primary bone tumors with image-guided percutaneous biopsy: experience with 110 tumors. Radiology 2002;223:731–7.
12. Carrino JA, Blanco R. Magnetic resonance—guided musculoskeletal interventional radiology. Semin Musculoskelet Radiol 2006; 10:159–74.
13. Douis H, Saifuddin A. The Imaging of cartilaginous bone tumours: Part 1—benign lesions. Skel Radiol 2012;41(10):1195–212.
14. Lee KC, Davies AM, Cassar-Pullicino VN. Imaging the complications of osteochondromas. Clin Radiol 2002;57:18–28.
15. Murphey MD, Flemming DJ, Boyea SR, et al. Enchondroma versus chondrosarcoma in the appendicular skeleton: differentiating features. Radiographics 1998;18:1213–37.
16. Robinson P, White LM, Sundaram M, et al. Periosteal chondroid tumors: radiological evaluation with pathologic correlation. Am J Roentgenol 2001;177:1183–8.
17. Kaim AH, Hugli R, Bonel HM, Jundt G. Chondroblastoma and clear cell chondrosarcoma: radiological and MRI characteristics with histopathological correlation. Skeletal Radiol 2002;31:88–95.
18. Maheshwari AV, Jelinek JS, Song AJ, et al. Metaphyseal and diaphyseal chondroblastomas. Skeletal Radiol 2011;40:1563–73.
19. Wu CT, Inwards CY, O'Laughlin S, et al. Chondromyxoid fibroma of bone: a clinicopathologic review of 278 cases. Hum Pathol 1998;29:438–46.
20. Atesok KI, Alman BA, Schemitsch EH, et al. Osteoid osteoma and osteoblastoma. J Am Acad Orthop Surg 2011;19:678–89.
21. Chai JW, Hong SH, Choi JY, et al. Radiologic diagnosis of osteoid osteoma: from simple to challenging findings. Radiographics 2010;30:737–49.
22. Allen SD, Saifuddin A. Imaging of intra-articular osteoid osteoma. Clin Radiol 2003;58:845–52.
23. Aynaci O, Turgutoglu O, Kerimoglu S, et al. Osteoid osteoma with a multicentric nidus: a case report and review of the literature. Arch Orthop Trauma Surg 2007;127:863–6.
24. Becce F, Theumann N, Rochette A, et al. Osteoid osteoma and osteoid osteoma-mimicking lesions: biopsy findings, distinctive MDCT features and treatment by radiofrequency ablation. Eur Radiol 2010;20:2439–46.
25. Liu PT, Kujak JL, Roberts CC, de Chadarevian JP. The vascular groove sign: a new CT finding associated with osteoid osteomas. Am J Roentgenol 2011;196:168–73.
26. von Kalle T, Langendörfer M, Fernandez FF, Winkler P. Combined dynamic contrast-enhancement and serial 3D-subtraction analysis in magnetic resonance imaging of osteoid osteomas. Eur Radiol 2009;19:2508–17.
27. Shukla S, Clarke AW, Saifuddin A. Imaging features of foot osteoid osteoma. Skeletal Radiol 2010;39:683–9.
28. Goto T, Shinoda Y, Okuma T, et al. Administration of non-steroidal anti-inflammatory drugs accelerates spontaneous healing of osteoid osteoma. Arch Orthop Trauma Surg 2011;131:619–25.
29. Vanderschueren GM, Taminiau AH, Obermann WR, et al. The healing pattern of osteoid osteomas on computed tomography and magnetic resonance imaging after thermocoagulation. Skeletal Radiol 2007;36:813–21.
30. Berry M, Mankin H, Gebhardt M, et al. Osteoblastoma: a 30-year study of 99 cases. J Surg Oncol 2008;98:179–83.
31. Mortazavi SM, Wenger D, Asadollahi S, et al. Periosteal osteoblastoma: report of a case with a rare histopathologic presentation and review of the literature. Skeletal Radiol 2007;36:259–64.
32. Taconis WK, Schutte HE, Heul RO. Desmoplastic fibroma of bone: a report of 18 cases. Skeletal Radiol 1994;23:283–8.
33. Mahnken AH, Nolte-Ernsting CC, Wildberger JE, et al. Cross-sectional imaging patterns of desmoplastic fibroma. Eur Radiol 2001;11:1105–10.
34. Smith SE, Kransdorf MJ. Primary musculoskeletal tumors of fibrous origin. Semin Musculoskelet Radiol 2000;4:73–88.
35. Mankin HJ, Trahan CA, Fondren G, Mankin CJ. Non-ossifying fibroma, fibrous cortical defect and Jaffe-Campanacci syndrome: a biologic and clinical review. Chir Organi Mov 2009;93:1–7.
36. Shimal A, Davies AM, James SL, Grimer RJ. Fatigue-type stress fractures of the lower limb associated with fibrous cortical defects/non-ossifying fibromas in the skeletally immature. Clin Radiol 2010;65:382–6.
37. Jee WH, Choe BY, Kang HS, et al. Non-ossifying fibroma: characteristics at MR imaging with pathologic correlation. Radiology 1998;209:197–202.
38. Ceroni D, Dayer R, De Coulon G, Kaelin A. Benign fibrous histiocytoma of bone in a paediatric population: a report of 6 cases. Musculoskelet Surg 2011;95:107–14.
39. Murphy MD, Nomikos GC, Flemming DJ, et al. From the archives of AFIP. Imaging of giant cell tumor and giant cell reparative granuloma of bone: radiologic-pathologic correlation. Radiographics 2001;21:1283–309.
40. Errani C, Ruggieri P, Asenzio MA, et al. Giant cell tumor of the extremity: A review of 349 cases from a single institution. Cancer Treat Rev 2010;36:1–7.
41. Bertoni F, Bacchini P, Staals EL. Malignancy in giant cell tumor of bone. Cancer 2003;97:2520–9.
42. Siebenrock KA, Unni KK, Rock MG. Giant-cell tumour of bone metastasizing to the lungs. A long-term follow-up. J Bone Joint Surg Br 1998;80:43–7.
43. Dumford K, Moore TE, Walker CW, Jaksha J. Multifocal, metachronous, giant cell tumor of the lower limb. Skeletal Radiol 2003;32:147–50.
44. Wenger DE, Wold LE. Benign vascular lesions of bone: radiologic and pathologic features. Skeletal Radiol 2000;29:63–74.
45. Rigopoulou A, Saifuddin A. Intraosseous haemangioma of the appendicular skeleton: imaging features of fifteen cases and a review of the literature. Skel Radiol 2012;41(12):1525–36.
46. Laffosse JM, Gomez-Brouchet A, Giordano G, et al. Intraosseous leiomyoma: a report of two cases. Joint Bone Spine 2007;74: 389–92.
47. Kapukaya A, Subasi M, Dabak N, Ozkul E. Osseous lipoma: eleven new cases and review of the literature. Acta Orthop Belg 2006; 72:603–14.
48. Campbell RS, Grainger AJ, Mangham DC, et al. Intraosseous lipoma: report of 35 new cases and a review of the literature. Skeletal Radiol 2003;32:209–22.
49. Yu JS, Weis L, Becker W. MR imaging of a parosteal lipoma. Clin Imaging 2000;24:15–8.
50. Ida CM, Scheithauer BW, Yapicier O, et al. Primary schwannoma of the bone: a clinicopathologic and radiologic study of 17 cases. Am J Surg Pathol 2011;35:989–97.
51. Parman LM, Murphey MD. Alphabet soup: cystic lesions of bone. Semin Musculoskelet Radiol 2000;4:89–101.
52. Kransdorf MJ, Sweet DE. Aneurysmal bone cyst: concept, controversy, clinical presentation, and imaging. Am J Roentgenol 1995; 164:573–80.
53. Mahnken AH, Nolte-Ernsting CC, Wildberger JE, et al. Aneurysmal bone cyst: value of MR imaging and conventional radiography. Eur Radiol 2003;13:1118–24.

54. Maiya S, Davies M, Evans N, Grimer J. Surface aneurysmal bone cysts: a pictorial review. Eur Radiol 2002;12:99–108.

55. Ilaslan H, Sundaram M, Unni KK. Solid variant of aneurysmal bone cysts in long tubular bones: giant cell reparative granuloma. Am J Roentgenol 2003;180:1681–7.

56. Wilkins RM. Unicameral bone cysts. J Am Acad Orthop Surg 2000;8:217–24.

57. Margau R, Babyn P, Cole W, et al. MR imaging of simple bone cysts in children: not so simple. Pediatr Radiol 2000;30:551–7.

58. Parekh SG, Donthineni-Rao R, Ricchetti E, Lackman RD. Fibrous dysplasia. J Am Acad Orthop Surg 2004;12:305–13.

59. Cabral CE, Guedes P, Fonseca T, et al. Polyostotic fibrous dysplasia associated with intramuscular myxomas: Mazabraud's syndrome. Skeletal Radiol 1998;27:278–82.

60. Jee WH, Choi KH, Choe BY, et al. Fibrous dysplasia: MR imaging characteristics with radiopathologic correlation. Am J Roentgenol 1996;167:1523–7.

61. Most MJ, Sim FH, Inwards CY. Osteofibrous dysplasia and adamantinoma. J Am Acad Orthop Surg 2010;18:358–66.

62. Khanna M, Delaney D, Tirabosco R, Saifuddin A. Osteofibrous dysplasia, osteofibrous dysplasia-like adamantinoma and adamantinoma: correlation of radiological imaging features with surgical histology and assessment of the use of radiology in contributing to needle biopsy diagnosis. Skeletal Radiol 2008;37(12):1077–84.

63. Azouz EM, Saigal G, Rodriguez MM, Podda A. Langerhans' cell histiocytosis: pathology, imaging and treatment of skeletal involvement. Pediatr Radiol 2005;35:103–15.

64. Song YS, Lee IS, Yi JH, et al. Radiologic findings of adult pelvis and appendicular skeletal Langerhans cell histiocytosis in nine patients. Skeletal Radiol 2011;40:1421–6.

65. Breuil V, Brocq O, Pellegrino C, et al. Erdheim–Chester disease: typical radiological bone features for a rare xanthogranulomatosis. Ann Rheum Dis 2002;61:199–200.

66. Gianfrancesco F, et al. J Bone Miner Res 2013;28(2):341–50. doi: 10.1002/jbmr.1750.

CHAPTER 4

Bone Tumours (2): Malignant Bone Tumours

A. Mark Davies • Steven L.J. James • Asif Saifuddin

CHAPTER OUTLINE

Introduction
Bone Metastases
PRIMARY MALIGNANT NEOPLASMS OF BONE
Chondroid Origin
Osteoid Origin

Fibrous Origin
Marrow Tumours
Notochordal Origin
Miscellaneous Tumours

INTRODUCTION

Bone tumours can be generally divided into two groups: benign, including tumour-like lesions (see Chapter 3), and malignant. The malignant category can be subclassified into primary, secondary and metastatic. In common parlance the terms secondary and metastatic are frequently used interchangeably. In the context of this chapter, however, the term secondary is reserved for those tumours arising from malignant transformation of a pre-existing benign bone condition.

BONE METASTASES

Bone metastasis or metastatic disease refers to the spread of a malignant tumour from its primary site to a non-adjacent part of the skeletal system. They are relatively common, frequently found on imaging to be multiple and are the commonest bone malignancy over 40 years of age. Approximately, 10% of carcinoma metastases will present as a solitary bone lesion. A solitary lesion in a middle-aged or elderly patient is, therefore, still more likely to be a metastasis than a primary malignant bone tumour. Post-mortem studies have shown that bone is the third commonest site of metastatic spread after the lung and liver.

Metastases are assumed to arise from venous tumour emboli, from the primary tumour or from prior disease spread to the regional lymph nodes or other metastases, e.g. in the lung. Venous embolisation of malignant cells is multifactorial but is particularly related to the vascularity of the primary tumour and/or access to a valveless venous plexus, e.g. Batson's vertebral plexus.

Bone metastasis is a relatively late occurrence in the natural history of malignant disease because the lungs trap most tumour emboli. It is recognised that bone metastases may occur without obvious evidence of pulmonary involvement due to:

1. Pulmonary lesions that are present but occult;
2. Transpulmonary spread of malignant cells;
3. Paradoxical embolisation via a patent foremen ovale; and
4. Retrograde venous embolism with involvement of the vertebral column.

Arguably, the incidence of truly occult pulmonary metastases is less these days due to the superior sensitivity of multidetector CT of the chest routinely used in cancer staging as compared with standard radiography or single slice CT employed in the past.

The most common primary malignancies metastasising to bone are carcinoma of the breast, bronchus, prostate, kidney and thyroid, making up over 80% of all patients with bone metastases. The overall incidence of bone metastases during life is uncertain and will depend on the sensitivity of the imaging technique employed. At the time of death the prevalence of bone metastases is approximately 80–85% for breast and prostate cancer, more variable for lung cancer with a quoted range of between 40 and 80%, 50–60% for thyroid cancer and 20–35% for renal cancer. With modern improved cancer management leading to longer survival times, bone metastases have become a fairly common occurrence in everyday medical practice.

Distribution of Bone Metastases

The commonest sites of metastatic involvement are those containing red bone marrow, explaining why the axial skeleton is affected more commonly than the appendicular skeleton in adults; hence, the predilection for the spine, pelvis, proximal femora and humeri, ribs, sternum and skull (Fig. 4-1). Spinal metastases occur most commonly in the thoracic vertebrae, but carcinomas arising

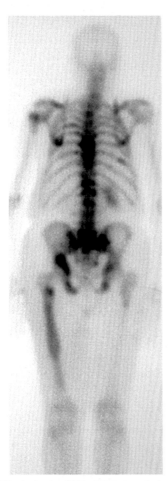

FIGURE 4-1 ■ Whole-body ⁹⁹ᵐTc-MDP (methylene diphosphonate) bone scintigram (posterior view) showing multiple regions of increased uptake due to prostatic carcinoma metastases. Involvement typically occurs in the spine, pelvis and ribs.

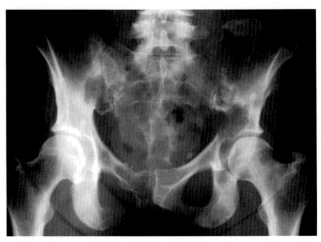

FIGURE 4-2 ■ AP radiograph of the pelvis showing multiple lytic breast metastases.

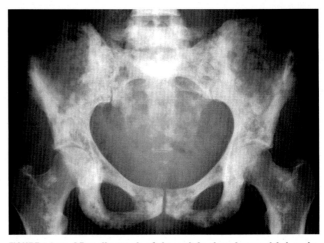

FIGURE 4-3 ■ AP radiograph of the pelvis showing multiple sclerotic breast metastases.

within the pelvis, particularly prostatic carcinoma, show a predilection for the lumbosacral spine.

Diagnosis of Bone Metastases

Clinical

Unexplained back or limb pain in a patient with a history of carcinoma may indicate a skeletal metastasis. Non-mechanical pain (i.e. bone pain at rest) is highly suggestive of tumour, be it primary or metastatic. A metastasis may present with a pathological fracture following minor trauma. Radiographs are necessary to reveal the pre-existing lesion. Elevation of the serum alkaline phosphatase is a non-specific finding and typically is not seen until multiple bone metastases have developed.

Radiological Features

Bone metastases may be lytic (most common) (Fig. 4-2), mixed lytic and sclerotic and predominantly sclerotic (Fig. 4-3). Small lytic lesions confined to the medullary bone can be difficult to identify on radiographs, particularly in complex anatomical areas such as the pelvis and

spine or where there is reduced bone density (osteopenia). It is much easier to detect a metastasis as and when there is evidence of cortical destruction. It is for this reason that vertebral metastases are frequently first detected on radiographs as showing destruction of the cortex of a pedicle even though cross-sectional imaging may reveal fairly extensive destruction of the medullary bone in the adjacent vertebral body (Fig. 4-4). As the destructive process increases, a soft-tissue mass may develop. A periosteal reaction may be seen but this is usually less pronounced than those seen in primary bone malignancies. Exceptions include some prostatic metastases and mucinous adenocarcinoma metastases from the colon. Some carcinomas, such as renal, almost always produce lytic metastases. Others, such as prostate, are most commonly osoteoblastic, while breast metastases may show a mixed appearance. It should be noted that the osteoblastic reaction reflects the response of the host bone to the metastasis rather than the production of tumour bone, which is a characteristic of osteosarcoma. Cortical-based metastases are less common than

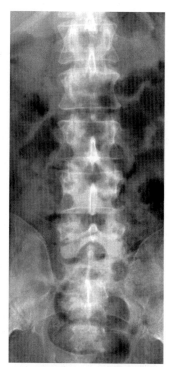

FIGURE 4-4 ■ **AP radiograph of the lumbar spine.** There is a renal metastasis destroying the left pedicle of the L1 vertebra.

medullary and tend to arise along the diaphyses of the long bones from lung, kidney and breast primaries (Fig. 4-5).

The importance of identifying multiple lesions cannot be overemphasised, as an individual metastasis may be indistinguishable from a primary malignant bone tumour. For this purpose, ^{99m}Tc-MDP bone scintigraphy is the most cost-effective method, although both whole-body MRI and ^{18}F-fluoride PET/CT are considered more sensitive. A variety of scintigraphic abnormalities are seen, with the most common being multiple foci of increased skeletal activity, predominantly in the axial skeleton (Fig. 4-1). Abnormal increased activity relies on an intact local blood supply and increased host bone osteoblastic activity. Metastases that have infarcted or stimulate no host osteoblastic response may appear as photopenic areas or 'cold spots', most commonly seen with larger renal metastases. Occasionally a combination of 'hot' and 'cold' lesions occurs. Diffuse osteoblastic metastatic disease, typically from breast or prostate carcinoma, may result in a 'superscan' appearance where there is generalised increase in skeletal activity with a relative paucity of renal activity.

It is important to recognise that not all foci of abnormally increased activity on bone scintigraphy, in a patient being investigated for suspected metastatic disease, need necessarily be due to metastases. Foci of activity in the ribs, particularly if contiguous, suggest old fractures, linear foci peripherally in the sacrum suggest insufficiency fractures and intense expanded foci of activity extending up to a joint margin may indicate Paget's disease. Any area of unexplained abnormal uptake should be correlated with further up-to-date imaging. Generally,

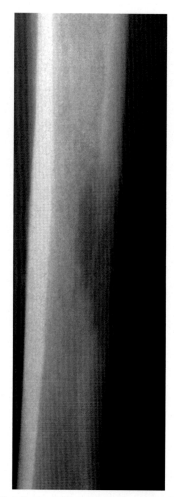

FIGURE 4-5 ■ **Detail of an AP radiograph of the tibia showing a cortically based metastasis from carcinoma of the bronchus.**

MRI is utilised as it is more sensitive than radiography, and more specific than scintigraphy. Most metastases are located within the medulla and show reduced signal intensity (SI) on T1-weighted sequences, with increased SI on T2-weighted or fat-suppressed sequences. The identification of a hyperintense 'halo' around a lesion is a feature highly suggestive of a metastasis on fluid-sensitive images. Both whole-body MRI and FDG-PET are being increasingly utilised in the detection and monitoring of bone metastases.[1,2] The efficacy of PET can be increased with fused anatomical imaging, e.g. PET/CT.[3]

Prostate. Prostatic metastases are typically osteoblastic (sclerotic) (Fig. 4-6) or mixed, with purely lytic lesions being very rare. Occasionally, long bone metastases may exhibit a prominent 'sunburst' periosteal reaction mimicking an osteosarcoma, a rare disease in this age group in the absence of Paget's disease or previous radiotherapy. Disseminated prostatic metastases may produce confluent sclerosis on radiographs, simulating other disorders such as myelofibrosis and Paget's disease, although the latter condition can usually be excluded by noting the absence of bony expansion. Assessment of the prostate serum antigen (PSA) level can be useful in determining the value of performing bone scintigraphy. If the PSA

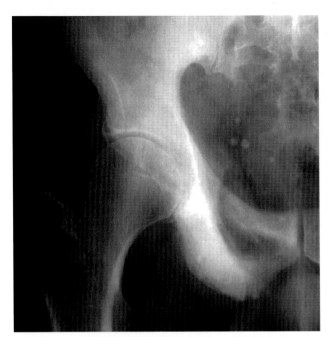

FIGURE 4-6 ■ AP radiograph of the hip showing a sclerotic prostatic metastasis in the ischium.

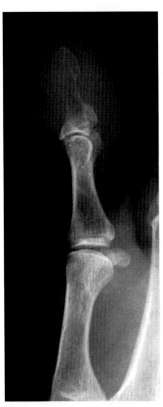

FIGURE 4-7 ■ Lateral radiograph of the thumb showing destruction of the terminal phalanx due to a bronchial carcinoma metastasis (acrometastasis).

level is <10 ng/mL the likelihood of positive bone scintigraphy is <1%. This increases to approximately 10% if the PSA level is 10–50 ng/mL and 50% with a PSA level >50 ng/mL. While ^{99m}Tc-MDP bone scintigraphy may be adequate for the initial identification of prostatic metastases, FDG-PET is preferred after treatment for distinguishing persistent active metastases from healing bone.

Breast. Most breast bone metastases are lytic (Fig. 4-2) but breast carcinoma is the commonest cause of osteoblastic metastases in women (Fig. 4-3). About 10% of metastases are purely osteoblastic and 10% mixed. Diffuse marrow infiltration may occur and only become radiographically visible when sclerosis develops after therapy. In this situation the sclerosis may be mistaken for disease progression rather than a response to treatment. Breast metastases have a predilection for the spine, pelvis and ribs. Patients may present with acute-onset vertebral collapse at one or more levels and positive neurology. In this clinical situation the differential diagnosis would include benign causes such as osteoporotic collapse and malignant causes such as metastases from other primaries, lymphoma and myeloma. Further investigation with MRI ± diffusion-weighted imaging would be mandatory. Bone scintigraphy is usually sufficient to confirm/exclude bone metastases when clinical or laboratory parameters are suspicious but after treatment, follow-up studies may show increased activity due to the 'flare phenomenon' secondary to the normal healing response of bone. Again, in this context FDG-PET may be preferred with increasing activity indicating a lack of response to treatment.

Lung. Lung metastasis to bone is common. Most spread to the axial skeleton and are typically lytic. Metastases to the hands and feet (acrometastases), although rare,

originate from a lung primary in approximately half of cases (Fig. 4-7).[4] Bronchogenic carcinoma is the commonest source of cortical-based metastases with large lesions showing the so-called 'cookie-bite' appearance (Fig. 4-5). It is also the commonest disorder associated with hypertrophic osteoarthropathy, formerly known as hypertrophic pulmonary osteoarthropathy. A single or multiple layer periosteal reaction along the distal long bones, including the hands and feet, characterises this condition. Bone scintigraphy will reveal symmetrical increased linear activity along the long bones, known as 'double stripe' or 'parallel tract' sign.

Kidney. Renal carcinoma is the commonest primary malignancy associated with solitary bone metastases. Solitary or multiple lesions are invariably lytic and may be expansile (blowout) and trabeculated. So-called expansile metastases may also be typically seen in thyroid metastases (Fig. 4-8) and less commonly in breast and lung. A similar radiographic appearance may be seen with plasmacytoma and, if subarticular, in a younger age group, giant cell tumour of bone. Renal metastases tend to be hypervascular, exhibiting multiple serpiginous signal voids within and around the periphery of the lesion on MRI.[5]

Melanoma. After extension to locoregional lymph nodes, malignant melanoma can spread to almost any part of the body, including the axial skeleton. It is important to appreciate that melanoma metastases may be

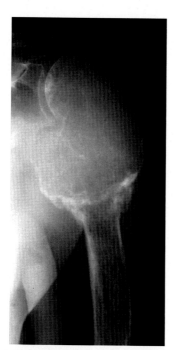

FIGURE 4-8 ■ **AP radiograph of the proximal humerus showing an expansile thyroid metastasis.**

TABLE 4-1 **Mirels' Rating System for Prediction of Pathological Fracture Risk of Metastases in Long Bones as Measured on Radiographs[6]**

Score	Site	Nature	Size[a]	Pain
1	Upper extremity	Blastic	$<\frac{1}{3}$	Mild
2	Lower extremity[b]	Mixed[c]	$\frac{1}{3}-\frac{2}{3}$	Moderate
3	Peritrochanteric	Lytic	$>\frac{2}{3}$	Severe

[a]Relative proportion of bone width involved with tumour.
[b]Non-perithrochanteric lower extremity.
[c]Mixed lytic and blastic.

clinically silent and that there can be a long latent period between treatment of the primary lesion and the development of the metastasis. Most bone metastases from melanoma are lytic. Melanin is paramagnetic and, depending on the concentration, the metastasis may show mild hyperintensity on T1-weighted MR images.

Radiological Investigation of Bone Metastases

When a known primary malignancy is established, the presence or absence of metastases is part of the routine surgical staging process. This will vary, depending on the nature of the primary and local/national guidelines. In most situations bone scintigraphy is adequate for assessing the whole skeleton (Fig. 4-1). Combining the study with SPECT may increase the sensitivity in detecting small lesions in anatomically complex areas such as the spine. Whole-body MRI may be preferred because of its increased sensitivity but it should be noted that if only coronal sequences are obtained both rib and spinal lesions may be overlooked.

When there is no history of prior malignancy then, in patients over 40 years of age, a CT study of the chest, abdomen and pelvis should be performed. Should the staging studies show the bone lesion to be solitary, then an image-guided needle biopsy will be required, irrespective of whether there is a documented prior history or current imaging evidence of a primary malignancy elsewhere. This is because the bone lesion need not necessarily be related to that other tumour and failure to establish the correct diagnosis could lead to inappropriate management prejudicial to the long-term prognosis for the patient. This biopsy should be performed so as to avoid contamination of uninvolved anatomical compartments in case the histology reveals a primary malignancy of bone rather than a metastasis. In cases with disseminated metastases to multiple organ systems, where palliative care is the only reasonable management, needle biopsy is arguably unnecessary. In patients with a suspected primary malignancy and bone metastases, a needle biopsy of the most accessible bone lesion may be the quickest and easiest way to establish a definitive tissue diagnosis.

An important cause of morbidity in patients with bone metastases is the development of pathological fractures. This is most common in the spine, with or without neurological compromise, and in the lower limbs because of weight-bearing. It is clearly advantageous for the patient if these debilitating fractures can be prevented with prophylactic fixation. In the long bones the Mirels' scoring system is widely employed to assess fracture risk (Table 4-1).[6]

In the past the identification of bone metastases usually meant an early demise for the patient; but nowadays modern therapies and improved surgical techniques are leading to longer survival times. Therefore, follow-up imaging to assess response of bone metastases to treatments is not uncommon. Such imaging can be difficult to interpret: while disease progression is usually obvious, it can be more problematic to confirm lack of progression. The 'flare phenomenon' on bone scintigraphy is an example where a good response to therapy may be misinterpreted as disease progression. It is also important to recognise that new bone lesions may not be further metastases but actually caused by the drugs administered. This includes bone infarction after chemotherapy and/or steroids and necrosis of the mandible and atypical stress fractures in the femora after bisphosphonate therapy.[7] It is likely that FDG-PET will have an increasing role in the assessment of the response of bone metastases to therapy.

Bone Metastases in Children

This is a distinctly less common occurrence than in adults. In the younger child the commonest disseminated neoplasms affecting bone are neuroblastoma and leukaemia, which may have identical radiographic appearances. The commonest paediatric soft-tissue sarcoma and also the commonest to metastasise to bone is rhabdomyosarcoma, with a 10% incidence identified at time of initial diagnosis. Retinoblastoma may involve bone by direct spread and blood-borne metastases. It is also one of a number of conditions associated with an increased incidence of osteosarcoma. Both osteosarcoma and Ewing sarcoma may present or develop local (skip) or distant bone metastases. The commonest intracranial neoplasm to metastasise to bone outside the skull is cerebellar medulloblastoma, typically after surgery to the primary tumour.

PRIMARY MALIGNANT NEOPLASMS OF BONE

Primary malignant tumours of the skeleton are rare, accounting for only 0.2% of all neoplasms, with an annual incidence of new diagnoses of approximately 1/100,000 population. Major advances in the past 40 years in chemotherapy and limb-salvage surgery have vastly improved the outcome, such that in specialist centres, the 5-year survival for appendicular osteosarcoma now exceeds 60%. The classification of these tumours, as described by the World Health Organisation, is based on their histopathological characteristics.[8] While the tumours themselves have remained unchanged over the years, the nomenclature has metamorphosed as successive generations of pathologists have attempted to refine and reclassify these disorders.

Radiographs remain of fundamental importance in the detection and diagnosis of a primary bone tumour, be it benign or malignant. Radiographic features suggestive of an aggressive and therefore more likely to be malignant lesion include a wide zone of transition (permeative or moth-eaten), an aggressive periosteal reaction (onion-skin, Codman angle or spiculated), cortical destruction and a soft-tissue mass.[9] Matrix mineralisation does not help to distinguish benign from malignant disorders but can be an indicator of the underlying histopathological origin, be it osteoid (i.e. bone-forming) or chondroid (i.e. cartilage-forming).

CHONDROID ORIGIN

Chondrosarcoma

Chondrosarcoma is a malignant cartilage-forming tumour accounting for 8–17% of all biopsied primary bone tumours and 20–25% of all biopsied malignant bone tumours. It is classified as central if arising within medullary bone (Fig. 4-9) and peripheral if arising from the surface of bone. It is further subclassified as primary if arising de novo or secondary if arising from a pre-existing bony lesion, usually an enchondroma (central type) or osteochondroma (peripheral type) either as a solitary occurrence or as part of the bone dysplasias of Ollier's disease (multiple enchondromatosis), Maffucci's syndrome (multiple enchondromatosis and soft-tissue angiomas) and hereditary multiple exostoses (diaphyseal aclasis) (Fig. 4-10). The incidence of malignant change in solitary enchondroma and osteochondroma is <1% and in hereditary multiple exostoses <5%. The incidence is somewhat higher, at approximately 20% in Ollier's disease and 30% in Maffucci's syndrome.

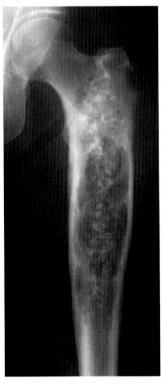

FIGURE 4-9 ■ **AP radiograph of the femur showing an extensive central chondrosarcoma with typical chondroid matrix, cortical expansion and thickening with endosteal scalloping.**

Chondrosarcoma is also classified according to its histological grade. These are defined as low grade (grade 1; 45–50% of cases), intermediate grade (grade 2; 30–40% of cases), high grade (grade 3; 10–25% of cases) and dedifferentiated, which refers to the development of areas of high-grade non-cartilaginous sarcoma within the chondrosarcoma (10% of cases), typically osteosarcoma or spindle cell sarcoma (Fig. 4-11).[10] Other distinct variants include mesenchymal and clear-cell chondrosarcoma.

Clinical Presentation

Most patients are above the age of 50 years, with the peak incidence in the fifth to seventh decades. Secondary chondrosarcoma tends to present at a slightly younger age in the fourth and fifth decades. Chondrosarcoma is sufficiently rare in children that the diagnosis should be seriously questioned if proffered by a pathologist based

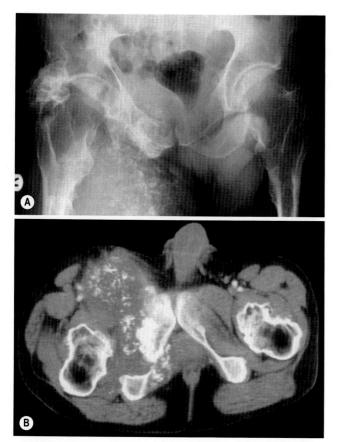

FIGURE 4-10 ■ (A) AP radiograph and (B) CT of the hips in a patient with hereditary multiple exostoses (diaphyseal aclasis). There is a large peripheral chondrosarcoma arising from the right pubis.

on a needle biopsy specimen. There is a minor male preponderance and the commonest site of occurrence is the pelvis (Fig. 4-10), proximal femur (Fig. 4-9) and proximal humerus. Approximately 9% of chondrosarcomas occur in the ribs, making this the most common primary malignancy, other than myeloma, to arise at this location. Chondrosarcomas in the hands and feet are rare in contradistinction to the high incidence of enchondromas at both these sites.

Imaging Features

The radiographic features of central chondrosarcoma are those of a lytic lesion, well-defined in low-grade cases and progressively increasingly ill-defined in higher-grade cases.[11,12] Chondroid calcification is visible in 75% cases, variously described as ring-and-arc, punctate, stippled or popcorn in appearance (Fig. 4-9). The relatively slow growth of the tumour allows for reactive change to occur in the adjacent normal bone. There is a combination of endosteal resorption producing endosteal scalloping and periosteal new bone formation. In time this leads to bony expansion with varying thickness of the replacement cortex. In the higher-grade cases, cortical destruction and soft-tissue extension reveal the aggressive nature of the process (Figs. 4.11A, 4.12A). CT can be helpful in

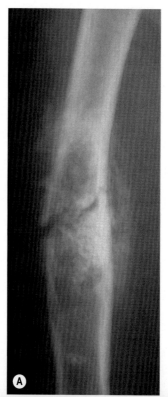

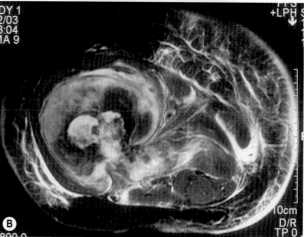

FIGURE 4-11 ■ (A) AP radiograph of the femur showing a pathological fracture through a dedifferentiated chondrosarcoma. (B) Axial T2-weighted fat-suppressed image showing soft-tissue extension with areas of low signal intensity indicative of malignant osteoid.

identifying occult chondroid matrix not visible on radiographs. MR imaging shows a typical hyperintense multilobular pattern on fluid-sensitive sequences with low signal intensity foci representing chondroid calcification on all pulse sequences (Fig. 4-12B). Most chondrosarcomas are poorly vacularised and enhancement after intravenous administration of a gadolinium chelate is limited, typically showing a peripheral or septal pattern. The identification on T2-weighted images of a mass of intermediate signal intensity adjacent to the hyperintense multilobular tumour is highly suggestive of dedifferentiation. Such areas should be targeted for image-guided

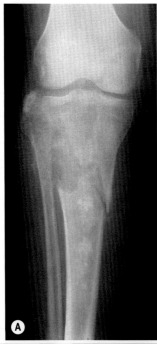

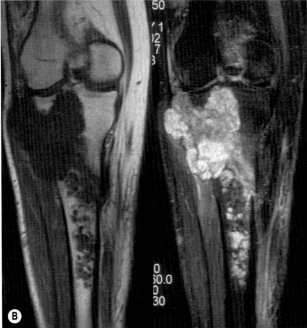

FIGURE 4-12 ■ (A) AP radiograph and (B) coronal T1-weighted and STIR images of the proximal tibia in a patient with Ollier's disease (multiple enchondromatosis). Typical features of benign enchondroma distally with an aggressive tumour destroying the cortex and soft-tissue extension proximally due to malignant transformation into a secondary central chondrosarcoma.

biopsy. A common diagnostic dilemma is the distinction of a low-grade chondrosarcoma from an enchondroma. This is an increasing problem with improved access to MR imaging. The incidence of 'incidental' central cartilage tumours around the knee in adults undergoing routine knee imaging is approximately 3%. There are no hard-and-fast-rules in this respect and the issue is compounded by the fact that pathologists often have as much

difficulty in the diagnosis of these borderline lesions as do the radiologists. Lesions in excess of 5 cm in length and with deep endosteal cortical scalloping (greater than two-thirds) are suggestive of chondrosarcoma as opposed to enchondroma. Bone scintigraphy cannot be reliably used to distinguish benign from malignant lesions, as up to 30% of enchondromas in adults may show some increased activity due to persistent endochondral ossification. However, as over 80% of chondrosarcomas show increased activity, normal background skeletal activity favours the diagnosis of enchondroma. Unenhanced and static contrast-enhanced MRI is also of limited value. Both dynamic contrast-enhanced MRI[13–15] and FDG-PET imaging have been claimed to be useful but many remain sceptical when the histological diagnosis, at least in low-grade lesions, remains somewhat subjective.

Identification of a secondary peripheral chondrosarcoma from an osteochondroma should be clinically suspected if pain develops or there is continued growth after skeletal maturity. Radiographic features of malignant change consist of destruction of part of the calcified cap or ossified stem of the osteochondroma with dispersal of the calcifications within a soft-tissue mass. The thickness of the cartilage cap cannot be reliably measured on radiographs but can be determined with ultrasound, CT or MRI. If the cartilage cap is less than 2 cm in thickness, then malignancy is unlikely. If it is greater than 2 cm, the likelihood of malignancy increases (Fig. 4-10B).[16] It is important that any measurement is made perpendicular to the bony component of the osteochondroma as tangential measurements from cross-sectional imaging may overestimate the thickness of the cartilage cap. Malignant transformation of an osteochondroma may be mimicked by other complications that are associated with the development of an overlying soft-tissue mass, including inflammatory bursa and pseudoaneurysm formation.[17,18]

Other Chondrosarcoma Variants

Periosteal Chondrosarcoma

Periosteal chondrosarcoma, also known as juxtacortical chondrosarcoma, is a rare tumour arising on the outer surface of long bones, commonly the metaphysis of the proximal humerus and distal femur. It is characterised by a cartilaginous mass usually greater than 5 cm in length with a variable degree of cartilage calcification. It can be distinguished from the other surface form of chondrosarcoma, the peripheral chondrosarcoma, by the lack of continuity with the underlying medullary bone.

Mesenchymal Chondrosarcoma

Mesenchymal chondrosarcoma occurs at a younger age than conventional chondrosarcoma, most commonly in the second and third decades. It is a high-grade malignancy comprising approximately 5% of all chondrosarcomas. It contains well-differentiated hyaline cartilage with more cellular malignant matrix than conventional chondrosarcoma. Radiographically, it is indistinguishable from central chondrosarcoma but there is a predilection for the mandible and ribs. Local recurrence and

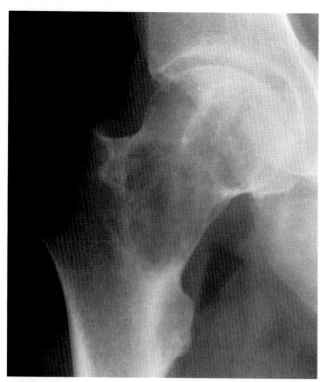

FIGURE 4-13 ■ **AP radiograph of the hip showing a clear-cell chondrosarcoma as a well-defined lytic lesion extending up to the articular margin.**

disseminated metastases occur early and more frequently than with conventional chondrosarcoma.

Clear Cell Chondrosarcoma

Clear cell chondrosarcoma accounts for approximately 2% of all chondrosarcomas. Most cases arise in the third to fifth decades. Radiographically, it appears as a well-defined, lytic subarticular lesion (Fig. 4-13). Matrix calcification is uncommon. It can mimic a chondroblastoma although the age group tends to be older. Growth tends to be slow and so it can be mistaken for a subchondral cyst/intraosseous ganglion.

OSTEOID ORIGIN

Osteosarcoma

Osteosarcoma is the commonest non-haematological primary bone malignancy, with an estimated annual incidence of approximately 4 per million population. Sixty per cent of cases present under the age of 25 years, with a minor male preponderance, and 75% of all cases are the high-grade medullary type frequently referred to as conventional osteosarcoma. The remainder are made up of other variants distinguished by site and histological grade.[19,20] Osteosarcoma may also occur secondary to Paget's disease, radiotherapy or as the dedifferentiated component of a lower-grade sarcoma such as chondrosarcoma and parosteal osteosarcoma. An association with several rare clinical syndromes is recognised. These include Li–Fraumeni syndrome, Rothmund–Thomson syndrome and familial retinoblastoma.

Central Osteosarcomas

Conventional Central Osteosarcoma

Clinical Presentation. This high-grade tumour is the commonest form of osteosarcoma. Approximately 80% present before 30 years of age, but it is uncommon under the age of 10 years and rare under 5 years. In the 10% of cases occurring over 40 years of age it is frequently secondary to a pre-existing disorder of bone, such as Paget's disease.

Presentation is typically with pain and a palpable mass not infrequently attributed to an unrelated previous incident of trauma. Osteosarcoma classically arises in the metaphyseal region of the growing end of long bones and about 50–75% are found in the distal femur or proximal tibia (Fig. 4-14). Diaphyseal osteosarcoma accounts for less than 10% cases. Other commonly affected sites include the proximal humerus and femur. Rarer sites include the ilium, ribs, scapula, vertebrae and jaw.

Imaging Features. Conventional osteosarcoma typically presents as a metaphyseal lesion with a moth-eaten or permeative pattern of bone destruction. The medullary component is lytic with a spectrum of tumour osteoid. This can produce mineralisation variously described as solid, amorphous, 'cloud-like' and 'ivory-like' (Fig. 4-14C). There is a spectrum of radiographic appearances from the entirely lytic (13% cases) through to the entirely sclerotic. Cortical destruction is common, resulting in the development of an eccentric extra-osseous soft-tissue mass, which commonly shows typical osseous amorphous matrix mineralisation. The density of the extraosseous mass is increased by periosteal new bone formation that is frequently complex, comprising perpendicular/spiculated, 'sunburst', lamellated/onion-skin with reactive Codman's angles at the margin of the tumour (Fig. 4-14).

Although MR imaging contributes little to the imaging diagnosis, it is mandatory for local surgical staging. It accurately defines the extent of the tumour within bone, in the soft tissues and any involvement of the adjacent joint and neurovascular structures. It is essential to have a least one MR sequence of the whole affected bone to confirm or exclude skip metastases (Fig. 4-15). These are foci of tumour, seen in approximately 5% of cases, arising within the same bone but separate from the main tumour or, on occasion, across the adjacent joint (trans-articular skip metastasis). Static sequences following the intravenous injection of a gadolinium chelate do not contribute to local staging. However, sequential dynamic contrast-enhanced sequences obtained pre- and post-adjuvant chemotherapy can be used to assess tumour response to therapy. FDG-PET has a complimentary role to other imaging in the initial staging of osteosarcoma but has an established role in the evaluation of response to adjuvant chemotherapy and for recurrent disease, both locally and remote. The natural history of osteosarcoma is for haematogenous spread with the production of pulmonary metastases. These are typically peripheral, may be mineralised and, rarely, may result in chronic pneumothorax.

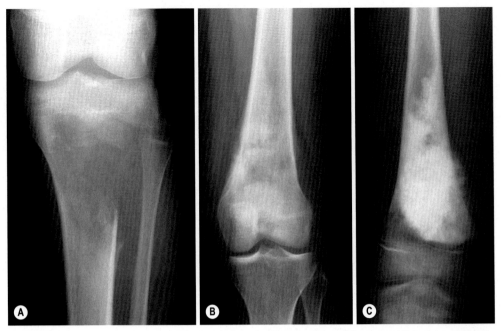

FIGURE 4-14 ■ AP radiographs of three cases of conventional central osteosarcoma arising around the knee: (A) lytic with a Codman angle distally; (B) mixed pattern with lysis and minor malignant osteoid with a lamellar (onion skin) periosteal reaction; and (C) sclerotic with dense amorphous malignant osteoid.

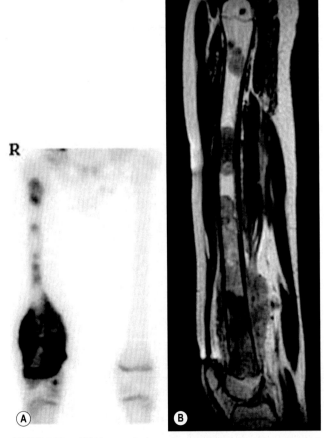

FIGURE 4-15 ■ (A) Bone scintigraphy and (B) sagittal T2-weighted MR images showing a large primary osteosarcoma of the distal femur with multiple proximal skip metastases.

If sufficiently large, the pulmonary metastases may show increased uptake on bone scintigraphy.

Other Varieties of Central Osteosarcoma. Primary multicentric osteosarcoma is the identification of multiple foci of intramedullary osteosarcoma in the absence of pulmonary metastases. It may be either synchronous or metachronous in presentation. The synchronous type typically consists of mutiple sclerotic metaphyseal lesions developing simultaneously, usually in children or adolescents. In the metachronous type, presentation is with a solitary lytic or sclerotic lesion in a long or flat bone with the development of a second or multiple lesions after a period of greater than 5 months. Some authorities question whether these lesions are truly multiple primaries or an unusual subset of metastatic disease.[21] Suffice to say that the prognosis for the synchronous manifestation is dismally similar to that of the patient presenting with metastatic disease, whereas the metachronous picture can be associated with a better outcome.

Telangiectatic osteosarcoma accounts for approximately 5% of all osteosarcomas and is twice as common in male patients, with a mean age at presentation of 24 years. It is characterised by the formation of multiple blood-filled cavities and hence may be mistaken for an aneurysmal bone cyst (ABC) on both imaging and histology. The femur, tibia and humerus are the most commonly involved bones. Radiographs show a predominantly lytic lesion ± bone expansion.[22] MR imaging reveals multiple fluid–fluid levels (Fig. 4-16) but the identification of solid areas within the tumour on post-contrast-enhanced sequences helps to differentiate telangiectatic osteosarcoma from an ABC.

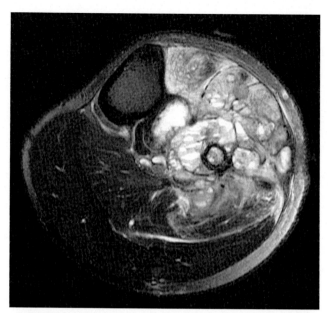

FIGURE 4-16 ■ Axial T2-weighted fat-suppressed image showing a large telangiectatic osteosarcoma arising in the proximal fibula. There are multiple cystic/haemorrhagic areas within the tumour containing fluid–fluid levels.

Small cell osteosarcoma accounts for approximately 1.5% of osteosarcomas. It is a histological variant but tends to show imaging features identical to those of conventional osteosarcoma.

Low-grade central osteosarcoma accounts for approximately 1% of cases of osteosarcoma. As the name implies it is a relatively indolent lesion affecting mainly the femur and tibia. It occurs in a slightly older age group than conventional osteosarcoma, with a mean age at presentation of 34 years. Four radiographic patterns have been described: lytic with coarse trabeculation; predominantly lytic; densely sclerotic; and mixed lytic and sclerotic. The imaging differential diagnosis includes benign fibro-osseous lesions such as fibrous dysplasia.

Surface Osteosarcomas. This designation refers to a group of tumours that arise from the surface of bone and includes parosteal, periosteal and high-grade surface osteosarcoma. All three types account for less than 10% of all osteosarcoma cases.

Parosteal Osteosarcoma. This is the commonest surface osteosarcoma and accounts for approximately 5% of all osteosarcomas. It is a low-grade malignancy, with 60% cases arising on the posterior aspect of the distal femur (Fig. 4-17) and less commonly the proximal humerus and tibia. It occurs at a slightly older age group than conventional osteosarcoma, with most patients affected in the third and fourth decades. The prognosis is excellent, with an over 90% 5-year survival unless there has been dedifferentiation to a high-grade osteosarcoma that occurs in approximately 20% of cases. The characteristic radiographic feature is of a densely sclerotic mass arising on and partially enveloping the posterior distal femoral metaphysis (Fig. 4-17A). Cross-sectional imaging will show that the mass is in part adherent to the underlying cortex with the more peripheral component

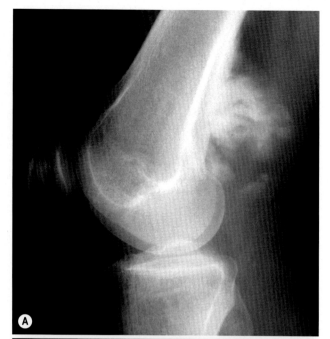

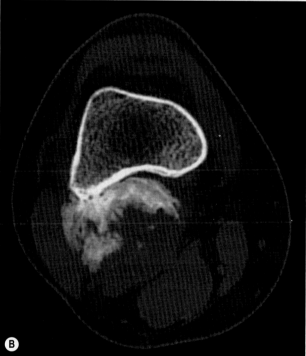

FIGURE 4-17 ■ (A) Lateral radiograph showing a sclerotic parosteal osteosarcoma arising on the posterior surface of the distal femoral metaphysis and (B) CT confirming the malignant osteoid attached in part to the underlying femoral cortex.

separated from the cortex by a thin radiolucent line (Fig. 4-17B). Medullary invasion may be seen in approximately 15% of cases. MRI typically shows the main lesion to be of low signal intensity on all sequences due to the sclerotic nature of the tumour. Should foci of intermediate T1- or increased T2-weighted signal intensity be identified at the periphery of the lesion, dedifferentiation should be considered and needle biopsy directed to these potentially higher-grade areas.[23]

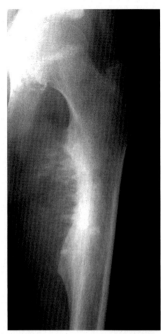

FIGURE 4-18 ■ **AP radiograph showing an extensive spiculated periosteal reaction from a periosteal osteosarcoma of the proximal femur.**

Periosteal Osteosarcoma. This intermediate-grade sarcoma accounts for less than 2% of all osteosarcomas. Its peak incidence is in the second and third decades with a slight male preponderance. It most commonly arises from the proximal tibial or distal femoral diaphyses. Two radiographic patterns may be seen; a surface lesion with cortical thickening or erosion and a perpendicular ('hair-on-end') periosteal reaction (Fig. 4-18) or a thin peripheral shell simulating a periosteal chondroma.[24] MR imaging may show lobulated hyperintensity on T2-weighted images, reflecting the chondroblastic nature of the tumour. Reactive marrow signal changes may be present but true marrow invasion is rare.

High-Grade Surface Osteosarcoma. This is the rarest of the surface osteosarcomas, accounting for less than 1% of all osteosarcomas. It has the same histological features as conventional central osteosarcoma. The imaging features can be similar to that of periosteal osteosarcoma but more aggressive in that the tumour is usually larger and there is a greater degree of cortical destruction and medullary extension (Fig. 4-19).

Secondary Osteosarcoma. Approximately 5–7% of osteosarcomas are secondary due to malignant transformation in a pre-existing bone lesion. Typical examples are in Paget's disease and following radiotherapy. Rarer examples include medullary infarction, fibrous dysplasia, osteogenesis imperfecta (OI) and chronic osteomyelitis. Care should be taken not to misinterpret hyperplastic callus formation well recognised in OI with malignant osteoid production.

Paget's Sarcoma. Of sarcomas arising in Paget's disease, 50% are osteosarcomas with the remainder spindle cell/pleomorphic sarcomas and uncommonly chondrosarcoma. Many osteosarcomas arising after the age of 50 years are secondary to Paget's disease of bone.[25]

There is a rare association between Paget's disease and giant cell tumour of bone that can be multifocal with a predilection for the maxillofacial skeleton. Malignant change to a sarcoma has been reported in 3–14% of patients with Paget's disease but the true prevalence is likely to be under 1% if one takes into account asymptomatic undiagnosed cases in the population. The incidence increases in older patients and the more extensive that Paget's disease is, although it can occur in monostotic disease. There is a decreasing incidence of Paget's disease worldwide and as a consequence the incidence of Paget's sarcoma also appears to be declining.[26] The sex incidence of Paget's sarcoma is similar to that of the primary disease, with men affected twice as often as women. Radiologically, the commonest sites for Paget's sarcoma are the pelvis, femur and humerus (Fig. 4-20). The spine is typically spared. Permeative bone destruction with cortical destruction and evidence of a soft-tissue mass are common features, best shown with CT and MRI (Fig. 4-21). MRI in uncomplicated Paget's disease will tend to show preservation of the medullary fat signal on T1-weighted images. Loss of the fat signal may indicate tumour infiltration as well as other complications such as pseudofracture formation with haemorrhage and oedema.[27] Bone scintigraphy is relatively insensitive to malignant transformation due to the avid, frequently multifocal, uptake of radionuclide in the underlying Paget's disease. Paradoxically, although most sarcomas are osteosarcomas, they may appear as relatively photopenic (cold) on bone scintigraphy (Fig. 4-21B). The prognosis for Paget's sarcoma is extremely poor, with most patients succumbing within a year of diagnosis. This is in part due to the late presentation of the disease, not infrequently already with pulmonary metastases, but also many of the affected patients are of an age that are too frail to undergo prolonged chemotherapy and major surgery. It is important to recognise that other malignancies, such as metastasis, lymphoma and myeloma, may occur in coincidence with Paget's disease, thereby mimicking sarcomatous transformation. Another mimicker of sarcoma is the rare pseudosarcoma, which may also present with a mineralised extraosseous mass.[28] Biopsy is therefore required to make the definitive diagnosis of Paget's sarcoma.

Post-Radiation Sarcoma. Post-radiation sarcoma (PRS), formerly known as radiation-induced sarcoma, refers to bone and soft-tissue sarcomas that develop following previous radiotherapy. They account for 0.5–5% of all sarcomas and the criteria for diagnosis include the following:[29]

1. A history of prior radiation therapy;
2. The development of a neoplasm within the radiation field typically peripheral;
3. A latent period of at least 3–4 years; and
4. Histological proof of a sarcoma, which differs significantly from the originally treated tumour.

The treated tumours most commonly associated with the development of PRS are breast carcinoma, lymphoma, head and neck and gynaecological malignancies. This accounts for the increased incidence in women. The mean age at presentation is in the sixth decade, with a mean latent period before development of PRS of 15

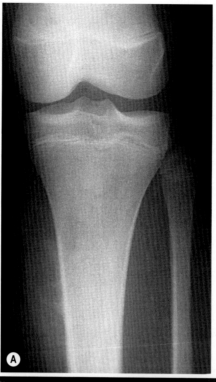

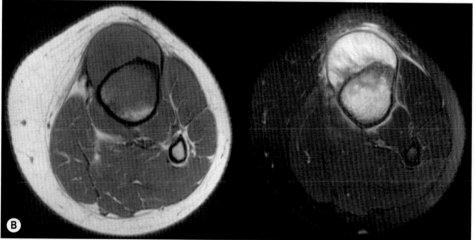

FIGURE 4-19 ■ (A) AP radiograph of a high-grade surface osteosarcoma of the tibia with a spiculated periosteal reaction. (B) Axial T1- and T2-weighted fat-suppressed images showing both the extra and intraosseous components.

years. PRS may be seen in younger individuals, as more paediatric patients undergoing radiotherapy are long-term survivors of their first malignancy. It is considered that a minimum dose of 30 Gy is required to induce a PRS and that the concurrent administration of chemotherapy may increase the risk. The commonest PRS is osteosarcoma, followed by spindle cell sarcoma. The commonest sites are the pelvic and shoulder girdle bones. Typical radiographic features include permeative bone destruction (>80% of cases), soft-tissue mass (>90% of cases) and varying degrees of matrix mineralisation and periosteal reaction (Fig. 4-22).[30] There may be evidence of underlying radiation change including patchy osteopenia, dystrophic calcification and radionecrosis (Fig. 4-23). The MRI appearances of PRS are those of an aggressive tumour destroying bone with soft-tissue extension of intermediate signal intensity on T1-weighted and hyperintense and heterogeneous signal intensity on T2-weighted images. As with Paget's sarcoma, the prognosis for PRS is poor.

FIBROUS ORIGIN

Malignant bone tumours of fibrous origin are classified histologically into those of fibrogenic (e.g. fibrosarcoma) and fibrohistiocytic (e.g. malignant fibrous histiocytoma/ MFH) origin. The nomenclature of fibrous tumours has changed over the years as pathologists have attempted to redefine these tumours. The terms fibrosarcoma and

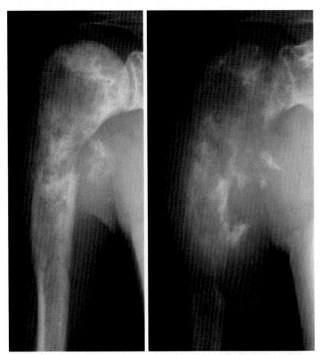

FIGURE 4-20 ■ AP radiographs of the proximal humerus obtained 6 weeks apart showing a rapidly progressive Paget's osteosarcoma.

MFH are less commonly used these days in favour of spindle cell sarcoma and more recently undifferentiated pleomorphic sarcoma (UPS). Because of the considerable overlap of these conditions they are considered as a single entity for the purposes of this chapter. They account for approximately 5% of all malignant bone tumours and occur in adults from 20 to 50 years of age. Up to 20% of cases can present with a pathological fracture. The lesions most commonly affect the long bones (70%), with 50% arising in the lower limb, particularly around the knee. On radiographs the tumours appear aggressive with cortical destruction but little periosteal new bone formation (Fig. 4-24).[31] In the younger age group they can be mistaken for a lytic osteosarcoma; in the third and fourth decades, if subarticular, a giant cell tumour and in the older age group a metastasis. Approximately 25% of cases arise in a pre-existing lesion, notably Paget's disease, post-radiotherapy, bone infarction (Fig. 4-24),[32] dedifferentiated chondrosarcoma, fibrous dysplasia[33] and chronic sinus tracts in osteomyelitis.[34]

MARROW TUMOURS

Malignancies arising from the marrow elements of bone include a group of malignant small round cell tumours comprising Ewing sarcoma, primitive neuroectodermal tumour (PNET), lymphoma, metastatic neuroblastoma and leukaemia, and plasmacytoma/myeloma. The imaging features of metastatic neuroblastoma, leukaemia and plasmacytoma/myeloma are covered in relevant sections elsewhere.

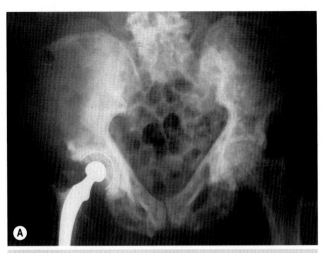

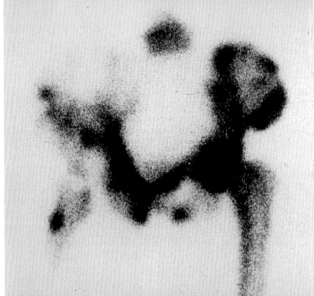

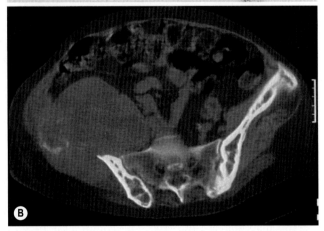

FIGURE 4-21 ■ (A) AP radiograph and (B) frontal image of bone scintigraphy and CT of the pelvis. There is extensive Paget's disease of the pelvis with a large Paget's osteosarcoma destroying the right ilium. The sarcoma appears relatively osteopenic on the scintigraphic image.

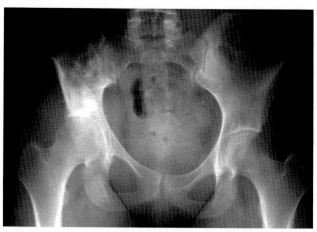

FIGURE 4-22 ■ AP radiograph showing a post-radiation osteosarcoma arising in the right ilium. There is malignant osteoid extending into the soft tissues laterally. The pelvic deformity and mild hypoplasia of the right ilium is secondary to radiotherapy in childhood as part of the treatment for a Wilms' tumour.

Ewing's Sarcoma and Primitive Neuroectodermal Tumour (PNET)

Both are malignant round cell tumours with varying degrees of neuroectodermal differentiation that exhibit similar imaging features and on cytogenetic analysis show specific constant reciprocal translocation between chromosomes 11 and 22. They account for approximately 8% of primary malignant bone tumours, with Ewing's sarcoma the second most common bone sarcoma in children after osteosarcoma. As many as 75% of patients are under the age of 20 years at presentation, most between 5 and 15 years, and 90% are under 30 years. The male-to-female patient ratio is 2:1 and 95% occur in Caucasians. Characteristically, presentation is with localised pain and swelling. The presence of systemic symptoms, including pyrexia and an elevated serum ESR, can simulate infection and may indicate disseminated disease. Usually a single bone is involved, but multiple lesions occur at presentation in 10% of cases and commonly later in the disease as Ewing's sarcoma readily metastasises to bone. In contradistinction to other bone sarcomas, most cases show involvement of the diaphyseal (35%) or the metadiaphyseal (60%) regions of a long bone and are typically central/medullary in origin (Fig. 4-25). The bones most commonly affected in order of frequency are

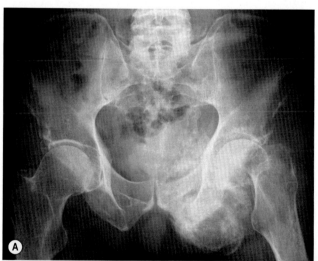

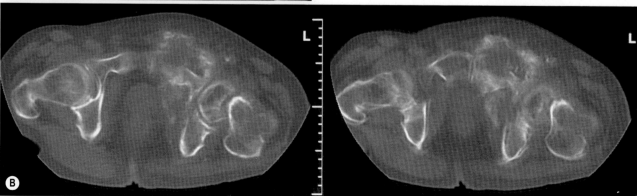

FIGURE 4-23 ■ (A) AP radiograph and (B) CT of the pelvis in a male patient 6 years following surgery and radiotherapy for a rectal carcinoma. There are three pathologies present. A post-radiation osteosarcoma arising from the left pubis, osteonecrosis with an ununited fracture of the femoral neck and a tumour distally in the left femoral neck which could have been a further sarcoma but biopsy proved it to be metastatic.

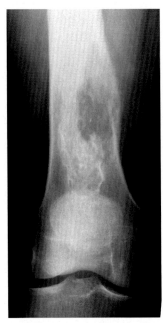

FIGURE 4-24 ■ **AP radiograph of the knee showing an undifferentiated pleomorphic sarcoma arising in association with medullary infarction in the distal femur.**

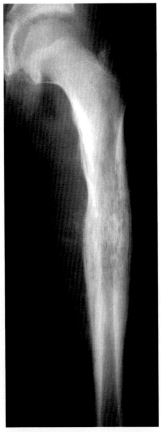

FIGURE 4-25 ■ **AP radiograph of an Ewing's sarcoma.** Typical features include a central diaphyseal location, permeative bone destruction, a lamellar (onion skin) periosteal reaction with spiculation medially.

the femur and humerus (31%), the pelvic bones (21%—most commonly the ilium) and ribs (<8%). The distal appendicular skeleton, including the hands and feet, is involved in 27% of cases. The Askin tumour is a rare PNET of the chest wall, occurring in children and young adults.[35]

Imaging Features

The radiographic features of Ewing's sarcoma are those of a permeative destructive lesion with a wide zone of transition (Fig. 4-25).[36] The most aggressive lesions may be difficult to identify on radiographs particularly if presentation is early. Soft-tissue extension is evident in 80% of cases. The classic multilamellar ('onion skin') periosteal reaction is uncommon. An interrupted periosteal reaction (Codman angle) is seen at the margins of the tumour in 27% of cases. A vertical 'hair-on-end'/spiculated periosteal reaction is also classic of Ewing's sarcoma seen in 50% of cases but can also be seen in osteosarcoma (Fig. 4-25). Occasionally, Ewing's sarcoma shows a mixed or mainly sclerotic appearance, especially in the flat bones and spine, thereby again mimicking an osteosarcoma (Fig. 4-26). This can be due to a combination of reactive sclerosis and visualisation of a spiculated periosteal reaction end on and is not due to tumour bone as malignant osteoid production is not a feature of this particular tumour. 'Saucerisation' of the outer bone cortex with a soft-tissue mass and eccentric lesions with a relatively small intraosseous component probably represent the rarer periosteal variant of Ewing's sarcoma. The radiographic differential diagnosis can include osteomyelitis, Langerhans cell histiocytosis and stress fracture. MRI accurately defines the medullary infiltration and soft-tissue extension that is of intermediate signal intensity on T1-weighted and intermediate/high signal intensity on T2-weighted and STIR sequences relative to skeletal muscle (Fig. 4-27). Skip metastases

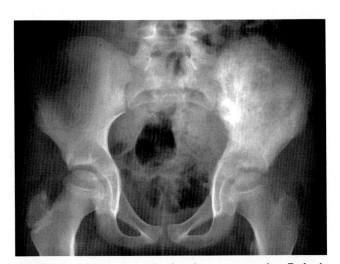

FIGURE 4-26 ■ **AP radiograph showing an extensive Ewing's sarcoma of the left ilium.** The increased density mimics an osteosarcoma and is due to reactive sclerosis and end-on periosteal new bone formation and not malignant osteoid.

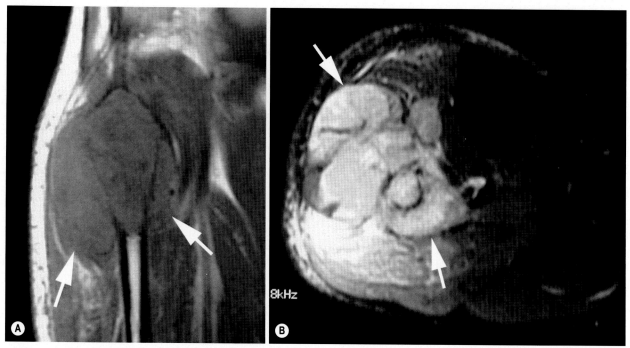

FIGURE 4-27 ■ **Ewing sarcoma of the proximal fibula.** (A) Coronal T1-weighted spin-echo and (B) axial STIR MR images show a large extraosseous mass (arrows).

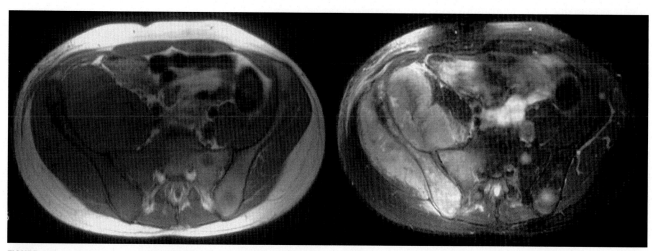

FIGURE 4-28 ■ Axial T1- and T2-weighted fat-suppressed images at initial presentation showing a primary Ewing's sarcoma infiltrating the right ilium with a large intra- and extrapelvic soft-tissue mass. There is also evidence of disseminated disease with foci in the sacrum and left ilium.

(12%) and distant metastases (<20%) in lungs and bone may be identified on initial imaging performed for surgical staging (Fig. 4-28). FDG-PET is more sensitive than bone scintigraphy in the detection of osseous metastases with a performance similar to that of whole-body MRI. FDG-PET may also be used in the assessment of response to adjuvant chemotherapy and detection of recurrence.

NOTOCHORDAL ORIGIN

Chordoma

Chordoma is a low-to-intermediate grade malignant tumour originating from ectopic cellular remnants of the notochord and as such arises from the midline of the axial skeleton. It accounts for 2–4% of all primary malignant bone tumours. Chordoma is the second commonest primary malignancy of the spine and accounts for over 50% of primary sacral tumours. The tumour has a predilection for the sacrococcygeal (50%) and clival (40%) regions, with other areas of the spine rarely involved. They most commonly present between 50 and 70 years of age with men more frequently affected in the older ages, particularly in the sacral region. Chordomas tend to be slow growing and symptoms of pain and related to pressure effects on adjacent structures are often prolonged before the tumour is detected. It is easy to overlook all but the largest of chordomas on radiographs of the pelvis or lumbosacral spine. Large tumours show bone destruction with occasional amorphous calcification. The soft-tissue mass is readily identified on CT or MRI extending anteriorly into the pelvis (Fig. 4-29). The midline origin of the tumour is a useful feature distinguishing it from other sacral tumours such as chondrosarcoma and metastases. The MRI features of intermediate-to-low signal intensity on T1-weighted and high signal on T2-weighted sequences are non-specific. A lobulated hyperintense pattern on T2-weighted images is suggestive of chordoma but can also mimic chondrosarcoma, as does septal enhancement following administration of a gadolinium chelate.[37] Wide excision is the treatment of choice, with radiotherapy reserved for inoperable cases or where wide resection is not possible.[38] Local recurrence, often multifocal, can be seen in up to 40% of cases presumed due to implantation at the time of surgery. Distant metastases are uncommon and death usually occurs due to complications from local extension of the disease. A benign counterpart of chordoma has recently been described, variously termed giant notochordal rest or benign notochord cell tumour.[39] These are benign non-progressive lesions arising at the same sites as chordoma. Whether this condition is a precursor of classic chordoma remains controversial.

MISCELLANEOUS TUMOURS

Malignant Vascular Tumours

Primary malignant vascular tumours of bone are rare. The terminology of endothelial tumours is somewhat confusing. Simplistically, there is a spectrum from the low-grade haemangioendothelioma through the extremely rare low-to-intermediate grade haemangiopericytoma to the highly malignant angiosarcoma. The radiographic appearances reflect the biological activity of the tumours from well-defined lytic lesions with no surrounding sclerosis in the low-grade to the permeative bone destruction in the high-grade lesions.[40,41] One important diagnostic feature seen in 25–40% of cases is a multifocal distribution (Fig. 4-30).[42] This is frequently confined to one limb (monomelic) but can be disseminated throughout the skeleton, thereby mimicking metastatic disease.

Adamantinoma

Adamantinoma of long bones is a rare tumour accounting for <0.5% of all primary malignant bone tumours. Although it has some histological resemblance to maxillofacial adamantinoma (ameloblastoma) the two conditions are not related. Most cases in the long bones occur between 10 and 50 years of age, with an average age of

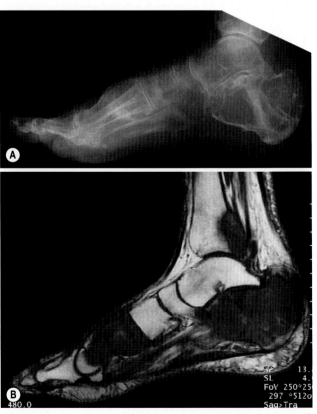

FIGURE 4-30 ■ (A) Lateral radiograph and (B) sagittal T1-weighted image of the foot showing multifocal low-grade haemangioendotheliomas involving the first metatarsal, calcaneus and distal tibia.

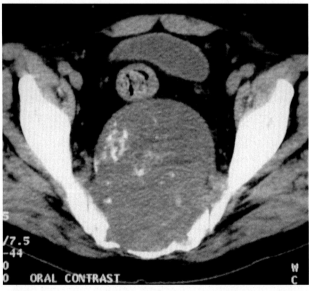

FIGURE 4-29 ■ **Sacral chordoma shown on axial CT as a predominantly lytic mass with foci of calcification.** The mass is shown to have considerable anterior extension into the pelvis.

marrow extension in 60% of cases, and extraosseous extension and multifocal distribution in 30% cases.[43] It is a locally aggressive tumour with a tendency to recur if incompletely removed. Metastases to the lung have been reported in approximately 10% of cases. The imaging appearances of adamantinoma can be indistinguishable from osteofibrous dysplasia, a benign tumour also with a predilection for the anterior tibial diaphysis. Histological similarities also exist between the two conditions, leading to the concept that osteofibrous dysplasia may be a precursor of adamantinoma. However, longitudinal studies have failed to show progression of osteofibrous dysplasia to adamantinoma. Another suggestion is that the two conditions represent the benign and malignant ends of a spectrum of the same condition.[44]

REFERENCES

1. Kwee TC, Takahara T, Katahira K, Nakanishi K. Whole-body MRI for detecting bone marrow metastases. PET Clinics 2010; 5(3):297–310.
2. Costelloe CM, Chuang HH, Madewell JE. FDG PET for the detection of bone metastases: sensitivity, specificity and comparison with other imaging modalities. PET Clinics 2010;5(3):281–96.
3. Cook JR. [18]Fluoride PET and PET/CT Imaging of skeletal metastases. PET Clinics 2010;5(3):275–80.
4. Flynn CJ, Danjoux C, Wong J, et al. Two cases of acrometastasis to the hands and review of the literature. Curr Oncol 2008; 15(5):51–5.
5. Choi JA, Lee KH, Jun WS, et al. Osseous metastasis from renal cell carcinoma: 'flow-void' sign at MR imaging. Radiology 2003; 228(3):629–34.
6. Mirels H. Metastatic disease in long bones. A proposed scoring system for diagnosing impending pathological fractures. Clin Orthop Rel Res 1989;249:256–64.
7. Chang ST, Tenforde AS, Grimsrud CD, et al. Atypical femur fractures among breast cancer and multiple myeloma patients receiving intravenous bisphosphonate therapy. Bone 2012;51(3):524–7.
8. WHO. World Health Organisation Classification of Tumours of Soft Tissue and Bone. 4th ed. Lyon: International Agency for Research on Cancer, IARC Press; 2013.
9. Kricun ME. Radiographic evaluation of solitary bone lesions. Orthop Clin North Am 1983;14:39–64.
10. Littrell LA, Wenger DE, Wold LE, et al. Radiographic, CT and MR imaging features of dedifferentiated chondrosarcomas: a retrospective review of 174 de novo cases. Radiographics 2004;24(5): 1397–409.
11. Murphey MD, Walker EA, Wilson AJ, et al. From the archives of the AFIP: imaging of primary chondrosarcoma: radiologic–pathologic correlation. Radiographics 2003;23(5):1245–78.
12. Douis H, Saifuddin A. The imaging of cartilaginous bone tumours. II. Chondrosarcoma. Skeletal Radiol 2012;42(5):611–26.
13. Geirnaerdt MJ, Hogendoorn PC, Bloem JL, et al. Cartilaginous tumors: fast contrast-enhanced MR imaging. Radiology 2000; 214(2):539–46.
14. Skeletal Lesions Interobserver Correlation among Expert Diagnosticians (SLICED) Study Group. Reliability of histopathologic and radiologic grading of cartilaginous neoplasms in long bones. J Bone Joint Surg Am 2007;89(10):2113–23.
15. Eefting D, Schrage YM, Geirnaerdt MJ, et al. Assessment of interobserver variability and histologic parameters to improve reliability in classification of central cartilaginous tumors. Am J Surg Path 2009;33(1):50–7.
16. Bernard SA, Murphey MD, Flemmin DJ, Kransdorf MJ. Improved differentiation of benign osteochondromas from secondary chondrosarcomas with standardized measurement of cartilage cap at CT and MR imaging. Radiology 2010;255(3):857–65.
17. Murphey MD, Choi JJ, Kransdorf MJ, et al. Imaging of osteochondroma: variants and complications with radiologic–pathologic correlation. Radiographics 2000;20(5):1407–34.
18. Douis H, Saifuddin A. The imaging of cartilaginous bone tumours. I. Benign lesions. Skeletal Radiol 2012;41:1195–212.

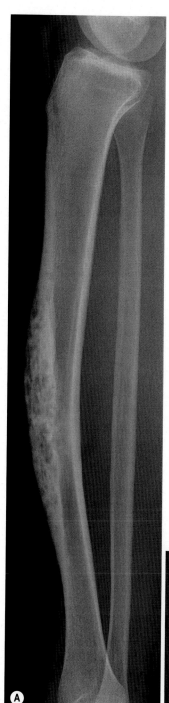
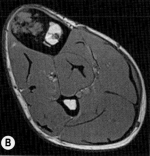

FIGURE 4-31 ■ (A) Lateral radiograph and (B) axial T1-weighted image showing an adamantinoma. Typical features include the anterior, diaphyseal location arising in the tibia.

35 years. There is a slight male preponderance but a higher female incidence is found at the younger end of the age range. Patients typically present with local pain and tenderness of several months to several year' duration. Ninety per cent of cases arise in the tibia, mostly in the mid-diaphysis, but almost as commonly towards either meta-diaphysis. The typical radiographic appearances are those of multiple well-defined lucencies with interspersed sclerosis eccentrically originating in the anterior cortex of the tibia (Fig. 4-31). MRI shows

19. Murphey MD, Robbin MR, McRae GA, et al. The many face of osteosarcoma. Radiographics 1997;17(5):1205–31.

20. Yarmish G, Klein MJ, Landa J, et al. Imaging characteristics of primary osteosarcoma: nonconventional types. Radiographics 2010;30(6):1653–72.

21. Daffner RH, Kennedy SL, Fox KR, et al. Synchronous multicentric osteosarcoma: the case for metastases. Skeletal Radiol 1997;26:569–78.

22. Discepola F, Powell TI, Nahal A. Telangiectatic osteosarcoma: radiologic and pathologic findings. Radiographics 2009;29(3):380–3.

23. Dönmez FY, Tüzün U, Basaran C, et al. MRI findings in parosteal osteosarcoma: correlation with histolopathology. Diagn Interv Radiol 2008;14(3):142–52.

24. Murphey MD, Jelinek JS, Temple HT, et al. Imaging of periosteal osteosarcoma: radiologic–pathologic correlation. Radiology 2004;233:129–38.

25. Lopez C, Thomas DV, Davies AM. Neoplastic transformation in Paget's disease of bone: pictorial review. Eur Radiol 2003;13:L151–63.

26. Mangham DC, Davie MW, Grimer RJ. Sarcoma arising in Paget's disease of bone: declining incidence and increasing age at presentation. Bone 2009;44(3):431–6.

27. Whitten CR, Saifuddin A. MRI of Paget's disease of bone. Clin Radiol 2003;58(10):763–9.

28. Tins BJ, Davies AM, Mangham DC. MR imaging in pseudosarcoma in Paget's disease of bone: a report of two cases. Skeletal Radiol 2001;30(3):161–5.

29. Sheppard DG, Libshitz HI. Post-radiation sarcomas: a review of the clinical and imaging features in 63 cases. Clin Radiol 2001;56(1):22–9.

30. O'Regan K, Hall M, Jagannathan J, et al. Imaging of radiation-associated sarcoma. Am J Roentgenol 2011;197:30–6.

31. Murphey MD, Gross TM, Rosenthal HG. From the archives of the AFIP. Musculoskeletal malignant fibrous histiocytoma: radiologic–pathologic correlation. Radiographics 1994;14(4):807–26.

32. Domson GF, Shahlaee A, Reith JD, et al. Infarct-associated bone sarcomas. Clin Orthop Relat Res 2009;467(7):1820–5.

33. Hoshi M, Matsumoto S, Manabe J, et al. Malignant change secondary to fibrous dysplasia. Int J Clin Oncol 2006;11(3):229–35.

34. Zlowodzki M, Allen B, Schreibman KL, et al. Case reports: malignant fibrous histiocytoma of bone arising in chronic osteomyelitis. Clin Orthop Relat Res 2005;439:269–73.

35. Sallustio G, Pironti T, Lasorella A, et al. Diagnostic imaging of PNET of the chest wall (Askin tumour). Pediatr Radiol 1998;28:697–702.

36. Kransdorf MJ, Smith SE. Lesions of unknown histiogenesis: Langerhans cell histiocytosis and Ewing sarcoma. Semin Musculoskelet Radiol 2000;4:1123–6.

37. Sung MS, Lee GK, Kang HS, et al. Sacrococcygeal chordoma: MR imaging in 30 patients. Skeletal Radiol 2005;34:87–94.

38. Fuchs B, Dickey ID, Yaszemski MJ, et al. Operative management of sacral chordoma. J Bone Joint Surg Am 2005;87(10):2211–16.

39. Kyriakos M. Benign notochordal lesions of the axial skeleton: a review and current appraisal. Skeletal Radiol 2011;40(9):1141–52.

40. Lomasney LM, Martinez S, Demos TC, Harrelson JM. Multifocal vascular lesions of bone: imaging characteristics. Skeletal Radiol 1996;25(3):255–61.

41. Errani C, Vanel D, Gambarotti M, et al. Vascular bone tumors: a proposal of a classification based on clinicopathological, radiographic and genetic features. Skeletal Radiol 2012;41:1495–507.

42. Wenger DE, Wold LE. Malignant vascular lesions of bone: radiologic and pathologic features. Skeletal Radiol 2000;29(11):619–31.

43. Khanna M, Delaney D, Tirabosco R, Saifuddin A. Osteofibrous dysplasia, osteofibrous dysplasia-like adamantinoma and adamantinoma: correlation of radiological imaging features with surgical histology and assessment of the use of radiology in contributing to needle biopsy diagnosis. Skeletal Radiol 2008;37(12):1077–84.

44. Most MJ, Sim FH, Inwards CY. Osteofibrous dysplasia and adamantinoma. J Am Acad Orthop Surg 2010;18(6):358–66.

CHAPTER 5

SOFT TISSUE TUMOURS

Paul O'Donnell

CHAPTER OUTLINE

Introduction
Imaging Characterisation of Soft Tissue
  Masses
**WORLD HEALTH ORGANIZATION
CLASSIFICATION OF SOFT TISSUE TUMOURS**
Lipomatous (Adipocytic) Tumours
Fibroblastic/Myofibroblastic Tumours

So-Called Fibrohistiocytic Tumours
Vascular Tumours
Chondro-Osseous Tumours
Tumours of Uncertain Differentiation
Tumours of Nerves
Non-Neoplastic Tumour Mimics

INTRODUCTION

Soft tissue masses are frequently referred for imaging assessment. The exact prevalence and the ratio of benign to malignant are impossible to estimate because:

- Many patients do not seek medical attention for masses that do not appear to be growing and do not impede activities of daily living.
- If medical attention is sought, indolent masses may not be biopsied or excised.
- Formal histological assessment of superficial masses may not be obtained and many are not entered into tumour registries.
- Benign (and some malignant) masses are occasionally excised without imaging.

Soft tissue tumours may be benign, malignant or non-neoplastic and all may present in a similar manner. Benign and non-neoplastic masses are more common, with benign lesions frequently said to occur approximately one hundred times more commonly than malignant.[1] Referrals to hospital will be biased towards clinically suspicious masses and data from tumour centres give a distorted picture. In a study of 358 soft tissue masses referred from primary and secondary care, 95% of cases were benign.[2] In a large study of consultation cases referred to the Armed Forces Institute of Pathology, 68.5% of nearly 40,000 tumours were benign.[3]

The characterisation of soft tissue masses on imaging remains challenging and the histological diagnosis of sarcomas based on imaging, with a few exceptions, is frequently unsuccessful, necessitating biopsy. Benign and non-neoplastic masses may show typical imaging features, but biopsy is often still required to confirm the diagnosis.

IMAGING CHARACTERISATION OF SOFT TISSUE MASSES

Radiographs

Radiographic assessment of a soft tissue tumour has a low diagnostic yield but may still be useful, either alone or as an adjunct to cross-sectional imaging.

The utility of plain radiography has been assessed in 454 soft tissue masses referred to a tumour centre (care is needed in the extrapolation of these results from a referral population to soft tissue tumours in general).[4] There was a positive finding in 62%. The most frequent finding was identification of a mass—most soft tissue tumours show similar density to muscle but a large mass may be seen, as may distortion (but preservation) of adjacent fat planes. In this study, a mass was seen in 31%. When seen on a radiograph, the lesion was more likely to be malignant although in part this depended on the location of the lesion, with visible tumours in the hands and feet more likely to be benign or non-neoplastic and tumours in the thigh, calf and arm more likely to be malignant.

If the mass is large and contains fat in sufficient quantity, its density will be lower than that of adjacent soft tissues. Fat was seen in 7% of the masses: 50% were well-differentiated liposarcomas/atypical lipomatous tumours (see below), with benign fat-containing lesions including lipoma, haemangioma, hibernoma and lipoblastoma.

Foreign bodies may be visualised on radiographs of a mass, as may a surrounding inflammatory reaction. Typically, glass and metal are visible but wood and plastic may not have sufficient density to be seen.

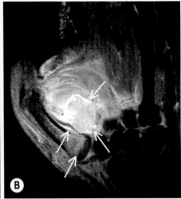
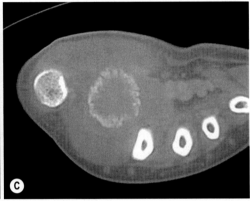

FIGURE 5-1 ■ Myositis ossificans. Radiograph of the hand (A) shows a soft tissue mass and periostitis on the palmar aspect of the thumb metacarpal (arrow). Coronal STIR MR image of the hand (B) shows a poorly demarcated hyperintense mass with surrounding soft tissue oedema (arrows). There is also marrow oedema and periosteal reaction in the thumb metacarpal (arrows). Axial CT (C) shows ossification at the periphery of the mass.

Mineralisation was present in 17% of the soft tissue masses in the study. Phleboliths, due to dystrophic mineralisation of thrombus in abnormal vessels, may be seen and are the hallmark of venous malformations. The pattern of calcification may give an indication of the underlying histological nature of the mass. Chondral calcification (for example in soft tissue chondral tumours and synovial chondromatosis) may take the form of punctate foci in comma shapes, rings and arcs, suggesting cartilage. Ossification (for example in myositis ossificans), when mature, forms trabeculae and a cortex, with density at the periphery greater than at the centre. When immature, it forms a rather amorphous, mineralised mass. The pattern of calcification does not always help with the diagnosis. Synovial sarcomas, approximately 30% of which are mineralised, may display chondroid or either type of osteoid matrix.[4]

Abnormality of a bone due to an adjacent soft tissue mass may take several forms. The study by Gartner et al. showed cortical erosion, periosteal reaction, scalloping, intramedullary extension and pathological fracture affecting approximately 14% of subjects,[4] and 39% of these were malignant. Changes were in general non-specific, with benign, non-neoplastic and malignant lesions capable of a wide range of interactions with the adjacent bone. Periosteal reaction was uncommon (4.4%), but 70% of cases showing it were non-malignant.

Computed Tomography (CT)

Evaluation of the soft tissue mass with CT is useful in some cases but, as with radiographs, it is often not tissue specific, as many masses show similar attenuation to muscle. The radiographic features of a soft tissue mass are demonstrated at least as well using CT and it is more sensitive for the identification of small amounts of fat and calcium. As an adjunct to MRI and radiographs, CT is useful for showing the peripheral ossification in myositis ossificans, confirming what may be a difficult MRI diagnosis (Fig. 5-1). CT angiography (and specifically arteriography) is helpful for the preoperative assessment of tumours close to vessels.

Ultrasound (US)

US has been shown to be a useful triage tool for masses referred from primary or secondary care.[2] It can play an important role in confirming a mass is present and not due to a normal anatomical structure or variant (such as an accessory muscle). It can also differentiate solid from cystic lesions. However, once a solid mass has been confirmed, further characterisation with US may be limited, often requiring further assessment with MRI and possible biopsy. As an adjunct to MRI, US can further characterise masses that show fluid signal intensity (cysts and solid myxoid masses), assess vascularity and compressibility (typically of venous malformations (Fig. 5-2)) and allows valuable clinical correlation by the examining radiologist.

Diagnostic features may be present in some lesions and these are more frequently benign or non-neoplastic. Examples include traumatic (muscle/tendon tear, haematoma), infective (abscess, pyomyositis), lipomatous

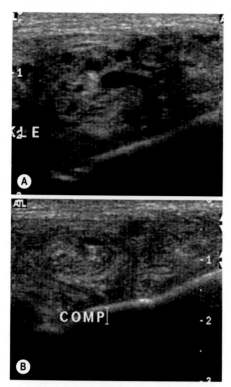

FIGURE 5-2 ■ **Venous malformation.** Ultrasound images without (A) and with (B) compression. A low-reflectivity mass contains tubular structures consistent with vessels, which rarely show blood flow on colour Doppler—occasionally, static or very slowly flowing blood can be seen on grey-scale images. With light probe pressure, the vascular and non-vascular elements are compressed.

(superficial and deep fatty masses—the latter usually need further assessment with MRI), vascular (thrombophlebitis, venous malformation, pseudoaneurysm) and neurogenic (nerve sheath tumours, nerve pseudotumours).

In the differentiation of a malignant from a benign solid mass, the grey-scale appearances are usually nonspecific. The assessment of tumour vascularity using colour/power and pulsed Doppler is possible with US and greater success has been claimed. Tumour neovascularity is an important feature of malignancy—tumour vessels are anatomically abnormal, lacking a muscular layer and showing irregular contour. This results in a heterogeneous network of abnormal vessels, often chaotically distributed within the tumour, with abnormal flow characteristics and morphology. A study of benign and malignant masses with high vascularity showed that the pattern of vessels within a mass was of limited value in the distinction of benign and malignant, but that in the presence of an organised pattern, a benign diagnosis was more likely.[5] An organised vascular pattern has been shown in 77% of benign and a disorganised pattern in 80% of malignant soft tissue tumours.[6] The atypical morphology of vessels in malignant masses may result in vessel trifurcations (rather than bifurcations), stenoses, occlusions and an anarchic rather than an hierarchical branching pattern.[7] Identification of any two of these

'major' criteria enabled malignant and benign masses to be distinguished.

Magnetic Resonance Imaging (MRI)

MRI is the technique of choice for local staging of a soft tissue mass, especially if it is in a deep location where US may be less able to assess tumour extent and relations. It is sensitive, can be tissue-specific and allows assessment of most masses, no matter where they are located. Despite this, MRI is often not sufficiently tissue specific to allow confident identification of some deep, solid masses; distinction of myxoid from cystic masses can be difficult without contrast medium and small calcific foci may not be seen. MRI also overlaps with radiography in its ability to identify fat, a foreign body and bone involvement in a soft tissue mass: differentiation of mineralisation and gas may require radiographs or CT, as both show hypointensity on T2-weighted (T2W) images and also on other fluid-sensitive sequences (see below).

Most tumours, and certainly most soft tissue sarcomas, are isointense to muscle on T1-weighted (T1W) images, of intermediate signal intensity on T2 images (similar to fat) and hyperintense on inversion recovery (STIR) or T2W images with fat saturation. As with US, specific diagnoses can sometimes be suggested based on the MRI appearances, more often with benign and non-neoplastic lesions, which may exhibit specific signal characteristics. Examples of MRI signal that allow characterisation and occasionally an MRI diagnosis (in combination with lesion morphology) include T1 hyperintensity, T2 hypointensity and T2 hyperintensity (fluid signal).

Hyperintensity on T1W imaging is commonly due to fat or subacute haemorrhage (methaemoglobin), but may also be due to melanin.

Hypointensity on T2W imaging may be due to calcification, fibrous tissue, chronic haemorrhage (haemosiderin), rapidly flowing blood (for example in an arteriovenous malformation or aneurysm) or gas. A radiograph is useful for excluding calcification as a cause.

Hyperintensity on T2W imaging may be seen in cystic masses, abscesses, myxoid masses (which include intramuscular myxomas, sarcomas and some nerve sheath tumours) and low-flow vascular malformations.

The presence of fluid–fluid levels is a non-specific sign in soft tissue masses: they are rare and equally common in benign and malignant lesions. The presence of haemorrhage is, however, useful—tumour necrosis is often seen in high-grade sarcomas; certain sarcomas (particularly synovial sarcoma) frequently show haemorrhagic foci (in synovial sarcomas up to 47%).

Staging of soft tissue sarcomas is best undertaken with MRI. This requires documentation of the size and local extent of the tumour, including any extracompartmental spread and the relationship of the tumour to adjacent structures such as bones, joints and neurovascular bundles. Initial staging will also usually require a chest radiograph and CT to exclude pulmonary metastases.

WORLD HEALTH ORGANIZATION CLASSIFICATION OF SOFT TISSUE TUMOURS[8]

The most recent version (2002) classified the following types of soft tissue tumours
- Adipocytic
- Fibroblastic/myofibroblastic
- So-called fibrohistiocytic tumours
- Smooth muscle tumours
- Pericytic/perivascular tumours
- Skeletal muscle tumours
- Vascular tumours
- Chondro-osseous tumours
- Tumours of uncertain differentiation

into the categories benign, intermediate and malignant. Several changes were made in this updated classification, including the recognition of two distinct types of intermediate malignancy ('locally aggressive' and 'rarely metastasising') and the reclassification of malignant fibrous histiocytoma, previously considered the commonest type of soft tissue sarcoma, as undifferentiated pleomorphic sarcoma. Many of the changes will be irrelevant to the imaging assessment of a soft tissue mass—the pathological diagnosis is being continually refined, particularly with the evolution of genetic techniques. It should be noted that peripheral nerve and skin tumours, both of which present as soft tissue masses, are considered in separate WHO classifications. Metastases to soft tissue and haematological malignancies, particularly lymphoma, may also present as a soft tissue mass.[9] Imaging is useful in the diagnosis of some of these soft tissue lesions and will be discussed below.

LIPOMATOUS (ADIPOCYTIC) TUMOURS

Lipomatous neoplasms are the most frequent mesenchymal tumours, with subcutaneous lipomas thought to represent up to 50% of all soft tissue tumours[10] and liposarcoma representing the commonest soft tissue sarcoma.[8]

Lipoma

This is a benign adipocytic tumour and the commonest mesenchymal neoplasm in adults. Lipomas typically occur in adults in the fifth to seventh decades with no sex predilection. They are rare in children and may be multiple.[8] Superficial (subcutaneous) tumours are common but lipomas may also occur in deep locations (intramuscular or intermuscular), or even adjacent to bone (parosteal), where they may stimulate a periosteal response. Subcutaneous lipomas are often diagnosed with great accuracy on clinical grounds alone, presenting as small (usually <5 cm), painless, firm, mobile masses.[11] Deep lipomas are often larger, but again usually painless. They cannot be diagnosed clinically and imaging is needed to confirm the diagnosis in deeper lesions. Atypical clinical presentation includes pain due to nerve compression in restricted spaces such as the carpal, tarsal and cubital tunnels.

Lipomas can contain other non-lipomatous elements contributing to a heterogeneous imaging appearance, vessels (angiolipoma), muscle (myolipoma), cartilage (chondrolipoma), bone (osteolipoma—following trauma or ischaemia) or extensive myxoid change (myxolipoma). Fibrous tissue and foci of fat necrosis can also cause a heterogeneous appearance.

Radiographs

Large lipomas are visible as areas of relative lucency (compared with soft tissue) (Fig. 5-3), but small lesions are not visible. Foci of mineralisation (calcification, ossification) are visible in 11%.[11]

Ultrasound

Subcutaneous lipomas are usually elliptical masses, often well-defined, with their long axis orientated parallel to the skin surface (Fig. 5-4). Their reflectivity is variable, while subcutaneous fat is usually low in reflectivity (unless previously inflamed or traumatised); lipomas are relatively reflective, often showing septation orientated along the long axis of the lesion. One study showed 29% had lower reflectivity than surrounding tissues and the

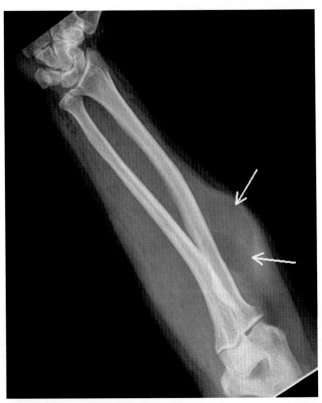

FIGURE 5-3 ■ Lipoma. AP radiograph shows an ovoid lucent mass (arrows) projected over the lateral aspect of the forearm.

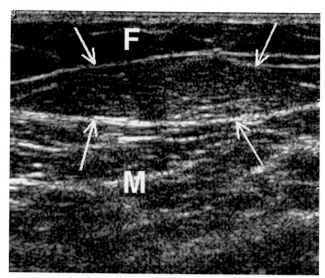

FIGURE 5-4 ■ **Subcutaneous lipoma.** Ultrasound image shows an elliptical mass (arrows), lower in reflectivity than adjacent muscle (M) but more reflective than subcutaneous fat (F). There are thin septations in the long axis of the mass.

remainder was of similar, greater or mixed reflectivity.[12] Light pressure with the ultrasound probe shows the lesions are compressible. They may appear encapsulated although many lipomas appear to blend with the surrounding tissues without evidence of a capsule.

Computed Tomography

This is rarely performed in the case of a subcutaneous lesion, but may show a mass of density similar to that of subcutaneous fat. Non-encapsulated lipomas may be occult. Deeper lesions are more likely to show heterogeneity (non-lipomatous elements, foci of mineralisation).

Magnetic Resonance Imaging

The mass is isointense to subcutaneous fat on T1- and T2W imaging, showing low signal intensity on STIR images and suppression of fat signal on T2W imaging with fat saturation. Fine septa (often immeasurable, typically less than 2 mm) are often seen, but the absence of thick or nodular septa is useful for differentiating a lipoma from a well-differentiated liposarcoma/atypical lipomatous tumour. Fine septa are also less likely to show gadolinium enhancement in benign lesions, which is also useful for differentiation.[13] Focal areas of non-adipose tissue (including fibrosis and necrosis) are not infrequent in benign tumours (particularly deep lesions) and make the distinction from a well-differentiated liposarcoma impossible on imaging alone. Mineralisation (calcification and ossification) may also be seen in benign tumours.

Intramuscular lipomas can be diagnosed with a high degree of confidence; an infiltrative margin and intermingled muscle fibres within and at the periphery of the lesion are features that make it possible to differentiate from other lipomatous tumours[14] (Fig. 5-5).

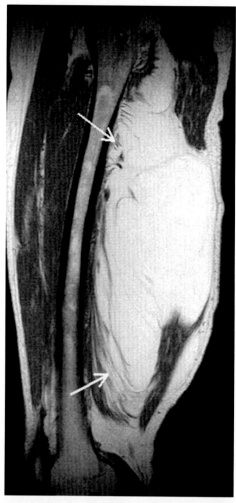

FIGURE 5-5 ■ **Intramuscular lipoma.** Sagittal T1-weighted MR image of the thigh: large, well-differentiated (predominantly fatty) lipomatous mass showing muscle fibres at the periphery (arrows).

Although they may be seen in simple lipomas, the following MRI features are atypical and should suggest the possibility of a well-differentiated liposarcoma:
- incomplete suppression of signal on fat-suppressed sequences
- thick, nodular septa (particularly if they enhance)
- focal non-lipomatous areas.

Other Benign Adipocytic Tumours

Lipoblastoma

Lipoblastoma is a tumour occurring in children—88% of patients are under 3 years old and the median age at onset is 1 year.[15] They usually occur in the extremities and consist of both mature and immature adipocytes (lipoblasts).[8] Lesions in younger patients contain prominent areas of myxoid tissue and MRI appearances may mimic a myxoid liposarcoma. However, they undergo a process of maturation, showing a tendency to develop into lipomas.[16] Imaging reveals a heterogeneous fatty mass on US, CT and MRI, due to myxoid and cystic areas, but, as both lipoma and liposarcoma are rare in young children, the diagnosis can be suggested in the presence of a heterogeneous fat-containing mass in a patient of the correct age.

Hibernoma

Hibernoma is a rare benign tumour composed of brown fat most frequently occurring in the thigh. The tumour appears lipomatous, but usually shows subtly different signal characteristics from those of subcutaneous fat, with hypointensity on T1W imaging and failure to suppress fully on fat-saturated images. Serpentine vessels may be identified within the highly vascular mass, a rare finding in an atypical lipomatous tumour/well-differentiated liposarcoma.[11]

Atypical Lipomatous Tumour/Well-Differentiated Liposarcoma (ALT/WDL)

These lesions are synonymous and classified as intermediate (locally aggressive) malignancies. They account for 40–45% of all liposarcomas and are the commonest subtype of liposarcoma.[8] ALT/WDL are well-differentiated tumours, often predominantly fatty, and show no capacity for metastasis unless dedifferentiation occurs (see below). Although ALT and WDL are identical morphologically and genetically, the term ALT is used for tumours in surgically accessible sites, such as the limbs and trunk, where complete excision is curative. WDL is usually used for tumours in inaccessible sites, such as the mediastinum and retroperitoneum, where complete

excision may not be possible and the disease may eventually be fatal following uncontrolled recurrence.

These tumours occur in middle age, most commonly in the sixth decade and there is no sex predilection. They arise in the deep soft tissues of the limbs, retroperitoneum, paratesticular area and mediastinum—rarely they occur subcutaneously.[8] Imaging shows a deep lipomatous mass with varying degrees of heterogeneity. The following features favour a diagnosis of a malignant rather than a benign tumour: lesion size >10 cm, thick, nodular septa, presence of globular or nodular non-adipose areas and fat content less than 75%[17] (Fig. 5-6). Incomplete fat suppression suggests a liposarcoma,[18] while septal enhancement is more likely if the lesion is malignant and may be more important than the thickness of the septa.[13,19] Although on imaging the differentiation of a lipoma in a deep location from ALT/WDL is unreliable, with considerable overlap in the appearances, it is largely irrelevant to initial management. Both are well-differentiated lipomatous neoplasms and would usually be treated by primary excision, with as wide a margin as possible, without prior biopsy.

Other Adipocytic Malignancies

The other major types of liposarcoma are dedifferentiated, myxoid and pleomorphic (pleomorphic liposarcoma is a very rare high-grade tumour). With higher grades of malignancy, fat becomes less conspicuous on MRI, such that there may be no suggestion of an adipocytic tumour in many liposarcomas.

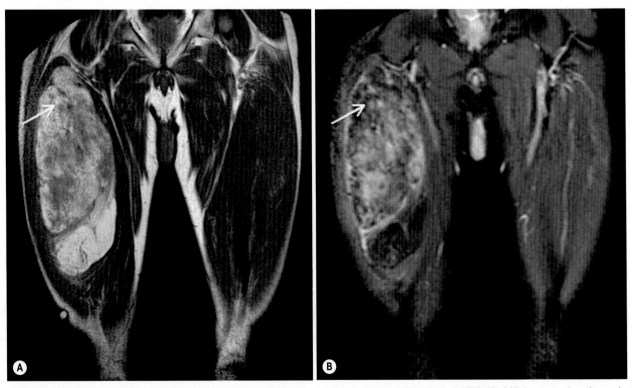

FIGURE 5-6 ■ **Atypical lipomatous tumour/well-differentiated liposarcoma.** Coronal T1 (A) and STIR (B) MR images showing a heterogeneous, partially fatty mass in the right thigh, with extensive areas of non-lipomatous signal, some small nodular foci superiorly (arrows) and thick septation.

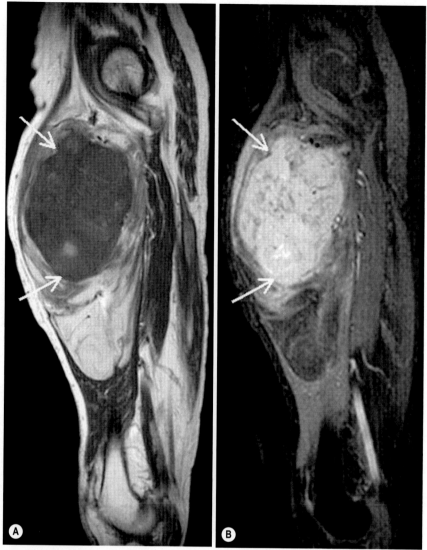

FIGURE 5-7 ■ **Dedifferentiated liposarcoma.** Sagittal T1 (A) and STIR (B) MR images showing a lipomatous mass. At the superior aspect of the mass there is a well-defined non-fatty tumour, corresponding to the dedifferentiated component (arrows).

Dedifferentiated Liposarcoma

Dedifferentiated liposarcoma results from the transition of ALT/WDL to a non-lipogenic sarcoma of variable grade and may occur in the primary tumour (90%) or in a recurrent lesion. The risk of dedifferentiation is greatest in retroperitoneal tumours and occurs in up to 10% of ALT/WDL—this may be time dependent rather than location dependent. It is usually a high-grade tumour, with the dedifferentiated component seen as a discrete non-lipomatous tumour within the fatty mass, reflected in both the histological and radiological appearances (Fig. 5-7). Occasionally, there is a gradual transition from lipomatous to non-lipomatous sarcoma.

Myxoid Liposarcoma

Myxoid liposarcoma is the second most common type of liposarcoma, accounting for approximately 10% of adult soft tissue sarcomas. The tumour consists of a myxoid stroma containing primitive non-lipogenic mesenchymal cells and a variable number of lipoblasts. An imaging diagnosis based on its MRI appearances is frequently possible and dependent on identifying the myxoid component, which resembles fluid, along with a fatty component, usually in the form of thin T1 hyperintense septa (often subtle) (Fig. 5-8). In the most recent WHO classification of soft tissue tumours, round cell liposarcoma, previously considered separately as the cellular, high-grade variant of myxoid liposarcoma, was reclassified as a synonymous lesion.

FIBROBLASTIC/MYOFIBROBLASTIC TUMOURS

Nodular Fasciitis (NF)

This is a fibrous proliferation that forms a rapidly growing mass, usually in the subcutaneous tissues, but is also found in intramuscular and intermuscular (fascial) sites.

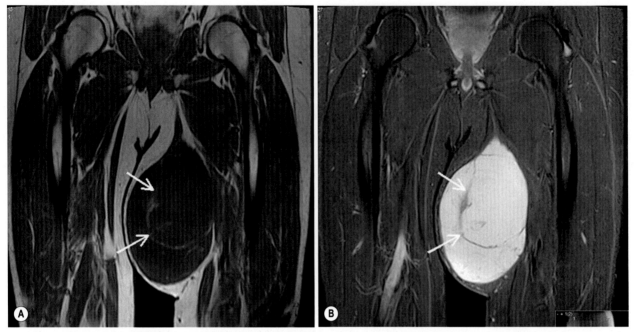

FIGURE 5-8 ■ **Myxoid liposarcoma.** Coronal T1 (A) and STIR (B) MR images showing a large mass at the medial aspect of the thigh with fluid signal characteristics, in keeping with a myxoid tumour, and thin fatty septa (arrows).

Owing to its rapid growth, cellular histology and frequent (although not atypical[8]) mitoses, inappropriately aggressive surgery may be performed. It is said to be the commonest lesion of fibrous origin,[20] occurring in all age groups, but most commonly affecting young adults,[8] with no sex predilection. The most frequent sites of involvement are the upper limb (48%) and trunk (20%),[20] although any site is possible. Imaging shows a mass, which is usually small (< 5 cm in maximum dimension, mean 2.2 cm diameter in one series[20]), and often poorly defined, whose MRI characteristics reflect the histology: the nodule undergoes a process of maturation, with early, cellular lesions containing myxoid tissue (near-fluid signal intensities, but slight T1 hyperintensity compared with muscle), later becoming fibrotic (hypointense on all sequences, including T1). NF has been treated, following confirmatory biopsy, with intralesional steroid injection and surgery, with few recurrences following excision.[21]

Elastofibroma (EF)

This is a tumour-like lesion (fibroelastic pseudotumour) occurring almost exclusively in elderly patients, consisting of mature adipose tissue entrapped within a fibrous mass, typically found adjacent to the inferior angle of the scapula. When typical in location and appearance on MRI, no biopsy is required and marginal resection suffices. The lesion is common and often bilateral. Over 50% of cases are said to be asymptomatic[22] and it is a frequent postmortem finding.[23] There is a reported prevalence of 2% in subjects >60 years undergoing chest CT for lung disease.[24] EF is thought to arise as a result of friction between the scapula and chest wall, possibly due to manual labour, resulting in collagen degeneration, but familial cases do exist.

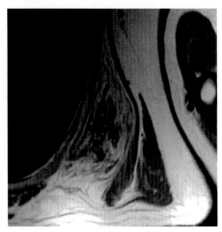

FIGURE 5-9 ■ **Elastofibroma.** Axial T1 image at the inferior aspect of the scapula, showing a soft tissue mass deep to serratus anterior. It consists of fatty (hyperintense) and fibrous (hypointense) striations.

Over 99% occur at the typical chest wall location, but other sites, including visceral sites, have been described.[8] US shows non-specific appearances but the mass can be revealed, sometimes fairly dramatically, with shoulder adduction. The appearances on CT and MRI reflect its fibroadipose contents. EF contains alternating striations of fat and fibrous tissue and is typically elliptical, located deep to serratus anterior (Fig. 5-9). The striations parallel the chest wall. Bilateral, symmetrical masses may cause confusion, as the mass may superficially resemble muscle.

Fibromatoses

These are intermediate-grade (locally aggressive) lesions[8] which are further classified as superficial (palmar/plantar) and desmoid-type fibromatosis.

Superficial Fibromatosis

Palmar Fibromatosis (Dupuytren's Disease). Palmar fibromatosis (Dupuytren's disease) is characterised by the development of fibrous nodules and subsequently cord-like bands within subcutaneous tissue, typically located on the ulnar aspect of the palm of the hand. They cause thickening and contraction of the skin and also affect the palmar aponeurosis and flexor tendons, usually of the ring and little fingers. A debilitating flexion deformity may result (Dupuytren's contracture) and it is the severity of the deformity and functional deficit that determines whether surgical resection is needed, although recurrence is frequent. Nodules show low reflectivity on US, but MRI may be more useful as signal characteristics within nodules and cords appear to correlate with cellularity. Cellular lesions (relatively hyperintense to the adjacent tendon on T1- and T2W imaging) are more likely to recur following excision.[25]

Plantar Fibromatosis (Ledderhose Disease). Plantar fibromatosis (Ledderhose disease) is histologically identical to palmar fibromatosis but involves the plantar aspect of the foot where nodules or larger masses arise in the plantar fascia, most often at its medial aspect. Nodules may be small, in which case they are often asymptomatic, and may be identified incidentally during US examination. Larger lesions may cause pain on prolonged standing and walking, and may be multiple. The appearances of a mass arising from the plantar fascia, showing low or intermediate MRI signal intensity, are frequently diagnostic (Fig. 5-10). Treatment is usually conservative, with excision reserved for large, debilitating lesions.[26]

Other Forms. Other forms of superficial fibromatosis include knuckle pads (fibrous masses at the dorsal aspects of the MCP and PIP joints) and Peyronie's (penile) fibromatosis. Superficial lesions in different sites may coexist.

Desmoid-Type Fibromatosis

This encompasses previously used terms such as deep, aggressive or musculoaponeurotic fibromatosis and extra-abdominal desmoid tumour. It is a clonal fibroblastic proliferation occurring in deep soft tissues, typically locally invasive but without the capacity to metastasise.[8] Young adults are most frequently affected, but the lesion may present at any age and in any location. The commoner sites include shoulder, chest wall and back, thigh and head and neck.[8] Abdominal wall and intra-abdominal involvement were previously considered as distinct subtypes.

When a mass occurs in a superficial site, it may appear very firm. Occasionally, this only becomes apparent at the time of needle biopsy, when it may be difficult to puncture the mass due to its consistency. Symptoms arise due to the infiltration or mass effect on adjacent structures, such as joints and nerves; the mass itself is usually painless. US shows a heterogeneous, solid mass which may be in a deep location, mimicking a sarcoma. CT is also usually non-specific, but densely collagenous lesions show higher attenuation, and the poorly defined nature of the mass may be appreciated.[26] The diagnosis may be apparent from MRI, although the appearances are highly variable. The hallmark of desmoid-type fibromatosis is low-signal bands of tissue which represent dense bundles of collagen (Fig. 5-11). Low signal intensity (SI) on T2W

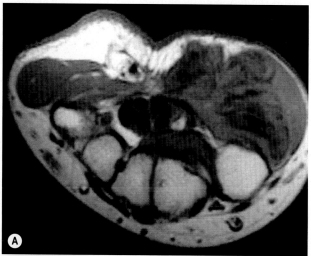
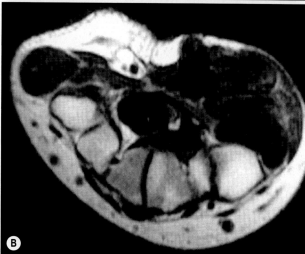

FIGURE 5-11 ■ Desmoid-type fibromatosis. Axial T1 (A) and T2 (B) MR images show a heterogeneous mass in the thenar eminence, which is mildly hyperintense to muscle on T1W imaging and hypointense on T2W imaging. Both sequences show prominent, thick striations of low signal due to bands of dense collagen.

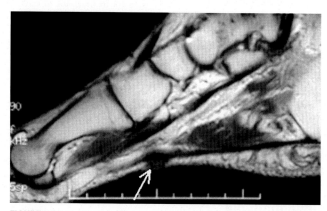

FIGURE 5-10 ■ Plantar fibroma. Sagittal T2 MR image showing a low-signal mass arising from the medial aspect of the plantar fascia (arrow).

imaging is thought to be due to a combination of high collagen content and low cellularity, with the latter possibly more important, as higher SI areas also show a high collagen content (but greater cellularity).[27] Signal elsewhere in the tumour is typically heterogeneous, but commonly intermediate on both T1- and T2W images.

Intra-abdominal tumours may occur sporadically or in association with Gardner's syndrome (an autosomal dominant condition of adenomatous intestinal polyps, multiple osteomas and desmoid-type fibromatosis).

Fibroma of the Tendon Sheath (FTS)

This typically presents as a painless, fibrous nodule related to flexor tendons, more often in the right hand.[8] The most frequently involved areas are the thumb, index and middle fingers, the palmar aspect of the hand and volar aspect of the wrist (these locations accounting for 80% of cases), but it also occurs in the knee and foot. Triggering of a finger may result, as may pressure symptoms if the lesion arises outside the fingers (for example median nerve pressure from a lesion in the carpal tunnel).[8] The lesion most commonly affects males in the fourth decade. T1- and T2W MRI shows a low-signal nodule or mass related to a tendon, which may have imaging appearances similar to those of giant cell tumour of the tendon sheath (see below), but does not show accentuation of low signal on T2* gradient-echo images ('blooming').

SO-CALLED FIBROHISTIOCYTIC TUMOURS

Pigmented Villonodular Synovitis (PVNS) and Giant Cell Tumour of the Tendon Sheath (GCTTS)

These terms encompass a number of related conditions, arising from the synovium of joints, tendon sheaths and bursae. It should be noted that giant cell tumour of tendon sheath described here is not related to the giant cell tumour of bone. Lesions may present as a localised mass related to a tendon sheath or bursa (GCTTS), as diffuse involvement of a joint or tendon sheath (pigmented villonodular synovitis (PVNS) or tenosynovitis) or as a localised intra-articular mass (localised intra-articular PVNS), most often in the knee.[28] Lesions in the tendon sheath present most commonly as a soft tissue mass.

Localised, mass-like GCTTS is usually painless, but may interfere with tendon function or cause local pressure effects. GCTTS is most often seen in adults with a male:female patient ratio of 2:1.[8] Although the lesion may occur at many sites, including the feet, wrists and ankles, most cases (around 85%) occur in the fingers (it is the second most common soft tissue tumour of the hand after ganglia), usually closely related to a tendon sheath (typically flexor). Radiographs are frequently abnormal and may reveal not only the mass but also

pressure erosion and cortical destruction (Fig. 5-12); they may also cause bone expansion with intraosseous growth. The lesions may occasionally cause a periosteal reaction and have been reported to show calcification. In one series of hand tumours, 11% of 133 cases showed an abnormality of the adjacent bone.[29]

On US the mass is usually homogeneous and of low reflectivity, showing internal vascularity. Cystic change is not usually seen but there may be posterior acoustic enhancement. The mass may just contact or completely encase the tendon, often extending between tendon and bone, but it does not move with the tendon due to the intervening tendon sheath. Bone erosions may be seen on US. On MRI, haemosiderin contained within the mass may give characteristically low signal intensity on all sequences, especially T2* gradient-echo images. A well-defined mass, showing low-to-intermediate signal on T1- and T2W images and exaggerated low signal on T2*, located on the flexor aspect of the fingers and related to the tendon, is highly suggestive of the diagnosis of GCTTS.

The localised intra-articular form of PVNS is a similar lesion to GCTTS, but is found almost exclusively at the knee and frequently in the infrapatellar (Hoffa's) fat pad.[30] It may also be seen in the suprapatellar pouch and intercondylar notch. Typically, there is a well-defined mass, which shows similar signal intensities on MRI to GCTTS (Fig. 5-13). The lesion may also contain fluid-signal linear foci. As with any predominantly low-signal mass in Hoffa's fat pad (or in any other location), radiographs are useful for excluding mineralisation—soft tissue chondromas also typically occur in this region. Simple excision of the mass is appropriate for typical GCTTS in the hand and localised nodular PVNS. Treatment of diffuse intra-articular PVNS may involve extensive synovectomy, with a much greater chance of recurrence.

Diffuse-Type Pigmented Villonodular Synovitis (Diffuse-Type Giant Cell Tumour)

This term encompasses PVNS, a diffuse synovial proliferation in a joint characterised by recurrent haemarthroses, and similar synovial processes in tendon sheaths (pigmented villonodular tenosynovitis).[8] PVNS presents as a chronic monoarthropathy in a large joint and this condition is further discussed in Chapter 7. Pigmented villonodular tenosynovitis may present as soft tissue swelling along the line of a tendon sheath which will be seen on MRI to contain fluid and synovitis; the latter may show evidence of haemosiderin with low signal intensity on all sequences.

VASCULAR TUMOURS

Haemangioma

The classification of benign vascular lesions is complex and may cause confusion. The International Society for

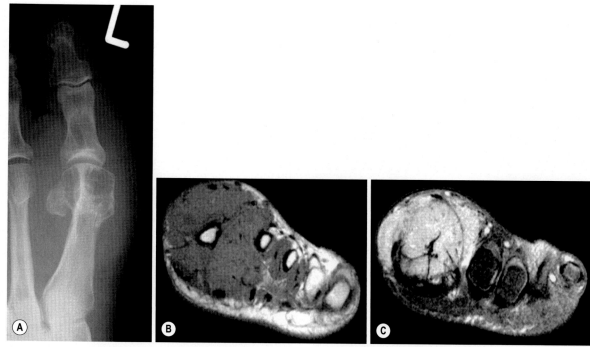

FIGURE 5-12 ■ **Giant cell tumour of the tendon sheath.** (A) Dorsoplantar radiograph shows a large mass in the region of the first metatarsophalangeal joint, with circumferential pressure erosion and lobular lucency in the metatarsal head. Axial T1 (B, slightly proximal) and STIR (C) MR images show a circumferential tumour invading bone at the metatarsal head.

the Study of Vascular Anomalies (ISSVA) differentiates vascular tumours, the most common of which is infantile haemangioma, and vascular malformations. The latter are subclassified into high-flow lesions, containing an arterial component (arteriovenous malformations (AVMs) and arteriovenous fistulas (AVFs)) and low-flow lesions (venous, lymphatic, capillary and mixed (capillary–venous and capillary–lymphatic–venous)).[31]

Haemangiomas are benign vascular tumours of infancy, usually presenting in the first few weeks of life and affecting 2–3% of children.[32] Following an initial period of rapid growth, there is a subsequent slow involution.

Malformations are congenital lesions consisting of dysplastic vascular channels, often unappreciated at birth but which enlarge with the patient and do not regress. High-flow (arteriovenous) malformations may present in childhood or adulthood. Clinical symptoms depend on location and size, but may include pain, tissue overgrowth (rapid growth can occur after minor trauma), bleeding or, with large AVMs, high-output cardiac failure. An abnormality is apparent in the skin, which may be pulsatile, with a palpable thrill and audible bruit.

Many of the lesions referred to as haemangiomas in adults are more accurately described as low-flow, frequently venous, vascular malformations. The WHO classification refers to these lesions as venous haemangiomas.[8] Venous malformations (VMs) account for half to two-thirds of low-flow vascular malformations;[33] lesions are usually purely venous, but may contain capillary or lymphatic elements. They are congenital, but are not always evident at birth. Occasionally, a patch of blue skin discoloration is visible with superficial lesions. With growth of

the patient, there is enlargement—fluctuation in size is often reported (depending on enlargement), but there is no significant local warmth of the skin or thrill. The tumour is soft and compressible, exerting no significant mass effect. Eventually, multiple tissue planes and anatomical structures may be affected (skin, fat, muscle, bone). Up to 40% of venous malformations occur in the head and neck, 20% in the trunk and 40% in the extremities.[34]

VMs consist of abnormal venous channels and variable amounts of hamartomatous stroma which contains adipose tissue. The vessels are dysplastic, post-capillary, thin-walled vascular channels which show patchy deficiency of mural smooth muscle—they dilate with time due to repeated stretching, allowing growth and infiltration of adjacent structures.[33] Thrombosis of vessels is frequent and dystrophic calcification within thrombus results in phleboliths. A localised coagulopathy develops within VMs due to consumption of clotting factors, increasing the risk of haemorrhage at surgery or if the lesions are traumatised.[35] Morbidity arises from pain and infiltration of local structures, leading to reduced mobility (muscle involvement and contracture), oedema, ulceration, bleeding and remodelling of the skeleton.[33] As there are no proliferating cellular elements, therapy is targetted at reducing blood flow[34] with techniques including percutaneous sclerotherapy. Imaging is often characteristic.

Radiographs

A lobular mass may be visible, depending on location. The radiographic hallmark of a VM is the phlebolith.

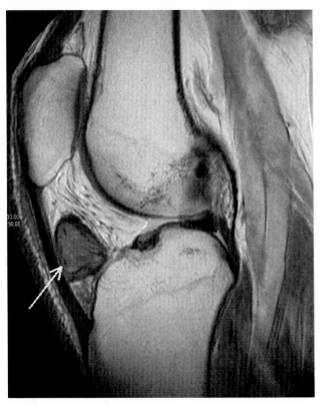

FIGURE 5-13 ■ Localised intra-articular PVNS. Sagittal proton density MR image showing a hypointense mass in Hoffa's fat pad (arrow).

These are not always seen, but may be numerous and are seen as a round focus of calcification, often with a lucent centre. Modelling deformity of adjacent bones may be seen (Fig. 5-14).

Ultrasound

Reflectivity is variable on US and the mass may show reflectivity similar to that of adjacent tissues (fat, muscle) and may not be immediately apparent. Low-reflectivity tubular structures suggesting vessels are seen, as are phleboliths. Colour or power Doppler will often show no flow within the mass, but when detected, flow is monophasic and of low velocity. Compressibility with probe pressure is a useful sign on US; the vascular structures and stroma of the mass are easily flattened, reflecting its consistency. Again, this is not a constant feature and depends to an extent on the location, depth and size of the VM, but helps to differentiate it from other soft tissue masses, particularly sarcomas, which in general do not compress (Fig. 5-2).

MRI

VMs show heterogeneous signals, but are generally mildly hyperintense to muscle on T1W imaging and are usually well-defined despite local infiltration. Focal T1 hyperintensity is also frequent, due to small amounts of fat within the lesion and also methaemoglobin (following haemorrhage/thrombosis). Serpiginous channels, which

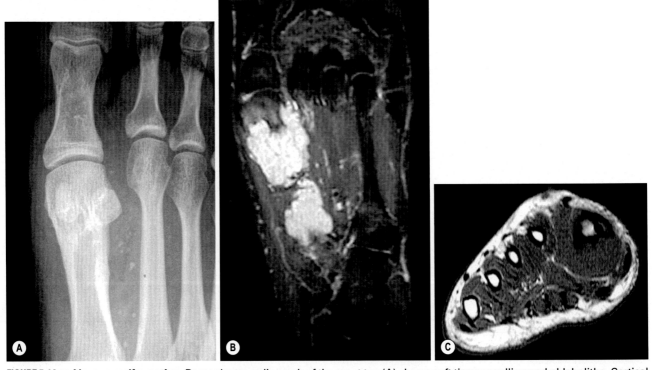

FIGURE 5-14 ■ Venous malformation. Dorsoplantar radiograph of the great toe (A) shows soft tissue swelling and phleboliths. Cortical thickening and subtle remodelling of the metatarsal is noted. Axial STIR MR image (B) shows a lobular, hyperintense mass with faint low-signal septation. Coronal T1W imaging (C) shows pressure erosion and cortical thickening of the plantar aspect of the metatarsal by a circumferential mass, which in this case is isointense to muscle.

TABLE 5-1	Syndromes Associated with Vascular Malformations

- Klippel-Trénaunay
- Sturge–Weber
- Maffucci
- Proteus
- Blue rubber bleb naevus

are hyperintense on T2W imaging, are interspersed between the solid, soft tissue matrix. Fluid–fluid levels are common in areas of static blood. Areas of signal void may be due to phleboliths, flowing blood or fibrous septa.[33] Enhancement can be seen on delayed images following intravenous injection of gadolinium contrast medium, but there is no arterial or early venous filling.[34] MRI with gadolinium contrast medium may be useful in differentiating a VM from a lymphatic malformation, the former showing delayed, diffuse enhancement and the latter septal enhancement in the walls of the cystic spaces.[33]

A summary of the features that should be assessed on MRI is:[33]

- classification into high flow (by presence of flow voids and arterial feeding vessels) or low flow;
- description of extent (focal, multifocal or diffuse);
- description of tissue involvement (skin, subcutaneous tissue, muscle, tendon, bone cortex, bone marrow); and
- connection with abnormal vessels (feeding arteries, draining veins).

There are several clinical syndromes associated with vascular malformations (Table 5-1).

CHONDRO-OSSEOUS TUMOURS

Soft Tissue Chondromas

These are benign tumours of hyaline cartilage, occurring outside bone, in extrasynovial locations and not attached to periosteum—other synonyms include extraskeletal chondroma and chondroma of soft parts.[8] They occur at any age but are commonest in adults aged 30–60 years. The commonest location is in the fingers, with 80% occurring in the hands and feet.[36] The masses are usually small (<3 cm diameter), lobular and solitary, and although showing no attachment to periosteum, they may be adherent to tendon sheath or joint capsule; proximity to bone may result in pressure erosion/remodelling[37] (Fig. 5-15). Imaging reflects their cartilaginous nature. Radiographs may show chondral mineralisation (punctate, curvilinear) or rarely ossification[36] and adjacent bone remodelling. MRI shows a lobular chondral mass; hyaline cartilage shows myxoid signal characteristics, with heterogeneous low-signal areas due to calcification. The radiographic differential includes periosteal chondroma (deep to the periosteum), synovial chondromatosis (affecting tendon sheath or arising from an adjacent

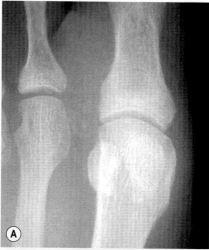
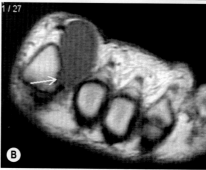

FIGURE 5-15 ■ **Soft tissue chondroma.** A mass between the first and second metatarsal heads contains punctate mineralisation (A). Coronal T1W imaging (B) shows subtle erosion of the lateral aspect of the first metatarsal head (arrow).

joint), traumatic and reactive lesions (myositis ossificans, bizarre parosteal osteochondromatous proliferation (BPOP)), tophi and calcification due to connective tissue disorders.[36]

Other benign chondral tumours occurring in soft tissue have been described,[38] including synovial chondromatosis (discussed in Chapter 7) and para-articular (intracapsular) chondroma. The latter represents cartilaginous metaplasia arising from a joint capsule or adjacent connective tissue, most frequently in Hoffa's fat pad, and may present as a mineralised mass. Calcification may progress to ossification, the lesion becoming a para-articular ossifying chondroma[39] or osteochondroma (without connection to bone).

TUMOURS OF UNCERTAIN DIFFERENTIATION

Myxoma

This is a benign soft tissue tumour composed of bland spindle cells in a stroma of abundant myxoid, gelatinous material, classified as a tumour of uncertain differentiation.[8] It is one of a number of myxoid tumours occurring

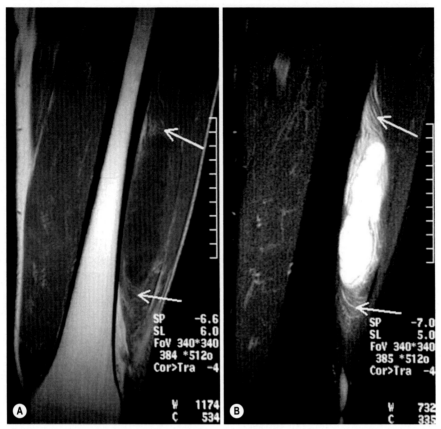

FIGURE 5-16 ■ **Intramuscular myxoma.** Coronal T1 (A) and STIR (B) MR images of the left thigh show an ovoid, poorly defined, heterogeneous mass which is hypointense on T1W imaging and hyperintense on STIR images. A small amount of fat is visible at the poles of the mass (arrows in (A)) and there is adjacent oedema (arrows in (B)).

in soft tissue, all consisting of a background matrix of mucoid material containing a variety of different cell types. While the cell type determines the clinical and biological behaviour, the imaging appearances of these lesions, determined by the myxoid stroma, are broadly similar. Differentiation can also be difficult for the histopathologist.

Most myxomas occur in intramuscular sites, although they may also be intermuscular, subcutaneous or juxta-articular;[40] myxomas also occur outside the musculoskeletal system. Women between the ages of 40 and 70 are most often affected and the most common location for this tumour is the thigh.[40] MRI is the most useful technique for assessment: myxoid tumours often resemble cysts, typically showing low SI on T1W imaging and high SI on T2W and fluid-sensitive sequences. The tumours may be homogeneous, or heterogeneous due to thin fibrous septa and may contain cystic areas; there may be surrounding soft tissue oedema.[40,41] A rind of fat may be seen, most prominently at the poles of the tumour, and this may simulate a 'split-fat sign', typically found in inter- rather than intramuscular tumours (Fig. 5-16). The surrounding fatty and oedematous signal changes reflect the infiltrative nature of the tumour, with fatty changes indicating adjacent muscle atrophy. Following administration of intravenous

contrast medium, internal enhancement can confirm that the lesion is not cystic, but occasionally the enhancement is purely peripheral with more prominent enhancement seen in tumours with greater cellularity and reduced myxoid content.[41] US and CT both show non-specific appearances.

The differential diagnosis includes cystic masses, some of which are synovial and para-articular including ganglia, synovial cysts, bursae and seromas. A rare variant of myxoma, the juxta-articular myxoma, can arise adjacent to joints, usually the knee.[42]

Soft Tissue Sarcomas (STSs)

Sarcomas are rare, malignant tumours of mesenchymal origin which account for less than 1% of all primary malignant tumours, but are still three to four times more common than primary bone sarcomas.[43] The greatest incidence is in older patients and in children and adolescents (under 20 years old); soft tissue sarcoma (STS) is very rare, with rhabdomyosarcoma (RMS) most common in younger subjects and non-RMS sarcomas commoner in older children. Many different types of STSs are classified as tumours of uncertain differentiation[8]. The most common STS of late adult life is the *pleomorphic undifferentiated sarcoma* (formerly malignant fibrous histiocytoma), which occurs most commonly in the extremities and retroperitoneum. As its name suggests, this tumour comprises STS which cannot be more precisely categorised.

Most STSs are poorly characterised by imaging. Initial attempts to differentiate benign from malignant soft tissue masses using MRI were unsuccessful and biopsy was recommended in most cases. Signs suspicious of malignancy have traditionally included a deep-seated, large mass with heterogeneous appearances on MRI.[43] More recently, the importance of tumour necrosis (non-enhancing areas, often haemorrhagic) and lesion size (greater than 5 cm at presentation) indicating a high grade lesion have been emphasised[44] (Fig. 5-17). A significant minority of sarcomas is known to arise superficially (in skin and subcutaneous fat). The relevance of lesion depth has been assessed in a referral population of 571 soft tissue tumours and was found to be unrelated to the final diagnosis, while patient age and size ≥5 cm were significant risk factors for malignancy.[45] Although the ability of imaging to reach a histological diagnosis has not advanced, the histopathological approach has been continuously refined using immunohistochemical and genetic techniques. Imaging features may assist in characterisation.

Synovial Sarcoma (SS)

Synovial sarcoma accounts for up to 10% of malignant mesenchymal tumours.[46] SS may be found at any age but most patients are aged 15–40 years. It is usually a slow-growing mass located in the extremities, often close to a joint and most commonly in the lower limb. Despite the name, less than 10% are said to be intra-articular. Although it is frequently a large, deep, multilobular and septated mass, it may also be small, homogeneous and slow growing, it is probably for these reasons that it was the malignant tumour most frequently diagnosed as benign using MRI in one study.[47] Imaging findings that may be useful in the diagnosis of SS include calcification (30% of cases) (Fig. 5-18), evidence of haemorrhage (44%), fluid–fluid levels (18%), 'triple signal'—areas of high, low and isointensity compared with fat on T2W imaging (indicating cystic/haemorrhagic elements, fibrous tissue and calcification and solid, non-necrotic tumour) (Fig. 5-19) and bone erosion or invasion (21%).

TUMOURS OF NERVES

Tumours of peripheral nerves are frequent causes of a soft tissue mass. They are classified by the WHO under lesions of the central nervous system, most recently in 2007.[48]

Two broad categories of nerve tumours exist: true neurogenic tumours and pseudotumours involving or arising from nerves. Clinical assessment and imaging are useful in conjunction in determining the nature of nerve lesions.

Benign Nerve Sheath Tumours

Schwannoma (*neurilemmoma*, NL) arises from the Schwann cells surrounding a nerve. They are typically small and slow growing and may arise in peripheral and central locations including sympathetic nerves. Although typically solitary, multiple tumours (schwannomatosis) may occur, either in association with neurofibromatosis type 2 or probably as a separate entity.

Neurofibroma (NF) accounts for slightly greater than 5% of benign soft tissue neoplasms. There are three types, all of which can be seen in neurofibromatosis type 1 (NF1): localised (the commonest type, accounting for >90%), diffuse and plexiform—the latter is one of the defining features of NF1.

- *Localised NF* is usually a slow-growing mass arising from a peripheral nerve, small nerve branch or larger central nerve. Most are solitary and not associated with NF1, but multiple neurofibromas can be found in patients with this condition.

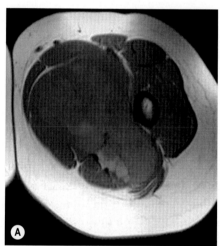

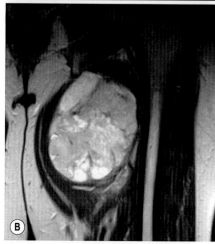

FIGURE 5-17 ■ **High-grade sarcoma.** Axial TW1 (A) and coronal T2W (B) imaging show a large heterogeneous, haemorrhagic mass in the adductor compartment of the left thigh.

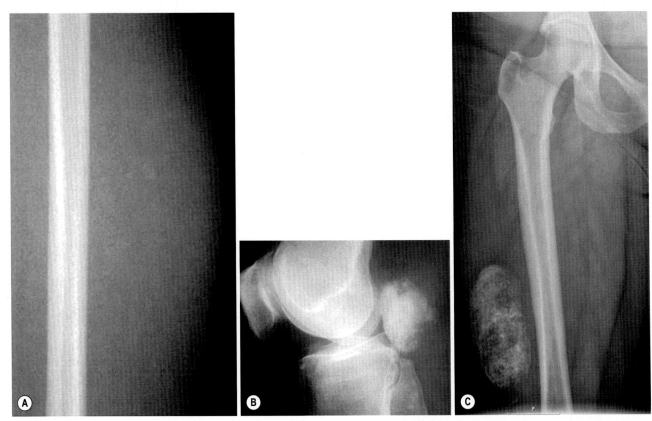

FIGURE 5-10 ■ Patterns of calcification of synovial sarcoma. (A) Faint punctate calcification; (B) heavy ossification; (C) bizarre diffuse mineralisation. There is some evidence to suggest that heavily mineralised or ossified synovial sarcomas have a better prognosis.

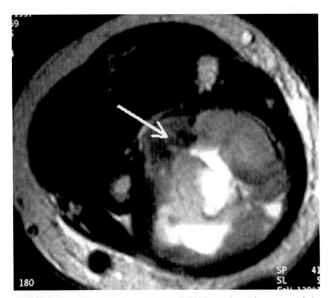

FIGURE 5-19 ■ Synovial sarcoma. T2W imaging shows a triple signal pattern: hyperintense haemorrhage, intermediate-signal solid tumour and low-signal mineralisation (arrow). Fluid–fluid levels are also seen.

- *Diffuse NF* presents as a diffuse area of thickening of the skin and subcutaneous tissues, again it is sporadic but can be associated with NF1 in approximately 10%.[49]
- *Plexiform NF* involves infiltration of a large nerve or plexus, with extension outside the nerve into adjacent tissues, resulting in a lobulated mass, loosely conforming to the morphology of the nerve, described as a 'bag of worms'. There may be associated bone and soft tissue overgrowth (Fig. 5-20).

There are a number of imaging features that suggest a benign nerve sheath tumour:

- *Relationship to a nerve*: The mass may arise in the anatomical location of a nerve, or an adjacent nerve may be visible on imaging studies. However, many arise from small peripheral nerves where no adjacent nerve is visible.
- *Nerve entering/leaving the mass*: Again, the utility of this sign depends on the size of the nerve. If visible, the location of the nerve relative to the mass may be useful in differentiating NLs and NFs. In NLs, the nerve may be eccentrically located relative to the mass, whereas in NF the nerve may enter and leave the mass centrally.
- *Fusiform morphology*.
- *Split-fat sign*: The neurovascular bundle travels in the intermuscular space, surrounded by fat, and an

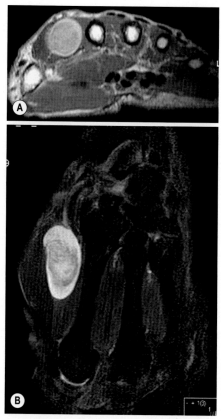

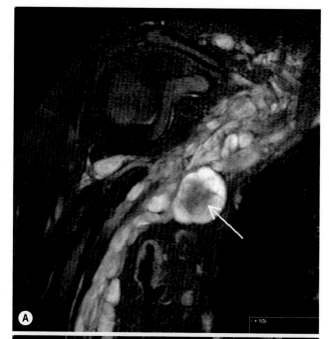

FIGURE 5-20 ■ **Schwannoma.** Axial proton-density (A) and coronal T2W imaging with fat saturation (B) show a well-defined, fusiform mass in the dorsum of the hand, between the thumb and index metacarpals. A fascicular sign is seen in (A) and a target sign in (B).

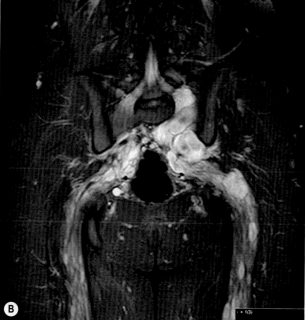

FIGURE 5-21 ■ **Plexiform neurofibromas of the right brachial plexus (A) and sciatic nerves (B).** Coronal STIR images showing marked lobular enlargement of major central nerves in a patient with neurofibromatosis type 1. A target sign is seen in the brachial plexus mass (arrow).

enlarging mass in this region, arising from any component of the neurovascular bundle, may show preservation of the surrounding rim of fat, with displacement of the adjacent muscle.

• *Distal muscle atrophy/denervation*: A variable sign depending on the impact on nerve function.
• *Target sign*: This refers to appearances on T2W imaging and US. On MRI, nerve sheath tumours often show central lower signal (reflecting a more fibrous content) and peripheral hyperintensity (more myxoid content). On US, the central portion shows hyperechogenicity with lower reflectivity in the periphery. This sign is seen most commonly in NFs but may also be seen in NLs (Figs. 5-20 and 5-21) and malignant peripheral nerve sheath tumours.
• *Fascicular sign*: Ring-like areas of hypointensity within the mass on proton-density or T2W imaging, which may correspond to fascicular bundles within the nerve sheath tumour (Fig. 5-21).

Despite the features outlined above, differentiation of NL from NF on US and MRI remains unreliable.

The imaging features of NL which have undergone a process of degeneration ('ancient' change) are often different and may obscure the neurogenic nature of the mass. A heterogeneous mass is usually seen, showing cavitation/cystic change, fluid–fluid levels/haemorrhage and calcification (Fig. 5-22).

Diffuse neurofibroma results in a plaque-like or infiltrative lesion, thickened skin and involvement of the subcutaneous tissues, with marked internal vascularity and enhancement following injection of gadolinium contrast medium.[49]

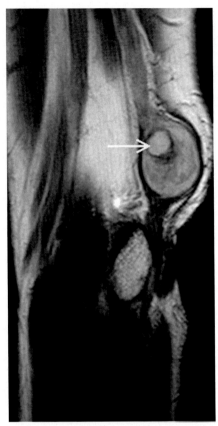

FIGURE 5-22 ■ **Ancient schwannoma of the ulnar nerve.** Sagittal T2W imaging shows continuity with an eccentric nerve and cyst formation within the tumour (arrow).

Malignant Nerve Tumours

Primary lesions are called malignant peripheral nerve sheath tumours, although several primary non-neurogenic or secondary malignancies may also arise in nerves.

Malignant Peripheral Nerve Sheath Tumours (MPNSTs)

Malignant peripheral nerve sheath tumours account for 5–10% of soft tissue sarcomas. In up to 50% of cases they occur in patients with NF1, affecting 2–5% of subjects with this condition who have an 8–12% lifetime risk of developing this malignancy.[50] MPNSTs in NF1 develop in deep plexiform NFS; the risk of transformation is greater in patients with large central lesions and varies with the precise nature of the genetic defect. In NF1 the tumours tend to be larger (possibly reflecting later presentation) and occur at an earlier age[51] and the prognosis of MPNST in NF1 is significantly worse when compared with that of the general population (5-year survival of 21% compared with 42%).[51]

MPNSTs may show some features of a neurogenic tumour but frequently are non-specific (Fig. 5-23); however, a heterogeneous mass arising from a nerve should raise suspicion, particularly if there is rapid enlargement, neurological deficit and nerve pain.[52] In NF1, there may be development of a mass from a plexiform NF and coincident new pain, change in consistency

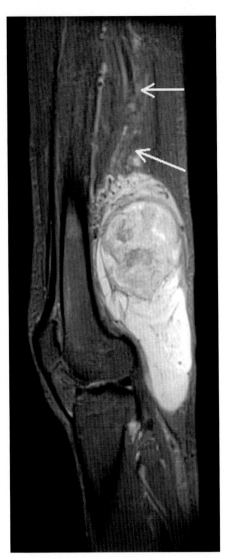

FIGURE 5-23 ■ **Malignant peripheral nerve sheath tumour (MPNST).** Sagittal STIR MR image: a large, heterogeneous but fusiform mass arises from a grossly enlarged sciatic/tibial nerve (arrows), in keeping with the development of an MPNST from a plexiform neurofibroma.

of the mass and neurological deficit. MRI features include a large, heterogeneous, lobular mass, lacking a target sign, with evidence of haemorrhage (T1 hyperintensity). Enhancement may be peripheral rather than the central enhancement seen in many benign PNSTs.[52] Positron emission tomography has been used to identify areas of malignant transformation within plexiform NFs, with a claimed high sensitivity and specificity.

Tumour-Like Lesions Arising from Nerves (Pseudotumours)

Nerve Sheath Ganglion (Intraneural Ganglion)

As might be expected, imaging shows a lobular area of fluid signal dissecting along a nerve. These lesions present with pain and nerve dysfunction, typically occurring at

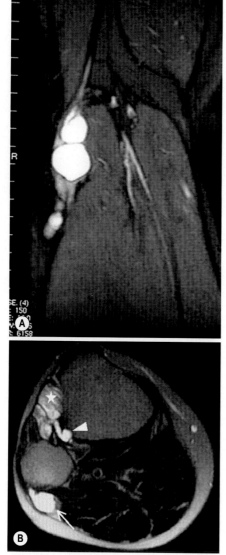

FIGURE 5-24 ■ **Intraneural ganglion.** Coronal STIR (A) and axial T2 with fat saturation (B) MR images of the right knee show a lobular, fluid–signal mass in the common peroneal nerve, compressing the hyperintense nerve (arrow in (B)). Continuation of the ganglion into the articular branch is seen (arrowhead in (B)). There is denervation of the extensor muscles (asterisk in (B)).

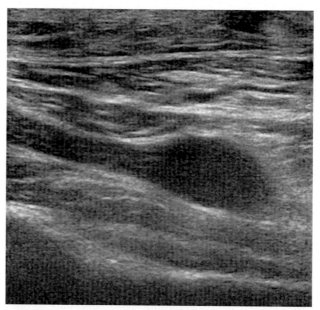

FIGURE 5-25 ■ **Amputation (traumatic) neuroma of the tibial nerve.** Longitudinal ultrasound image showing bulbous mass at the termination of the tibial nerve, which is rather thickened, some years following transtibial amputation.

the knee (common peroneal nerve, tibial nerve) but have also been described at other locations. Fluid decompresses from a degenerate joint through a capsular defect, dissecting along the epineurium of the articular branch and subsequently into the nerve itself, causing compression of nerve fascicles. In addition to the lobular, elongated, intraneural cystic mass, there may be signs of denervation (Fig. 5-24). Extraneural ganglia may also cause nerve compression but show a different morphology and relationship to the tibiofibular joint[53]—in addition to decompression of the nerve, the degenerate joint may need to be excised to prevent recurrence.

Traumatic Neuroma

Traumatic neuromas usually present with pain, which may be elicited by percussion of the nerve (Tinel's test).

They are most frequently found in the lower limb after amputation. Within hours of a nerve injury, there is distal degeneration of axons. Attempted repair by macrophages and Schwann cells, if unsuccessful, results in a fusiform (or occasionally laterally located) pseudotumour. Imaging reveals a bulbous mass at the termination of the severed nerve and frequently proximal nerve thickening[54] (Fig. 5-25).

Morton's Neuroma

Morton's neuroma is a common pseudotumour occurring on interdigital nerves in the web space of the forefoot. A small mass develops as a result of perineural fibrosis at the plantar aspect of the web space between the heads of the metatarsals. The lesion is most commonly seen between the third and fourth and, slightly less frequently, the second and third metatarsal heads, usually in middle-aged women. Ultrasound rarely identifies a nerve entering the mass, but does show a well-defined area of low reflectivity in the plantar aspect of the web space, which can be expelled with compression of the forefoot. MRI shows the neuroma best on images coronal to the web space and its low signal intensity reflects its fibrotic nature. T1 images are particularly useful as there is high contrast between the mass and adjacent web space fat.

Lipomatosis of Nerve

Lipomatosis of a nerve was formerly referred to as fibrolipomatous hamartoma or lipofibroma and is classified as an adipocytic soft tissue tumour by the WHO. Involvement of a variety of nerves has been described, but it most frequently affects the median nerve, resulting in a mass and features of neuropathy; and there may be associated macrodactyly. Imaging is characteristic on US and MRI

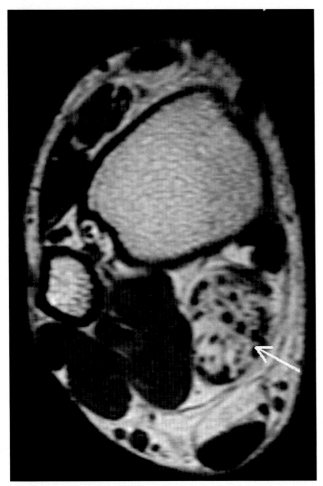

FIGURE 5-26 ■ **Lipomatosis of the tibial nerve.** Axial T1W imaging of the distal right calf shows enlargement of the tibial nerve (arrow). Nerve fibres are thickened and there is intervening hyperintense tissue consistent with fat.

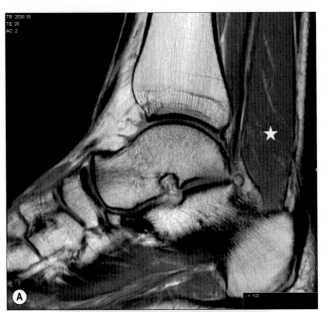

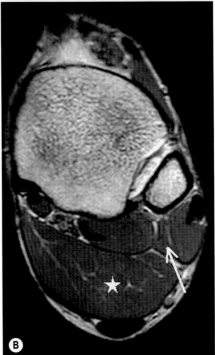

FIGURE 5-27 ■ **Accessory soleus muscle.** Sagittal (A) and axial (B) proton density MR images show the accessory muscle (asterisk) in the posterior calf between the flexor hallucis longus and the tendo Achilles. Another accessory muscle, the peroneus quartus, is also present in this subject (arrow).

demonstrating thickened nerve fascicles surrounded by adipose tissue within a grossly enlarged nerve (Fig. 5-26).

NON-NEOPLASTIC TUMOUR MIMICS

Many non-neoplastic lesions present as soft tissue masses. In general, imaging can offer a more accurate diagnosis than is often possible for many neoplasms, particularly sarcomas. 'Pseudotumours' are normal variants or non-neoplastic masses that mimic tumours—some examples are given below.

Accessory Muscles

A large number of these exist, but it is the accessory soleus that presents most frequently as a soft tissue mass (Fig. 5-27). The remainder tend to be small and impalpable, but may be identified on cross-sectional imaging examinations. Ultrasound and MRI can be reassuring, showing normal muscle tissue at the site of the mass.

Traumatic Lesions

These are frequent causes of a soft tissue mass. They include muscle tears, fascial hernias (Fig. 5-28), haematomas, fat necrosis and aneurysms. The *Morel-Lavallée lesion* is characteristic in site and appearance (Fig. 5-29). It is due to a closed degloving injury, resulting in shearing of the deep subcutaneous fat from the underlying fascia and causes a chronic haematoma, most frequently located over the lateral aspect of the hip and proximal thigh. An

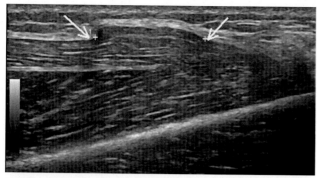

FIGURE 5-28 ■ Muscle fascial hernia. Longitudinal ultrasound image showing herniation of peroneal muscle through a fascial defect (arrows) in the distal lateral calf.

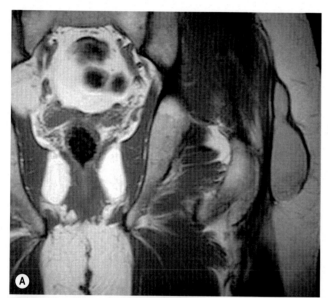

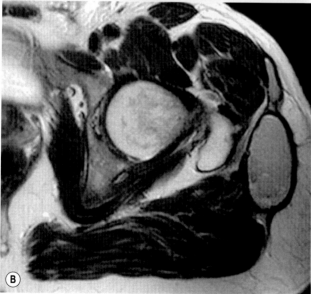

FIGURE 5-29 ■ Morel–Lavallée lesion. Coronal T1 (A) and axial T2W imaging (B). There is an elliptical mass whose appearances suggest chronic haemorrhage (hyperintense on T1W imaging, intermediate SI on T2W imaging with a surrounding rim of low signal), in a characteristic location in the deep subcutaneous fat at the lateral aspect of the hip.

elliptical mass, which frequently shows a low-signal rim and heterogeneous contents in keeping with chronic haemorrhage, is seen on MRI.[55] *Myositis ossificans* is classified by the WHO under fibroblastic/myofibroblastic tumours, but as a localised, self-limiting reactive process.[8] There may be no history of trauma in a significant number, despite representing ossification in the walls of a haematoma following muscle injury. In the early stages, an unmineralised soft tissue mass is apparent and MRI appearances may show extensive oedema around a heterogeneous lesion: careful inspection of the images often shows a characteristic low-signal rim at the margin of the mass and this is diagnostically useful. With time, the mass matures, with progressive peripheral ossification and resolution of pain, but in the early stages, US or CT is useful for identifying subtle mineralisation which may not be visible on radiographs (Fig. 5-1).

Infection/Inflammation

Pyomyositis (infective inflammation before the development of an abscess) causes a diffuse muscle swelling. US may identify a change in reflectivity within the muscle, small microabscesses and surrounding hyperaemia on colour Doppler, whereas on MRI soft tissue abscesses are hyperintense but heterogeneous on T2W imaging with surrounding oedema. Non-infective inflammatory myositis and foreign body reactions may also present as soft tissue masses.

Synovial Disorders

These are frequent causes of a soft tissue mass. Possible lesions include synovial cysts, ganglia, bursae, tenosynovitis. A *popliteal (Baker's) cyst* is one of the most common masses at the knee and often shows characteristic appearances, but it may be complicated by any process that involves the joint, including infection, haemorrhage, inflammatory arthritis and neoplasms.

REFERENCES

1. Enzinger F, Weiss S. Soft Tissue Tumors. 2nd ed. St. Louis: Mosby; 1988. pp. 1–18.
2. Lakkarajua A, Sinhaa R, Garikipati R, et al. Ultrasound for clinically suspicious soft-tissue masses. Clin Radiol 2009;64:615–21.
3. Kransdorf M. Malignant soft tissue tumours in a large referral population: distribution of diagnoses by age, sex and location. Am J Roentgenol 1995;164:129–34.
4. Gartner L, Pearce C, Saifuddin A. The role of the plain radiograph in the characterisation of soft tissue masses. Skeletal Radiol 2009;38:549–58.
5. Griffith J, Chan D, Kumta S, et al. Does Doppler analysis of musculoskeletal soft-tissue tumours help predict tumour malignancy? Clin Radiol 2004;59:369–75.
6. Belli P, Costantini M, Mirk P, et al. The role of color Doppler sonography in the assessment of musculoskeletal soft tissue masses. J Ultrasound Med 2000;19:823–30.
7. Bodner G, Schocke M, Rachbauer F, et al. Differentiation of malignant and benign musculoskeletal soft tissue tumors: combined color and power Doppler ultrasound and spectral wave analysis. Radiology 2000;223:410–16.
8. Fletcher C, Unni K, Mertens F, editors. Pathology and Genetics of Tumours of Soft Tissue and Bone, International Agency for Research on Cancer (IARC). Lyon: IARC Press; 2002.
9. Suresh S, Saifuddin A, O'Donnell P. Lymphoma presenting as a musculoskeletal soft tissue mass: MRI findings in 24 cases. Eur Radiol 2008;18:2628–34.

10. Myhre-Jensen O. A consecutive 7 year series of 1331 benign soft tissue tumours. Acta Orthop Scand 1981;52:287–93.

11. Murphey M, Carroll J, Flemming D, et al. Benign musculoskeletal lipomatous lesions. Radiographics 2004;24:1433–66.

12. Fornage B, Tassin G. Sonographic appearances of superficial soft tissue lipomas. J Clin Ultrasound 1991;19:215–20.

13. Ohguri T, Aoki T, Hisaoka M, et al. Differential diagnosis of benign peripheral lipoma from well-differentiated liposarcoma on MR imaging: is comparison of margins and internal characteristics useful? Am J Roentgenol 2003;180:1689–94.

14. Matsumoto K, Hukuda S, Ishizawa M, et al. MRI findings in intramuscular lipomas. Skeletal Radiol 1999;28:145–52.

15. Chung E, Enzinger F. Benign lipoblastomatosis: an analysis of 35 cases. Cancer 1973;32:482–92.

16. Ha T, Kleinman P, Fraire A, et al. MR imaging of benign fatty tumors in children: report of four cases and review of the literature. Skeletal Radiol 1994;23:361–7.

17. Kransdorf M, Bancroft L, Peterson J, et al. Imaging of fatty tumours: distinction of lipoma and well-differentiated liposarcoma. Radiology 2002;224:99–104.

18. Galant J, Marti-Bonmati L, Saez F, et al. The value of fat-suppressed T2 or STIR sequences in distinguishing lipoma from well-differentiated liposarcoma. Eur Radiol 2003;13:337–43.

19. Hosono M, Kobayashi H, Fujimoto R, et al. Septum-like structures in lipoma and liposarcoma: MR imaging and pathologic correlation. Skeletal Radiol 1997;26:150–4.

20. Leung L, Shu S, Chan A, et al. Nodular fasciitis: MRI appearance and literature review. Skeletal Radiol 2002;31:9–13.

21. Bernstein K, Lattes R. Nodular (pseudosarcomatous) fasciitis, a nonrecurrent lesion. Cancer 1982;49:1668–78.

22. Kransdorf M, Meis J, Montgomery E. Elastofibroma: MR and CT appearance with radiologic-pathologic correlation. Am J Roentgenol 1992;159:575–9.

23. Jarvi O, Lansimies P. Subclinical elastofibromas in the scapular region in an autopsy series: additional notes on the aetiology and pathogenesis of elastofibroma pseudoneoplasm. Acta Pathol Microbiol Scand 1975;83:87–108.

24. Brandser E, Goree J, El-Khoury G. Elastofibroma dorsi: prevalence in an elderly patient population as revealed by CT. Am J Roentgenol 1998;171:977–80.

25. Yacoe M, Bergman A, Ladd A, et al. Dupuytren's contracture: MR imaging findings and correlation between MR signal intensity and cellularity of lesions. Am J Roentgenol 1993;160:813–17.

26. Murphey M, Ruble C, Tyszko S, et al. Musculoskeletal fibromatoses: radiologic-pathologic correlation. Radiographics 2009;29:2143–76.

27. Sundaram M, McGuire M, Schajowicz F. Soft tissue masses: histologic basis for decreased signal (short T2) on T2-weighted MR images. Am J Roentgenol 1987;148:1247–50.

28. Murphey M, Rhee J, Lewis R, et al. Pigmented villonodular synovitis: radiologic-pathologic correlation. Radiographics 2008;28:1493–518.

29. Uriburu I, Levy V. Intraosseous growth of giant cell tumors of the tendon sheath (localized nodular tenosynovitis) of the digits: report of 15 cases. J Hand Surg 1998;23A:732–6.

30. Huang GS, Lee CH, Chan W, et al. Localized nodular synovitis of the knee: MR imaging appearance and clinical correlates in 21 patients. Am J Roentgenol 2003;181:539–43.

31. Enjolras O. Classification and management of the various superficial vascular anomalies: hemangiomas and vascular malformations. J Dermatol 1997;24:701–10.

32. Ernemann U, Kramer U, Miller S, et al. Current concepts in the classification, diagnosis and treatment of vascular anomalies. Eur J Radiol 2010;75:2–11.

33. Fayad L, Hazirolan T, Bluemke D, et al. Vascular malformations in the extremities: emphasis on MR imaging features that guide treatment options. Skeletal Radiol 2006;35:127–37.

34. Flors L, Leiva-Salinas C, Maged I, et al. MR imaging of soft-tissue vascular malformations: diagnosis, classification and therapy follow-up. Radiographics 2011;31:1321–40.

35. Mazoyer E, Enjolras O, Bisdorff A, et al. Coagulation disorders in patients with venous malformation of the limbs and trunk: a case series of 18 patients. Arch Dermatol 2008;114:861–7.

36. Zlatkin M, Lander P, Begin L, et al. Soft-tissue chondromas. Am J Roentgenol 1985;144:1263–7.

37. Woertler K. Soft tissue masses in the foot and ankle: characteristics on MR imaging. Semin Musculoskelet Radiol 2005;9:227–42.

38. Helpert C, Davies AM, Evans N, et al. Differential diagnosis of tumours and tumour-like lesions of the infrapatellar (Hoffa's) fat pad: pictorial review with an emphasis on MR imaging. Eur Radiol 2004;14:2337–46.

39. Singh V, Shah G, Singh P, et al. Extraskeletal ossifying chondroma in Hoffa's fat pad: an unusual cause of anterior knee pain. Singapore Med J 2009;50:e189–92.

40. Murphey M, McRae G, Fanburg-Smith J, et al. Imaging of soft-tissue myxoma with emphasis on CT and MR and comparison of radiologic and pathologic findings. Radiology 2002;225:215–24.

41. Luna A, Martinez S, Bossen E. Magnetic resonance imaging of intramuscular myxoma with histological comparison and a review of the literature. Skeletal Radiol 2005;34:19–28.

42. King D, Saifuddin A, Preston H, et al. Magnetic resonance imaging of juxta-articular myxoma. Skeletal Radiol 1995;24:145–7.

43. Kransdorf M, Murphey M. Imaging of Soft Tissue Tumours. 2nd ed. Lippincott Philadelphia: Williams and Wilkins; 2006. pp. 1–47.

44. Chen CK, Wu HT, Chiou HJ, et al. Differentiating benign and malignant soft tissue masses by magnetic resonance imaging: role of tissue component analysis. J Chin Med Assoc 2009;72:194–201.

45. Datir A, James S, Ali K, et al. MRI of soft-tissue masses: the relationship between lesion size, depth and diagnosis. Clin Radiol 2008;63:373–8.

46. Cadman N, Soule E, Kelly P. Synovial sarcoma: an analysis of 134 tumors. Cancer 1965;18:613–27.

47. Berquist T, Ehman A, King B, et al. Value of MR imaging in differentiating benign from malignant soft-tissue masses: study of 95 lesions. Am J Roentgenol 1990;155:1251–5.

48. Ohgaki H, Wiestler O, Cavenee W. WHO Classification of Tumours of the Central Nervous System. 4th ed. International Agency for Research on Cancer (IARC). Lyon: IARC Press; 2007.

49. Hassell D, Bancroft L, Kransdorf M, et al. Imaging appearance of diffuse neurofibroma. Am J Roentgenol 2008;190:582–8.

50. Ferner R, Golding J, Smith M, et al. [^{18}F]2-fluoro-2-deoxy-D-glucose positron emission tomography (FDG PET) as a diagnostic tool for neurofibromatosis 1 (NF1) associated malignant peripheral nerve sheath tumours (MPNSTs): a long-term clinical study. Ann Oncol 2008;19:390–4.

51. Evans D, Baser M, McGaughran J, et al. Malignant peripheral nerve sheath tumours in neurofibromatosis 1. J Med Genet 2002;39:311–14.

52. Ogose A, Hotta T, Morita T, et al. Tumors of peripheral nerves: correlation of symptoms, clinical signs, imaging features and histologic diagnosis. Skeletal Radiol 1999;28:183–8.

53. Spinner R, Luthra G, Desy N, et al. The clock face guide to peroneal intraneural ganglia: critical 'times' and sites for accurate diagnosis. Skeletal Radiol 2008;37:1091–9.

54. Gruber H, Glodny B, Bendix N, et al. High-resolution ultrasound of peripheral neurogenic tumors. Eur Radiol 2007;17:2880–8.

55. Mellado J, Perez de Palomar L, Diaz L, et al. Long-standing Morel-Lavallée lesions of the trochanteric region and proximal thigh: MRI features in five patients. Am J Roentgenol 2004;182:1289–94.

CHAPTER 6

METABOLIC AND ENDOCRINE SKELETAL DISEASE

Thomas M. Link • Judith E. Adams

CHAPTER OUTLINE

BONE PHYSIOLOGY AND PATHOPHYSIOLOGY

OSTEOPOROSIS

PARATHYROID DISORDERS

RICKETS AND OSTEOMALACIA

OTHER METABOLIC BONE DISORDERS

MISCELLANEOUS

BONE PHYSIOLOGY AND PATHOPHYSIOLOGY

Though bone appears rigid and inert, it is a highly metabolically active tissue, which is constantly remodelled with osteoblasts building bone and osteoclasts resorbing bone. This dynamic process allows the bone to be an extremely strong tissue that withstands the load-bearing requirements of the skeleton. Bone consists of crystals of hydroxyapatite embedded within an organic matrix, principally consisting of triple helical fibres of Type I collagen. Bones are generally divided into flat and tubular bones. Tubular bones are designed for weight bearing. Flat bones protect internal organs. Anatomically, bone is found in two forms:

- **compact (cortical) bone**, which forms the outer shell of bones,
- **trabecular (cancellous) bone**, which is found mainly in vertebral bodies, the pelvis and the distal regions of long bones.

Bones remodel from birth to maturity, maintaining their basic shape, repairing following fracture and responding to mechanical stresses throughout life. The strength of bone is related not only to its hardness and other physical properties but also to the architectural arrangement of the compact and trabecular bone. The skeleton contains 99% of the total body calcium and therefore plays a vital role in the maintenance of calcium homeostasis.

Bone Cells

Osteoblasts are bone-forming cells, which synthesise and secrete Type I collagen and mucopolysaccharides to form layers of bone matrix (osteoid) which subsequently becomes mineralised. Osteoblasts also synthesise collagenase, prostaglandin E_2 (PGE_2), and bone-associated proteins, osteocalcin and osteonectin. Osteoblasts have receptors for parathyroid hormone, vitamin D, prostaglandin E_2 and glucocorticosteroids.

Osteocytes are derived from the osteoblast and are initially present on the surface of bone but subsequently become encased within bone. Each osteocyte lies within a lacuna and is interconnected to other osteocytes and osteoblasts by cytoplasmic extensions within canaliculi. The osteocyte has a role in maintenance of bone matrix, which is facilitated by the transport of material and fluid via these canaliculi. Osteocytes respond to biomechanical loading, calcitonin and parathyroid hormone, and so play an important role in maintaining constant levels of calcium within the body fluids.

Osteoclasts are multinuclear giant cells that resorb both calcified bone and cartilage and derive from the mononuclear phagocytic cell line of haematopoietic stem cells. Osteoclasts lie on the surface of bone, causing active resorption and forming Howship's lacunae. Osteoclasts in contact with bone develop motile microvilli, which cause the cell to adhere to the bone surface and result in a microenvironment between the osteoclast and the mineralised bone. This brush border of microvilli increases with activation by such factors as prostaglandin, vitamin D and parathyroid hormone. Osteoclasts secrete acid hydrolases and neutral proteases, which degrade the bone matrix following its demineralisation. Figure 6-1 shows the different bone cells and their function in remodelling the bone.

Bone Formation and Turnover

Bone formation (osteoblastic activity) and bone resorption (osteoclastic activity) constitutes bone turnover, a process, which takes place on bone surfaces and continues throughout life (Fig. 6-1). Bone formation and resorption are linked in a consistent sequence under normal circumstances. Precursor bone cells are activated at a particular skeletal site to form osteoclasts, which erode a fairly constant amount of bone. After a period of time the resorption stops and osteoblasts are recruited to fill the eroded space with new bone. This coupling of osteoblastic and osteoclastic activity constitutes the basal

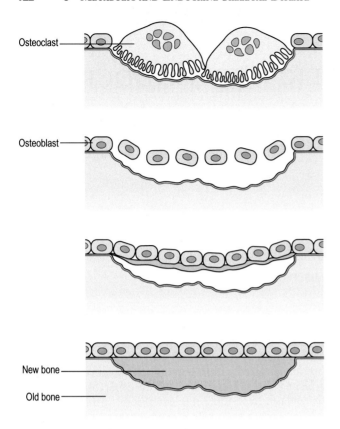

Osteoclast

Osteoblast

New bone

Old bone

FIGURE 6-1 ■ **Bone cells and basal metabolic unit (BMU).** Bone turnover continues throughout life so that old bone is replaced by stronger new bone; osteoclasts erode a pit of bone (top) and subsequently osteoblasts are recruited and fill the eroded pit with osteoid, which becomes mineralised. Normally this process is in balance and takes about 3–4 months to complete. If the process becomes uncoupled and erosion is excessive or the pit is incompletely filled with bone, there will be a net loss of bone over time (osteoporosis). Increase in both resorption and formation results in a high turnover state, e.g. Paget's disease.

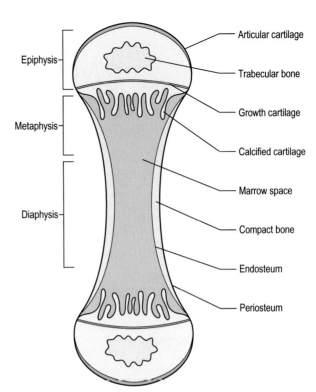

Epiphysis

Metaphysis

Diaphysis

Articular cartilage

Trabecular bone

Growth cartilage

Calcified cartilage

Marrow space

Compact bone

Endosteum

Periosteum

FIGURE 6-2 ■ **Tubular bone growth.** Tubular bones consist of an outer shell of cortical bone with inner trabecular bone, particularly at the ends of the bones, and haematopoietic marrow. They grow in length by endochondral ossification, which takes place at the physis (growth plate) between the distal epiphysis and the metaphysis.

multicellular unit (BMU) of bone. In healthy young adults the resorptive phase of the turnover cycle lasts about 30 days and the formation phase about 90 days. The length of the turnover cycle increases in later life and the rate of bone turnover is reduced. Uncoupling of the process (excessive osteoclastic resorption or defective osteoblastic function) results in a net loss of bone (**osteoporosis**). If there is both increased bone resorption and formation, this constitutes increased bone turnover. Woven immature, instead of mature lamellar, bone is laid down, as in Paget's disease of bone. Increased activation frequency of resorption units also results in high turnover state (hyperparathyroidism, postmenopausal bone loss). Bisphosphonate therapy reduces the activation of resorption units by inhibiting osteoclasts, and the reversal in the mineral deficit contributes to increase in bone mineral density (BMD).

Defective osteoclastic function prevents normal bone resorption, which is essential to maintain bone health by continuous slow renewal throughout life. Defective osteoclastic function in some diseases (i.e. osteopetrosis) can result in abnormal bone modelling and sclerosis on radiographs; these bone are more brittle and susceptible to fracture. Bone resorption by osteoclasts is a single-stage process in which collagen and mineral are removed together. Bone formation is a two-stage process: osteoblasts lay down osteoid, which subsequently becomes mineralised. Prerequisites for normal mineralisation are vitamin D ($1,25[OH]_2D_3$), normal levels of phosphorus and alkaline phosphatase, adequate intake of calcium and a normal pH. Defects in the mineralisation process will result in rickets or osteomalacia.

Bone Growth and Development

Early in fetal development the framework of the skeleton is in place but without mineralisation. At about 26 weeks of gestation the long bones assume their future shape and proportion. Bones grow in size and change in shape during childhood and adolescence, particularly during the pubertal growth spurt. Skeletal growth occurs primarily by endochondral ossification at the metaphyses and epiphyses (Fig. 6-2). The primary centre of ossification in the tubular bones is in the centre of the cartilaginous template. The secondary, later developing, centres (epiphyses) are located at the ends of the developing bones. In endochondral ossification there is hypertrophy of cartilage cells and glycogen accumulation. Subsequently, these cells undergo degeneration and become calcified (the provisional zone of calcification). The deeper perichondrial cells transform into osteoblasts through a process of intramembranous ossification. These osteoblasts, and vascular tissue, invade the cartilaginous matrix

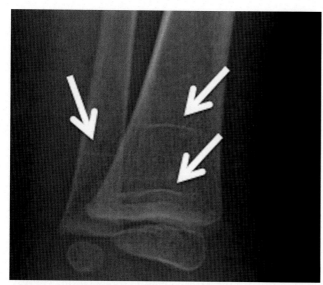

FIGURE 6-3 ■ **Growth arrest lines at the distal tibia (arrows).** If endochondral ossification ceases for any reason (e.g. period of illness, hypothyroidism), the zone of provisional calcification is left as a thin, horizontal, dense white line when the bone is at that particular stage of development.

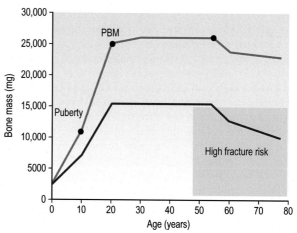

FIGURE 6-4 ■ **Bone gain and loss during life.** During childhood and adolescence there is accumulation of mineral in the bones which are growing in length and size, particularly at the time of puberty. Bones are larger and heavier in men than in women. Peak bone mass (PBM) is reached in the 20s and remains constant until about 35 years. At the time of the menopause, women lose bone due to oestrogen lack; both men and women lose bone with age. Maximising PBM and minimising bone loss by lifestyle factors such as regular exercise and good nutrition (adequate calcium and vitamin D) and avoiding risk factors (e.g. smoking, excess alcohol consumption) will prevent osteoporosis. Blue line, normal individual; red line, individual failing to achieve potential for skeletal mass. (Adapted from Heaney RP, Abrams S, Dawson-Hughes B, et al. Peak bone mass. Osteoporos Int. 2000;11(12):985–1009.)

and lay down osteoid, which becomes mineralised. Osteoblasts become trapped within the developing bone and transform into osteocytes.

Increase in bone length takes place at the metaphyses of long bones, which adjoin the cartilaginous growth plate. This cartilaginous growth plate remains between the ossification primary and secondary centres until growth ceases and skeletal maturity is reached. The remnant of the cartilage of the epiphyses adjacent to the articular surface becomes the articular cartilage of the adjacent joint. If endochondral ossification ceases for some reason (illness, nutritional deprivation) then the zone of provisional calcification present at that particular stage of skeletal development may remain as a thin white line (Harris growth arrest line) on radiographs (Fig. 6-3).

Bones consist of an outer shell of compact (cortical) bone with a central cavity which contains the marrow space, and 'lace-like' trabecular bone which is prominent in the axial skeleton and at the ends of long bones. Compact cortical bone constitutes about 80% of skeletal mass. Cancellous (trabecular) bone constitutes 20% of total skeletal mass, but contributes importantly to skeletal strength. The bone trabeculae are arranged to resist tensile deforming stresses, either from weight bearing or muscular activity. The number, thickness and distribution of trabeculae are related to biomechanical loading. Trabeculae provide a large surface area on which metabolic processes can take place and have a higher rate of turnover and richer blood supply than compact bone. Around the cortex of the bone is a layer of periosteum and adjacent to the marrow cavity is its endosteal surface. Excessive osteoclastic activity (e.g. in hyperparathyroidism) causes resorption of cortical bone, which may be visible radiologically (cortical 'tunnelling' and erosions) and is indicative of increased bone turnover. Resorption and formation takes place not only within the cortex of bone but also at the periosteal and endosteal surfaces.

As we age, more bone is removed at the endosteal surface than is replaced, resulting in a net loss of bone at this site. This causes the marrow cavity to enlarge and the bony trabeculae to become thinner—some may ultimately disappear. At the periosteal surface, resorption takes place, which is important in maintaining the normal shape of bones as they grow in length. There is a net gain of bone at the periosteal surface throughout life, so that tubular bones progressively increase in width as age advances.

The bones grow during the first two decades of life with a pubertal spurt during adolescence (Fig. 6-4). Skeletal maturity is achieved at an earlier age in girls (16–18 years) than in boys (18–20 years). Some disorders (hypothyroidism, chronic ill health) may retard skeletal development. Skeletal maturation is assessed radiologically from a non-dominant hand radiograph which is then compared with an atlas of hand radiographs of normal American Caucasian boys and girls of different ages[1] or using the Tanner and Whitehouse bone score (TW2) method, which assesses changes in presence, size and shape of certain bones with age.[2]

Following attainment of skeletal maturity, bone is consolidated and peak bone mass is achieved. For cortical bone this is reached at about 35 years of age, and a little earlier for trabecular bone (Fig. 6-4). Although the long bones grow in length at the metaphyses, they are remodelled in shape during development by endosteal resorption and periosteal apposition.

The size and shape of the skeleton and its individual bones are determined by genetic factors, but are influenced by endocrine and local growth factors, nutrition and physical activity. Remodelling allows the skeleton to adjust to mechanical forces to which it is exposed. There is considerable variation in skeletal size and weight, both within and between races. Black races have larger and heavier bones than whites, and Chinese tend to have lower skeletal mass and smaller size. Although genetic factors are important, they are modified by environmental differences such as diet and physical activity.

In mature healthy adults, bone turnover for the whole skeleton is about 2% per year, with maintenance of a constant bone mass. Bone formation is increased during periods of rapid growth and stimulated by physical activity, growth hormone and thyroid hormone. Bone formation is decreased as a consequence of immobilisation, undernutrition, deficiencies of thyroid and growth hormone and glucocorticoid excess. After the attainment of peak bone mass, bone loss, particularly of trabecular bone, is believed to occur from the third decade of life. Bone loss is a phenomenon, which occurs in all races (Fig. 6-4). Generally both men and women lose bone as they grow older, but women lose more than men. Women lose approximately 15–30% of their total bone mass between maturity and the seventh decade, whereas men lose only about half this amount. After the age of 35, women lose bone at an annual rate of approximately 0.75–1.0%, which increases to a rate of 2–3% in the postmenopausal period. This loss affects both cortical and trabecular bone, but the effect on trabecular bone predominates. In contrast, cortical bone is well preserved until the fifth decade of life when there is a linear loss in both sexes, such that men lose about 25% of their cortical bone whilst women lose about 30%. Low bone mineral density may be the result of either low peak bone mass attainment or subsequent accelerated bone loss.

The most common metabolic disorders of bone are: **osteoporosis**, in which there is a deficiency of bone mass leading to insufficiency (low-trauma) fractures; **rickets and osteomalacia**, in which there is a defective mineralisation of bone osteoid due to vitamin D deficiency, hypophosphataemia, lack of alkaline phosphatase or calcium, or severe acidaemia; and **hyperparathyroidism**, in which a tumour or hyperplasia of the parathyroid glands causes increase in parathyroid hormone production and stimulation of osteoclasts. Other metabolic bone disorders include osteogenesis imperfecta, hyperphosphatasia and osteopetrosis. Paget's disease is not strictly a metabolic bone disease, since it can be monostotic or polyostotic and does not involve the entire skeleton, but because it involves increased bone turnover it is often included in this group of disease.

OSTEOPOROSIS

Definition and Epidemiology

Osteoporosis is the most common metabolic bone disease, with increasing significance as the population ages. Fragility fractures due to osteoporosis are one of the most significant challenges to public health worldwide. The elderly represent the fastest-growing age group, and the yearly number of fragility fractures will increase substantially with continued ageing of the population.[3] Approximately 50% of women and 20% of men older than 50 years will have a fragility (insufficiency) fracture in their remaining lifetime in Caucasian populations.[4]

Osteoporosis is defined as a skeletal disorder characterised by compromised bone strength predisposing a person to an increased risk of fracture.[5] Bone strength primarily reflects the integration of bone mineral density (BMD) and bone quality.[5] BMD is expressed as grams of mineral per area or volume, and in any given individual is determined by peak bone mass and amount of bone loss. Bone quality refers to architecture, turnover, damage accumulation (e.g. microfractures), and mineralisation.[5]

Though BMD is only in part responsible for bone strength, dual energy X-ray absorptiometry (DXA) measurements of BMD have been universally adopted as a standard to define osteoporosis in terms of bone densitometry. In 1994 the World Health Organization (WHO)[6] used T-scores to classify and define BMD measurements. A T-score is the standard deviation of the BMD of an individual patient compared to a young, healthy reference population, matched for gender and ethnicity. According to the WHO, normal, osteopenic and osteoporotic BMD are differentiated.

Normal: BMD above (≥) –1 standard deviation (SD) of the young adult reference mean (peak bone mass).

Osteopenia: BMD between (<) –1 and (>) –2.5 SD below that of the young adult reference mean.

Osteoporosis: BMD more than (≤) –2.5 SD below the young adult reference mean.

It should be noted that even in the absence of osteoporotic BMD the *presence of one or more low-impact fragility fractures* is considered as a sign of severe osteoporosis[7] and that not infrequently in these patients the BMD measured with DXA may be in the normal or osteopenic range.

The osteoporosis/osteopenia definition is also applied to older men, but it is not used in men younger than 50, premenopausal women and children or adolescents who have not yet reached peak bone mass. In these patient groups, low bone mass would appropriately be defined as a BMD which is more than 2 standard deviations below the mean BMD matched for age, gender and ethnicity (http://www.iscd.org/visitors/positions/OP-Index.cfm and).[8–10] The WHO definition is *not applicable* to other bone densitometry techniques (quantitative computed tomography, QCT; quantitative ultrasound, QUS) or other anatomical sites (e.g. calcaneus).

Osteoporosis should not be considered as a single disease entity, but rather an end result of many disease processes (Table 6-1). It may result from defective skeletal accretion during bone growth and development. Alternatively, it may result from disease processes in which bone resorption exceeds new bone formation, resulting in a net loss of bone mass and consequent compromise to skeletal strength.

Radiological Features

Osteoporosis is radiographically characterised by decreased radiodensity of bone (Fig. 6-5). However, it

TABLE 6-1	**Main Causes of Osteoporosis**

Primary
Juvenile
Idiopathic of young adults
Postmenopausal
Senile

Secondary
Endocrine
Glucocorticoid excess
Oestrogen/testosterone deficiency
Hyperthyroidism
Hyperparathyroidism
Growth hormone deficiency (childhood onset)
Nutritional
Intestinal malabsorption (e.g. coeliac disease)
Chronic alcoholism
Chronic liver disease
Partial gastrectomy
Vitamin C deficiency (scurvy)
Hereditary
Osteogenesis imperfecta
Homocystinuria
Marfan's syndrome
Ehlers–Danlos syndrome
Haematological
Thalassaemia
Sickle-cell disease
Gaucher's disease
Leukaemia in children
Other
Rheumatoid arthritis
Haemochromatosis

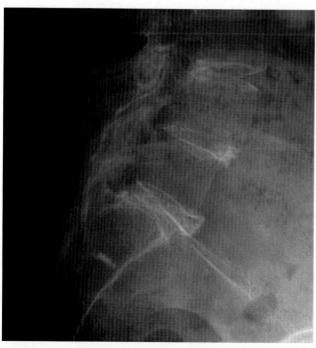

FIGURE 6-5 ■ **Osteopenia.** Lateral radiograph of the lumbar spine showing severe, diffuse osteopenia with degenerative changes of the lumbar spine.

should be noted that radiographs are very limited in assessing the amount of bone loss[11] and only advanced bone loss can be identified. Descriptive terms that have been used to describe reduced bone density in the absence of fragility fractures are 'osteopenia' or 'demineralisation'. The latter is an incorrect term since mineral and collagen are both reduced in osteoporosis. Reduced bone density is often more prominent in areas of the skeleton rich in trabecular bone, particularly in the axial skeleton (vertebrae, pelvis, ribs and sternum). Eventually, changes may also be evident in the bones of the appendicular skeleton. Trabeculae become thin and may disappear completely; they may be sparse, but those that remain may become thickened due to stresses to which the skeleton is exposed (Fig. 6-6). The cortex becomes reduced in width through endosteal bone resorption, and in states of increased bone turnover there will be intracortical tunnelling and porosity.

Osteoporotic bone is less able to withstand the stresses to which the skeleton is exposed compared to normal bone, and this leads to the cardinal clinical feature of low trauma fractures. Such fractures can occur at any skeletal site, but they are most common in sites of the skeleton rich in trabecular bone, particularly the vertebrae, the distal forearm and the proximal femur. These fractures may be associated with considerable pain and deformity. In individuals who suffer hip fractures 20% will die within the next year and 20% will require permanent nursing home care.[4] Even if age-adjusted incidence rates for hip fractures remain stable, the estimated number of hip fractures worldwide will rise from 1.7 million in 1990 to 6.3 million in 2050.[3] It is important to identify patients with osteoporosis and at increased risk of fracture as there are now therapies available (bisphosphonates, selective oestrogen receptor modulators (SERMs), strontium ranelate; teriparatide (parathyroid hormone) and denosumab) which cause relatively small increases in bone mineral density (4–12%) but more importantly reduce future fracture risk by between 40 and 70%.[12,13]

Spine in Osteoporosis

Related to biomechanical forces through the spine, as trabeculae are lost, the process of osteoporosis particularly involves the horizontally orientated secondary trabeculae. The vertical trabeculae actually become more prominent and thickened.[14] This results in a vertical 'striated' appearance to the vertebral body on lateral spinal radiographs and cross-sectional imaging studies. Figure 6-6 shows this pattern in sagittal and coronal reformations of CT images, which was also termed hypertrophic atrophy. This feature is generally seen in several, or all, of the vertebrae when it is related to osteoporosis, which serves to distinguish a similar appearance in a single vertebral body when it is related to haemangioma.

Vertebral fractures are the most common of osteoporotic fractures (Fig. 6-7). The anterior and central mid portion of the vertebrae withstand compression forces less well than the posterior and outer ring elements of the vertebrae, resulting in wedge or end-plate fractures or, less commonly, crush fractures.[15] Vertebral fractures can be graded as mild (20–25% change in shape;

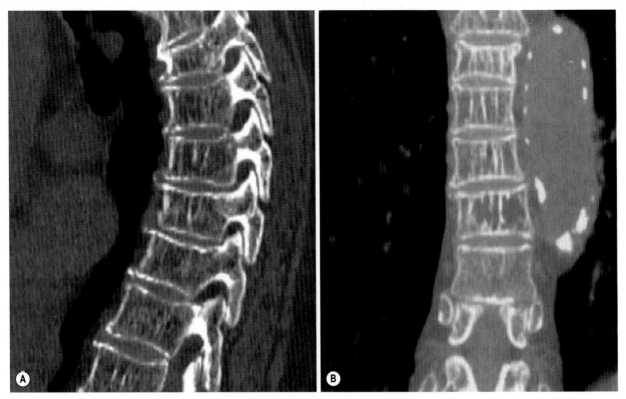

FIGURE 6-6 ■ **Hypertrophic atrophy in osteoporosis.** Sagittal (A) and coronal (B) CT MPRs of the thoracic spine showing diffuse bone loss with prominent vertical trabeculae resulting in a striated appearance.

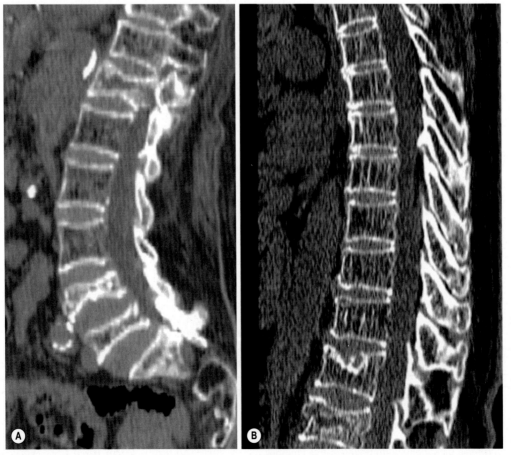

FIGURE 6-7 ■ **Osteoporosis—vertebral osteoporosis and fracture.** Sagittal reconstructions of CT data sets of the thoracolumbar spine showing moderate to severe osteoporotic fractures at T12, L4 and L5 (A) and at the lower thoracic spine with multilevel prominence of the vertical trabeculae and a striated appearance due to loss of the horizontal trabeculae (B).

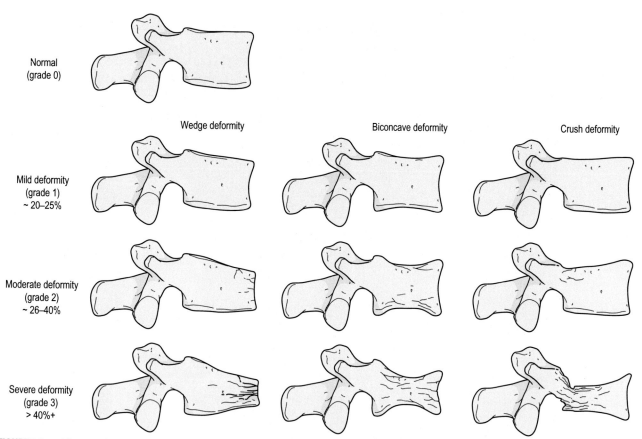

Normal
(grade 0)

Wedge deformity   Biconcave deformity   Crush deformity

Mild deformity
(grade 1)
~ 20–25%

Moderate deformity
(grade 2)
~ 26–40%

Severe deformity
(grade 3)
> 40%+

FIGURE 6-8 ■ **The semiquantitative method of grading of Genant et al,[16] which is widely used in epidemiology and pharmaceutical studies.** Vertebral fractures are strong predictors of future fractures (×5 for vertebral fracture; ×2 for hip fracture). The higher the grade of vertebral fracture, the higher the risk of future fracture.

grade 1), moderate (26–40% change in shape; grade 2) and severe (>40% change in shape; grade 3)[16] (Fig. 6-8). This semi-quantitative grading (SQ) method is the one currently most frequently applied to define the prevalence and incidence of vertebral fractures in epidemiology studies and pharmaceutical trials of the efficacy of new osteoporosis therapies.

The more severe the grade of vertebral fracture, the greater the risk of future fracture. Vertebral fractures are powerful predictors of future fracture (hip ×2; vertebral ×5). If vertebral fractures are present it is therefore extremely important that they are accurately and clearly reported by radiologists as fractures; other terms such as 'deformities', 'collapse', must be avoided. There is evidence that vertebral fractures are being under-reported by radiologists, with the result that patients who should be receiving treatment to reduce their risk of future fractures are not being identified.[17–19] As a consequence, a joint initiative was launched in 2002 between the International Osteoporosis Foundation (IOF) and the European Society of Skeletal Radiology (Osteoporosis Group) to improve the sensitivity and accuracy of reporting of vertebral fractures by radiologists. Vertebral fractures may occur as an acute event related to minor trauma and be accompanied by pain, which generally resolves spontaneously over 6–8 weeks. This resolution of symptoms serves to distinguish osteoporotic vertebral fractures from similar events due to more sinister abnormalities,

such as metastases, in which the symptoms are more protracted. However, 30% or more of vertebral fractures may be present in asymptomatic patients. Osteoporotic fractures occur most commonly in the thoracic and thoracolumbar regions and result in progressive loss of height in affected individuals. Osteoporotic fractures are uncommon above T7; if fractures are present above this anatomical region, metastases should be considered. Also if the posterior aspect of the vertebral body is fractured metastases or myeloma should be the first differential diagnosis. Wedging of multiple vertebral bodies in the thoracic spine can lead to increased kyphosis (dowager hump) which, if severe, may result in the ribs abutting on the iliac crests with compromise of respiratory function and reduced quality of life.

Vertebroplasty and Kyphoplasty

Vertebroplasty and kyphoplasty have selected application in patients with osteoporotic vertebral fractures that are persistently painful.[20] The technique is performed mostly by radiologists and orthopaedic surgeons. Vertebroplasty is the injection of cement (methylmethacrylate) into a fractured vertebral body as a means of treating pain. Injection is generally made by passing the introduction needle through the pedicles. Kyphoplasty is the injection of cement into the fractured vertebral body after a balloon has been used to form a cavity and to decompress the

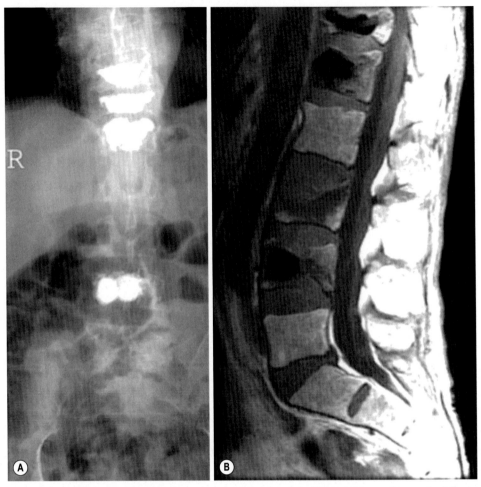

FIGURE 6-9 ■ **Osteoporosis—vertebroplasty/kyphoplasty.** In selected cases, pain from osteoporotic vertebral fractures which has not responded to conservative (analgesics) and bisphosphonate therapy may be treated by injection of cement (methylmethacrylate) into the vertebral body. The cement is radio-opaque so that it can be visualised during injection, and is seen in the frontal radiograph of the thoracolumbar spine at T11, T12, L1 and L4 (A) and the T1-weighted sagittal MR image at T12, L1 and L4 (B). In kyphoplasty a balloon is introduced through a needle passed through the pedicle and used to increase the height of the vertebral body. A cavity is thus created for the injection of the cement. The cement has rounded configuration in kyphoplasty (seen at L1 and L4) compared to vertebroplasty where the cement is simply injected into the vertebral body (T12).

fracture and correct some of the deformity[21] (Fig. 6-9). Both techniques are intended to relieve pain in patients who have not responded to conservative measures. It has been suggested that vertebroplasty/kyphoplasty should be performed in the first 4–6 weeks after presentation with pain, which requires opiates for pain relief and/or hospital admission.[22] Certainly patients with proven osteoporosis should always be commenced on bone protective/ bone enhancing therapy when vertebroplasty is to be performed. Patient selection is crucial to the outcome of the procedure. The pain should arise from vertebral fractures that are temporally related to the onset of symptoms. Magnetic resonance imaging (MRI) with fluid-sensitive sequences and fat suppression can aid the identification of more acute fractures showing bone marrow oedema, typically along the end-plates, in acute and subacute fractures with ongoing bony remodelling.

Two recent trials comparing vertebroplasty with a sham procedure suggested that improvements in pain and pain-related disability associated with osteoporotic compression fractures in patients treated with vertebroplasty were similar to the improvements in a control group.[23,24] Conversely a study published in 2010 concluded that pain relief after vertebroplasty was immediate, sustained for at least a year, and was significantly greater than that achieved with conservative treatment, at an acceptable cost.[25] The chance of successful pain relief by vertebroplasty for osteoporotic fracture is between 70 and 95%.[26] In a previous study kyphoplasty and vertebroplasty demonstrated similar good clinical outcomes during the 12-month follow-up; but kyphoplasty offered a higher degree of spinal deformity correction and resulted in less cement leakage than vertebroplasty.[27]

There are potential risks of vertebroplasty; these may be needle related (pedicle fracture, needle breakage, pneumothorax, haemorrhage, infection), cement related (root compression, cord compression, pulmonary cement emboli), procedure related (pulmonary fat emboli, rib or vertebral fracture), sedation related (respiratory arrest, airway injuries, cardiac arrest) or drug related (allergy). The overall complication rate from reports suggests that symptom-inducing or potentially serious complications occur in approximately 2% of patients treated for osteoporotic fracture.[28]

Most cases are treated under conscious sedation with analgesia, but in some patients general anaesthesia is required. For needle placement, high-quality fluoroscopy in either a biplane or C-arm configuration is recommended. Needles, injector sets and cements are now manufactured specifically for vertebroplasty. Care should be taken to ensure a sterile environment. All patients treated by vertebroplasty or kyphoplasty for osteoporotic compression fractures should be under the care of a clinician with special interest in osteoporosis management and on appropriate medical therapy to reduce future fracture risk.[13]

Osteoporotic Fractures

Fractures that occur in osteoporosis generally heal well with satisfactory callus formation. In some sites the presence of multiple micro-fractures and callus formation can cause osteosclerosis on a radiograph; this must be distinguished from other pathologies such as bone metastases. These insufficiency fractures occur in particular anatomical sites, including the symphysis pubis, the sacrum, pubic rami and calcaneus. Other sites involved are the sternum, supra-acetabular area and elsewhere in the pelvis, femoral neck, humerus and proximal and distal tibia. Some of these fractures may be accompanied by considerable osteolysis, particularly those involving the symphysis pubis. Fragility fractures of the pelvis have been misinterpreted as neoplastic lesions and several previous studies[29-31] focused on the importance of correctly diagnosing sacral fractures to avoid misguiding patient management, which may produce dangerous and costly interventional procedures. Cross-sectional imaging techniques (CT and MR imaging) may help to differentiate insufficiency fractures from other pathologies (Fig. 6-10). On radionuclide bone scintigraphy there is increased uptake in regions of acute insufficiency fractures.

When the sacrum is involved, there is often a characteristic H pattern (Honda sign) of radionuclide uptake. CT and MRI are particularly helpful in defining the fracture lines of insufficiency fractures involving the sacrum (fractures usually occur parallel to the sacroiliac joint) and in the calcaneus. In these sites fractures may not be identified on radiographs because of complex anatomy and overlying structures. MRI is helpful in differentiating vertebral fractures resulting from osteoporosis from those caused by other pathologies (myeloma, metastases). It should be noted that MR is more sensitive than CT in diagnosing pelvic insufficiency fractures.[30]

During the past decade a number of publications focused on osteoporotic insufficiency fractures and demonstrated that findings previously defined as osteonecrosis are actually insufficiency fractures.[29,30,32-35] Previously, the term' spontaneous osteonecrosis of the knee (SONK), was used to describe an osteochondral lesion which was typically observed at the medial femoral condyle but which is now considered to be an insufficiency fracture. Both insufficiency fractures at the medial femoral condyle of the knee and femoral head are frequent findings in older individuals and indicate increased fragility of the skeleton (Fig. 6-11).

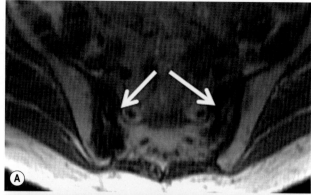

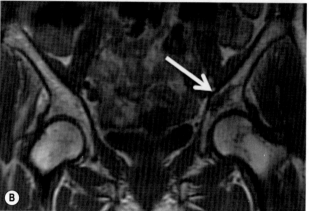

FIGURE 6-10 ■ **Pelvic insufficiency fractures.** Axial and coronal T1-weighted FSE sequences of the pelvis in a 72-year-old woman with bilateral sacral insufficiency fractures (arrows in A) and a left supra-acetabular fracture (arrow in B). T1-weighted sequences frequently show fracture lines best.

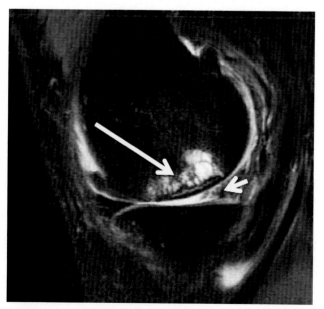

FIGURE 6-11 ■ **Medial femoral condyle insufficiency fracture.** Sagittal intermediate-weighted fat-saturated MR image of the knee in a 65-year-old man showing a medial femoral condyle insufficiency fracture (long arrow) with meniscal maceration (short arrow).

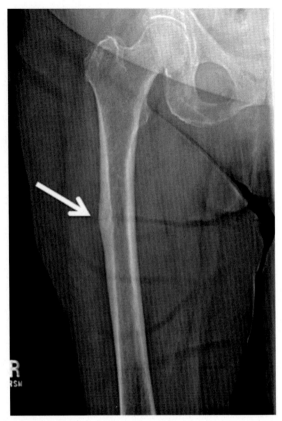

FIGURE 6-12 ■ **Atypical proximal femur fracture after bisphosphonate therapy.** Radiograph of the right proximal femur showing an atypical, incomplete femoral diaphysis fracture (arrow) after long-term bisphosphonate therapy (arrow).

Recently atypical subtrochanteric and femoral shaft fractures have been reported in older individuals and on long-term bisphosphonate therapy.[36–38] Coexisting factors have been discussed in the aetiology of these fractures such as co-morbidities (e.g. vitamin D deficiency, chronic obstructive airways disease, rheumatoid arthritis, diabetes) and other drugs (e.g. glucocorticoids, proton pump inhibitors).[36–38] The task force of the American Society for Bone and Mineral Research[38] identified a number of major and minor clinical and imaging features of these fractures which include location in the subtrochanteric region and femoral shaft, transverse or short oblique orientation, minimal or no associated trauma, a medial spike when the fracture is complete, absence of comminution, focal cortical thickening and a periosteal reaction of the lateral cortex (Fig. 6-12). There may be prodromal symptoms such as dull or aching pain in the groin or thigh. As these stress fractures may be bilateral in up to 50% of patients and occur anywhere in the femoral shaft, if suspected, imaging should include both femora in their entirety. These fractures are increasingly diagnosed, can occur in bisphosphonate naïve patients and not infrequently only lateral cortical thickening is evident. This may progress to a complete fracture and is therefore a critical finding, which needs to be communicated to the clinician. These incomplete stress fractures are treated with prophylactic internal fixation surgery. The relation of this complication with long-term bisphosphonate

therapy has led to consideration of a drug 'holiday' at 5-year review. If the BMD T-score is above –2.5, treatment may be discontinued for two years and then the necessity for recommencement is considered; however, there are no scientific data on which to base such recommendations.

Aetiology

Osteoporosis can be classified as generalised, regional (involving a segment of the skeleton) or localised.

Regional Osteoporosis

This can occur in disuse and reflex sympathetic dystrophy (RSD/regional pain syndrome) following fracture, or related to other pathologies (primary and secondary tumours). Chronic disuse is characterised by a uniform pattern of bone loss; acute immobilisation causes more focal and irregular bone formation and resorption. This results in different patterns of bone loss, which include diffuse osteopenia, linear translucent bands, juxta-articular speckled radiolucent areas and cortical bone resorption.[39] MRI findings in disuse osteopenia are also typical and include accentuation of vertical trabecular lines, presence of subchondral lobules of fat, horizontal trabecular lines, prominence of blood vessels, and dotted and patchy areas of high signal intensity on fluid-sensitive sequences[40] (Fig. 6-13).

RSD/complex regional pain syndrome is a clinical syndrome that can occur in children and adults and may be precipitated by a variety of processes. There is overactivity of the sympathetic nervous system, initially causing pain, soft-tissue swelling and hyperaemia, with excessive bone resorption (probably stimulated by cytokines), which occurs particularly in a peri-articular distribution and may simulate malignant disease. The diagnosis of RSD/complex regional pain syndrome relies on clinical evaluation and radiographs. MRI may provide a differential diagnosis between RSD and other bone pathologies as it demonstrates diffuse signal abnormalities with soft-tissue and bone marrow oedema pattern.[41]

There are also conditions which cause focal or migratory and transient osteoporosis, usually in the region of large joints (hip, knee), the aetiology of which is uncertain. Transient osteoporosis of the hip occurs in younger and middle-aged individuals and middle age, more frequently in men than women. Also, it is typically found in women in the third trimester of pregnancy. There is sudden onset of pain without preceding trauma. Radiographically there is reduction in density of the proximal femur. There may be an underlying abnormality of perfusion of the marrow, which is oedematous. MRI is sensitive in demonstrating bone marrow oedema pattern without focal abnormalities before any radiographic abnormality is evident (Fig. 6-14).[42,43]

Generalised Osteoporosis

There are many causes of osteoporosis, falling into four categories:

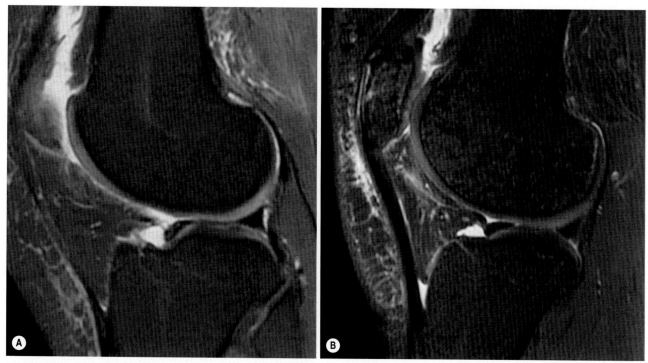

FIGURE 6-13 ■ **Disuse osteopenia.** Sagittal intermediate-weighted fat-saturated MR image of the knee in a 35-year-old man with an ankle fracture showing normal bone marrow signal at the time of the fracture.

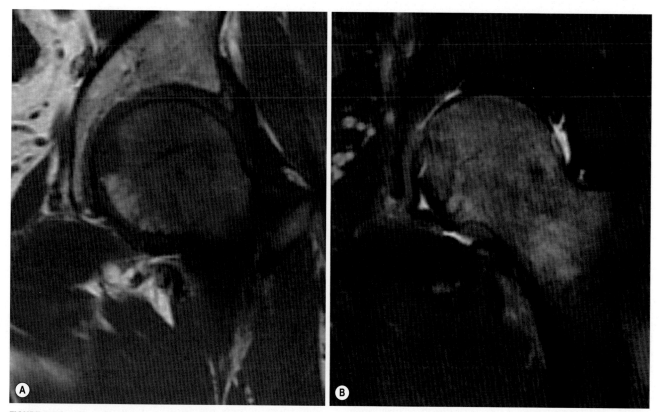

FIGURE 6-14 ■ **Transient osteoporosis of the hip.** Coronal T1-weighted FSE (A) and STIR (B) images of the left hip in a 42-year-old man with transient osteoporosis. Note homogeneous bone marrow oedema pattern without focal linear signal abnormalities, which would suggest a fracture, or deformities as might occur in avascular necrosis of the femoral head with subchondral fracture.

1. Factors which reduce peak adult bone mass
2. Age-related bone loss
3. Bone loss associated with menopause or hypogonadal state
4. Bone loss that is secondary to other medical conditions and drugs (Table 6-1).

Idiopathic Juvenile Osteoporosis (IJO). This self-limiting form of osteoporosis occurs in prepubertal children and must be differentiated from osteogenesis imperfecta and other forms of juvenile osteoporosis. IJO is a rare disorder, first described by Dent and Friedman,[44] and occurs in children aged between 8 and 14 years who have previously been healthy. The disease runs an acute course over a period of 2–4 years, during which there is growth arrest and fractures. There is a wide spectrum of severity, and both cortical and trabecular bone are affected. In the mild form, only one or two vertebral fractures may be present, but in more severe cases fractures involve all the vertebrae and the extremities, particularly the metaphyseal region of the distal tibia. A few affected patients may develop severe kyphoscoliosis, deformities of the extremities, and even die from respiratory failure due to thoracic deformity. The disease is reversible and remits spontaneously. Affected patients may be left with only a mild or moderate kyphosis, short stature and some bone deformity following fractures.[44] Investigations indicate uncoupling of the two components of bone turnover due to both increase in resorption and decrease in formation. The important differential diagnosis in children with vertebral fracture is hypercortisolism and leukaemia. Affected patients do not have the blue sclerae characteristic of osteogenesis imperfecta.

Osteoporosis of Young Adults. This heterogeneous condition occurs equally in young men and women.[45] The disease generally runs a mild course with multiple vertebral fractures occurring over a decade or more, with associated loss in height. Fractures of metatarsals and ribs are also common, and hip fractures may occur. The cause of the condition is uncertain and in some patients it may simply be that inadequate bone mass has been accrued during skeletal growth. Some affected individuals may have a mild variant of osteogenesis imperfecta. Rarely, osteoporosis may present during pregnancy, but whether this is a causal or coincidental association is unknown.

Postmenopausal Osteoporosis. At the time of the menopause, lack of oestrogen will result in some women losing trabecular bone at a rate three times greater than is usual (2–10% per annum). The condition, previously referred to as type I osteoporosis, characteristically becomes clinically evident in women 15–20 years after the menopause. Fractures occur in sites of the skeleton rich in trabecular bone, including the vertebral bodies and distal forearm (Colles' fracture).

Senile Osteoporosis. This condition, previously referred to as type II involutional osteoporosis, occurs in both men and women of 75 years or older and is due to age-related bone loss. This occurs as a consequence of age-related impaired bone formation associated with secondary hyperparathyroidism caused by reduced intestinal calcium absorption due to decreased levels of $1,25(OH)_2D$ production in the elderly.[46] There is reduction in both cortical and trabecular bone. The syndrome manifests mainly as hip fractures and wedge fractures of the vertebrae, but fractures may also occur in the proximal tibia, proximal humerus and pelvis.

Secondary Osteoporosis. A large number of conditions may lead to osteoporosis (Table 6-1). Radiologically these may be indistinguishable from age-related osteoporosis. However, some may have specific and diagnostic radiological features (i.e. subperiosteal erosions of the phalanges in primary hyperparathyroidism). In glucocorticoid excess (endogenous and exogenous), there is reduced bone formation due to a direct effect on the osteoblast, and increased osteoclastic activity, probably mediated through secondary hyperparathyroidism, stimulated by reduced gastrointestinal absorption of calcium. There is also evidence that glucocorticoids induce premature apoptosis of both osteoblasts and osteoclasts. The effect is primarily on trabecular bone. Fractures occur particularly in the vertebral bodies and ribs; the latter may heal with profuse callus formation. Fractures may appear relatively rapidly after starting oral glucocorticoid medication, in particular with high doses and in younger patients (Fig. 6-15).

Osteogenesis Imperfecta

A number of inherited disorders of connective tissue may result in osteoporosis. Osteogenesis imperfecta (OI), or brittle bone disease, results from mutations affecting either the *COL1A1* or *COL1A2* gene of Type I collagen.[47] Although the disease is usually apparent at birth or in childhood, more mild forms of the disease may not become apparent until adulthood, when affected individuals may present with insufficiency fractures and osteopenia (Fig. 6-16). Radiographic features vary according to the type of disease and its severity and include osteopenia and fractures, which may heal with florid callus formation, mimicking osteosarcoma. Bones are thin and over-tubulated (gracile), normal in length or shortened, thickened and deformed by multiple fractures. Intrasutural (Wormian) bones can be identified on skull radiographs. In severe forms of osteogenesis imperfecta the diagnosis may be made before birth by detailed ultrasound in the second trimester. Diagnostic features include cranial enlargement, reduced echogenicity of bone and deformity and shortening of limb bones as a result of intrauterine fractures.

Osteogenesis imperfecta is classified based on distinct characteristics, including blue sclerae, the severity of the disorder and the mode of inheritance (dominant, recessive, sporadic/new mutation).[48] However, accurate classification is difficult because of phenotypic overlap.[47]

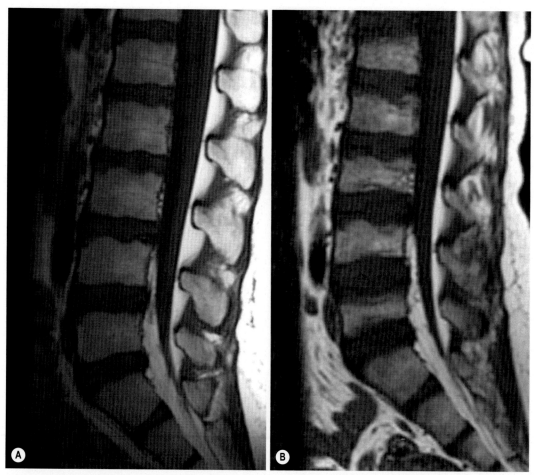

FIGURE 6-15 ■ **Glucocorticoid Induced Vertebral Fractures.** Sagittal T1-weighted MR images of the lumbar spine in an 11-year-old child at the time of glucocorticoid therapy initiation (A) and 3 months later (B) with multiple vertebral fractures having occurred.

Affected subjects who do not have dental involvement are designated as group A. Subjects with dentinogenesis imperfecta are designated as group B.

Type I

This is the mildest and most prevalent form of the disease and may only become apparent in adulthood. There is a history of fractures, generally dating back to childhood. In children the fractures may become radiographically and clinically apparent as the child becomes more active (5+ years), and may take the form of overt fractures or micro-fractures involving the metaphyses. In infancy these features may resemble those found in non-accidental injury.[49] The differential diagnosis can usually be resolved by the presence of associated extraskeletal manifestations of osteogenesis imperfecta (blue sclerae, dentinogenesis imperfecta), or evidence of a family history of the condition. Bone biopsy for diagnosis is rarely required. Affected patients are short in stature, only 10% being of normal height, with joint laxity, blue sclerae and presenile hearing loss. Transmission is by autosomal dominant trait. Radiologically the bones are usually reduced in radiodensity, although some patients may have normal bone density. Bones may be gracile, or modelled normally. Vertebral fractures often occur in the fourth decade and when scoliosis is present, it is mild.

Type II (Lethal Perinatal)

Affected infants are small for dates with deep blue sclerae and shortened and deformed limbs due to multiple fractures. Fractures involve the ribs and death is usually the result of pulmonary insufficiency. Survival is rare beyond the first three months of postnatal life. Other complications include brain and spinal cord injury. Radiologically, multiple fractures are present with a characteristic 'concertina' deformity of the lower limbs. The ribs may appear 'beaded' due to multiple rib fractures, which can occur in utero. The cranial vault is severely undermineralised and may be distorted by moulding, with Wormian (intrasutural) bones in the occipital and parietal region. Platyspondyly is present. Histology reveals defective endochondral ossification at the metaphyses and epiphyses, which appear disorganised with persistent islands of calcified cartilage and under-mineralised bone. There is defective transformation of woven bone to lamellar bone in both the cortical and trabecular skeletal components. Membranous ossification is also deficient, accounting for the marked calvarial thinning.

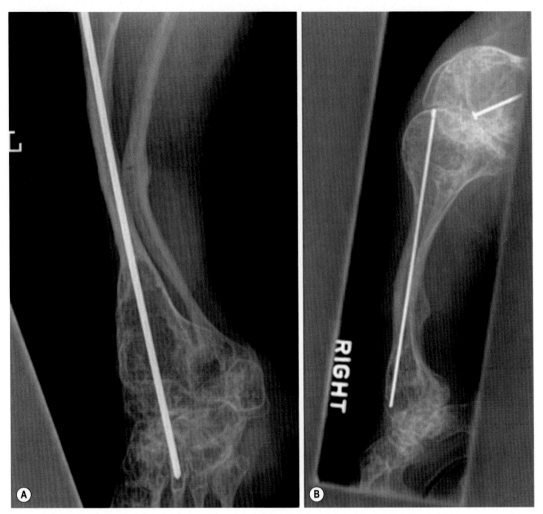

FIGURE 6-16 ■ **Osteogenesis imperfecta.** AP (A) and lateral (B) radiographs of the left distal lower extremity in a 10-year-old child with extensive deformity, incomplete healing fractures and internal fixation with rods. Findings are those of osteogenesis imperfecta, a disorder caused by genetic mutations in Type I collagen resulting in osteoporosis and low-trauma insufficiency fractures (brittle bone disease). The different types vary in clinical presentation and severity.

Type III (Severe Progressive)

This is inherited as an autosomal recessive trait. Fractures are usually present at birth and involve the long bones, clavicles, ribs and cranium, leading to deformity. Although size at birth is normal, growth retardation is evident in the first year of life and many affected patients only reach 0.9–1.2 m (3–4 ft) in height. As growth proceeds, increasing deformity of the calvarium occurs, with associated facial distortion, dental malocclusion and mild prognathism, basilar invagination and progressive hearing loss. Sclerae are blue at birth but this diminishes with age, and sclerae are white in adults. Vertebral fractures occur at an early age and contribute to the progressive and severe kyphoscoliosis, which develops during childhood. Affected patients tend to be wheelchair bound because of the progressive deformities resulting from fractures. Complications include progressive pulmonary insufficiency due to thoracic distortion. Radiologically, the bones may be slender or broad due to recurrent fractures. Epiphyses are abnormal, with expansion and islands of calcified ('popcorn') cartilage. As with other forms of

osteogenesis imperfecta, the incidence of fractures declines following puberty.

Type IV (Moderately Severe)

This is inherited as an autosomal dominant trait, can vary in severity and is sometimes confused with either type I or type III OI. There is generally more severe osteopenia and more extensive bone deformity than in type I. The sclerae are blue in children and while this may persist into adulthood, they may also fade to white. Individuals are short in stature with abnormal moulding of the calvarium and basilar invagination in a high proportion of patients. Bones in the axial and appendicular skeleton are osteoporotic and dysplastic, resulting in scoliosis and deformity, particularly of the pelvis. Joint laxity can result in dislocation, particularly of the ankle or knee.

Type V OI resembles type IV disease in terms of frequency of fractures and degree of skeletal deformity. It dominantly inherited or may develop spontaneously and is characterised by development of hypertrophic callus at sites of fractures or surgical intervention. Ossification of the interosseous ligament between radius and ulna may restrict movement in this site.

Quantitative Assessment of the Skeleton

The most important technique to quantify bone mineral density (BMD) is dual energy X-ray absorptiometry (DXA); additional techniques have been used which include quantitative CT, quantitative ultrasound and radiogrammetry. Six-point morphometry is used to quantify change in vertebral shape (deformity) and has an increasing role, with DXA being used to image the whole spine for vertebral fracture assessment (VFA).[50] BMD is the single most important determinant of fracture, accounting for approximately 70% of bone strength. Reduced BMD is a useful predictor of increased fracture risk. The lower the peak bone density, the higher the risk of fracture in later life. Methods of measuring bone density are therefore relevant to the study of skeletal development, the detection of osteopenia and assessment of efficacy of treatment of osteoporosis. Such methods for measuring BMD should be accurate, precise (reproducible), sensitive both to small changes with time and to differences in patient groups (i.e. fracture compared to non-fracture), inexpensive and involve minimal exposure to ionising radiation.

Accuracy expresses how close the measurements made are to the actual BMD measured by chemical analysis. All the quantitative methods available have some inaccuracies caused by variable fat content, either within the marrow of trabecular bone (single energy quantitative computed tomography, QCT) or by the fat content of extra-osseous soft tissue (other photon absorptiometric techniques, DXA). Changes in body composition or marrow fat may introduce errors in the measurement depending upon the technique and measurement site used.

Precision assesses the reproducibility of the measurement technique and is usually expressed as a percentage of coefficient of variation (CV%). A high precision (low CV% in the region of 1%) is essential in longitudinal studies to detect small changes in BMD over reasonable periods of time. Short-term precision principally reflects repositioning errors, whilst long-term precision using calibration phantoms reflects machine instability. Change in BMD is best evaluated by calculating the percentage change; the least significant change from two measures ($p = 0.05$) is given by $2.77 \times$ precision error of the method.[51] As changes in BMD are generally small, an interval of at least 18–24 months should be used between quantitative measures.

Dual Energy X-ray Absorptiometry (DXA)

DXA was introduced in 1987 and is the most widely available bone density technique. It utilises two X-ray beams with differing kVp (30–50 and >70 keV) to enable subtraction of the soft-tissue component allowing measurement of BMD in a given area of bone ('areal' BMD) measured in g/cm^2. This is typically done in the lumbar spine (L1–4), proximal femur (femoral neck and total)

and distal radius. Original machines had a pencil beam and coupled detector and acquired data in a rectilinear fashion. Modern systems have a fan beam X-ray source and banks of detectors allowing rapid data acquisition with improved spatial resolution (1 to 0.5 mm). The accuracy of DXA is between 3 and 8%, with precision (CV%) better than 1% in PA spine and total femur, and 1–2% in femoral neck. Radiation dose is low (1–6 µSv for BMD; up to 50 µSv if performed with VFA).[52]

Proximal femur and lumbar spine measurements are performed most frequently. Using an automatic segmentation, which is checked and corrected by the operator, the L1–4 vertebral bodies, femoral neck, intertrochanteric and trochanteric regions are measured. The total femur region of interest is derived from femoral neck, intertrochanteric and trochanteric regions. In addition to areal density values in g/cm^2, DXA provides T- and Z-scores. Z-scores are standard deviations (SD) compared to an age-matched reference population, while T-scores are SD compared to a young adult reference population. Whole-body DXA with regional analysis gives information not only on total and regional BMD but also on body composition (lean muscle mass and fat mass).

In postmenopausal women and men over 50 DXA BMD is used to define osteoporosis (T-score at or below −2.5) and osteopenia (T-score between −1.1 and −2.4).[6] This definition was originally only established for BMD of the proximal femur (neck and total femur regions of interest), but is currently also used for lumbar spine (postero-anterior projection) and distal radius (1/3 radius region of interest) DXA (Fig. 6-17). In premenopausal women, men younger than 50 and children Z-scores are used comparing individual BMD measurements to an appropriate age-matched reference population.[8-10] A Z-score lower than −2 is defined as 'below the expected range for age'. It should be noted that osteoporosis cannot be defined using DXA BMD alone in these populations.

Guidelines for DXA referral vary internationally and were generally performed on a case finding (high fracture risk) strategy, as population screening is not cost-effective. DXA was indicated in women aged 65 and over and in younger and perimenopausal women with risk factors for insufficiency fractures.[9] DXA was also advocated in men 70 years and older and younger men with risk factors for fracture.

Although the T-score of −2.5 was satisfactory as a definition of osteoporosis, it was never appropriate as a level for therapeutic intervention, largely because age is such a strong independent predictor of fracture. In 2008 the WHO introduced the 10-year fracture risk prediction tool (FRAX) which can be accessed at http://www.shef.ac.uk/FRAX/. This tool uses clinical risk factors and the presence of secondary causes of osteoporosis with or without DXA femoral neck BMD to calculate the risk of hip, and other major, osteoporotic fractures.[53,54] With the use of appropriate guidelines,[55,56] which may vary between different nations, FRAX should lead to a more appropriate utilisation of DXA and its results, and more cost-effective intervention strategies.[57]

Individuals being considered for osteoporotic bone protective/bone-enhancing therapy and those already on

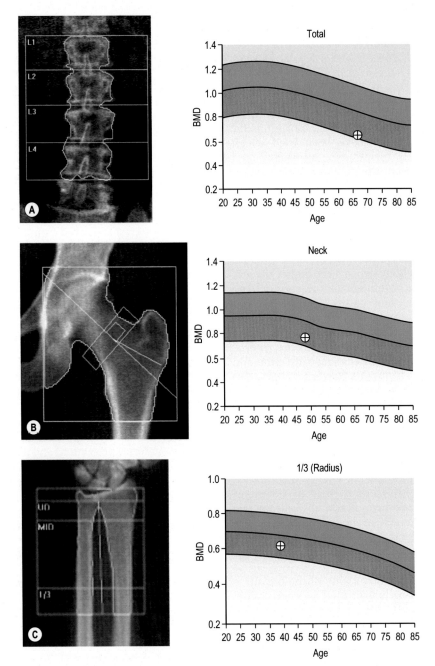

FIGURE 6-17 ■ **DXA images of the lumbar spine (A), proximal femur (B) and distal radius (C).** DXA provides 'areal' BMD (g/cm²) and is currently the 'gold standard' method for diagnosis of osteoporosis by bone densitometry in adults (WHO definition T-score –2.5 or below). The blue band shows range of two standard deviations above normal age-matched BMD and the purple band demonstrates range of two standard deviations below the normal age-matched BMD.

therapy should be examined with DXA.[9] Follow-up DXA every 1–2 years is used in clinical practice to verify response to treatment, although measuring serum bone turnover markers will confirm response to bisphosphonate therapy in a shorter period (3–4 months).

DXA has some limitations which need to be considered:

1. It is a 2D image of a 3D bone, which measures density/area (in g/cm²) of integral (cortical and trabecular) bone and not the volumetric density (in mg/cm³) as is provided by quantitative CT. Areal BMD is dependent on bone size and will thus overestimate fracture risk in short individuals with small

bones, who will have lower areal BMD than normal-sized individuals.

2. Spine and hip DXA are sensitive to artefacts caused by degenerative changes and individuals with significant degenerative disease will have falsely increased areal BMD, which will indicate a lower fracture risk than is actually present. DXA is limited in elderly patients in whom degenerative changes are commonly present (60% in those aged 70 years or more) (Fig. 6-18).

3. All structures overlying the spine such as aortic calcifications, or morphological abnormalities of the vertebrae such as fractures (false elevation of

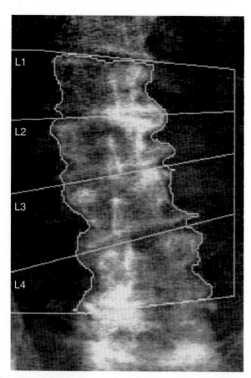

FIGURE 6-18 ■ DXA images of degenerated lumbar spine. DXA image of the lumbar spine demonstrating degenerative changes with sclerosis leading to falsely elevated BMD.

BMD) or laminectomy (false reduction) will affect DXA BMD measurements.

Other causes of falsely high BMD on DXA include vertebral fracture, Paget's disease of bone, sclerotic metastases, vertebral haemangioma, spinal metallic pinning or plating, calcified lymph nodes, residual Myodil and navel rings. Such artefacts require the results from affected individual vertebral bodies to be excluded from analysis, but a minimum of two vertebrae must be available for interpretation.

Treatment with strontium ranelate causes artefactual elevation of BMD, approximately 50% of the increase being due to the high-atomic-number strontium in the bones. DXA can be used for examining peripheral sites: for instance, the distal 1/3 radius is a site consisting predominantly (95%) of cortical bone and measurement here may be helpful in patients with primary or secondary hyperparathyroidism. It can also be used to study regional bone density around a prosthesis following hip arthroplasty.

Quantitative Computed Tomography (QCT)

QCT uniquely allows for the separate estimation of trabecular and cortical BMD and provides a true volumetric density in mg/cm³. To perform QCT a standard CT unit with a bone equivalent calibration phantom under the patient is used. Density values, measured in Hounsfield units, are transformed into BMD, measured in mg hydroxyapatite/cm³ using the phantom. Typically, the L1–3 vertebral bodies are measured; either single-slice mid-vertebral 10-mm slice or volumetric MDCT

methods can be used to measure BMD (Fig. 6-19); volumetric MDCT techniques are also available to measure proximal femur BMD.

In addition to the true volumetric measurements provided by QCT, the technique has several other important advantages over DXA. QCT can provide separate measures of cortical and trabecular BMD. Trabecular BMD is more sensitive to monitoring changes with disease and therapy, as trabecular bone is more metabolically active than cortical bone.[58] Cross-sectional studies have shown that QCT BMD of the spine allows better discrimination of individuals with and without vertebral fractures.[59,60] QCT is also better suited to examining obese patients as DXA makes assumptions about body composition and so has limitations in measuring BMD in patients with a body mass index over 25 kg/m². In such obese patients superimposed soft tissue will falsely elevate measured BMD due to attenuation of the X-ray beams and beam hardening artefact.[61–63]

Limitations of QCT are a higher radiation dose (0.06–2.9 mSv depending on whether lumbar spine or hip is being assessed), although lower doses are utilised for QCT compared with conventional CT[52] and the presence of only a small number of longitudinal studies assessing how QCT predicts fractures. The WHO T-score of –2.5 defining osteoporosis is not applicable to QCT. A T-score threshold of –2.5 for QCT would identify a much higher percentage of apparently osteoporotic subjects and QCT has therefore never been established for clinical use. Currently volumetric QCT techniques are preferred over single-slice techniques[64–67] and in clinical practice absolute measurements of BMD have been defined to characterise fracture risk: 110–80 mg/cm³ = mild increase in fracture risk; 80–50 mg/cm³ = moderate increase in fracture risk; and below 50 mg/cm³ = severe increase in fracture risk. According to the American College of Radiology (ACR) Guidelines for QCT a BMD range of 120–80 mg/cm³ is defined as osteopenic and values below 80 mg/cm³ as osteoporotic.[68]

Recommendations for the appropriate use of QCT instead of DXA are (i) very small or large individuals, (ii) older individuals with expected advanced degenerative disease of the lumbar spine or morphological abnormalities and (iii) if high sensitivity to monitor change in BMD is required, such as in patients treated with parathyroid hormone or oral glucocorticoids. A recent study comparing DXA and QCT in older men with diffuse idiopathic skeletal hyperostosis (DISH) demonstrated that QCT was better suited to differentiate men with and without vertebral fractures.[69]

Although QCT is usually applied to the spine and proximal femur, dedicated peripheral QCT units (pQCT) have been developed which allow separate analysis of cortical and trabecular bone in the non-dominant forearm and in other sites of the skeleton, including the tibia. In bone shafts, cortical thickness and cross-sectional bone area can be measured, from which certain biomechanical parameters (stress strain index; moment of inertia) can be extracted. Cross-sectional muscle area and muscle density can also be measured, relevant to studies investigating the interaction of muscle and bone and in sarcopenia.

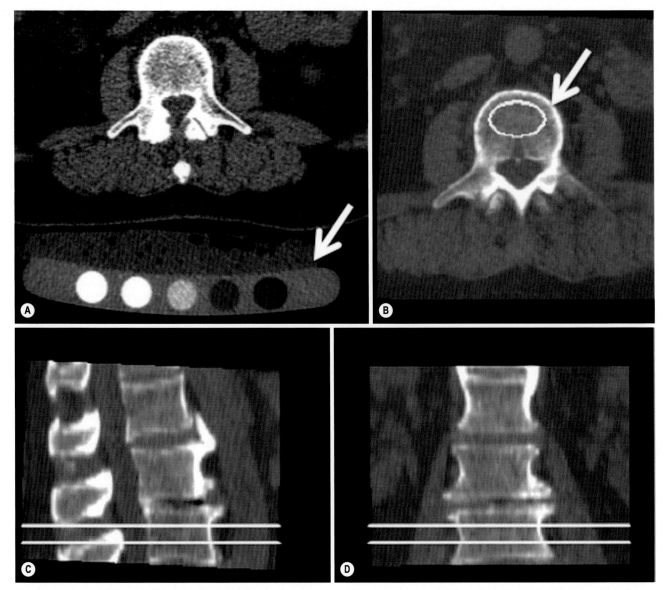

FIGURE 6-19 ■ **Volumetric QCT of the L3 vertebral body.** BMD calibration phantom is shown below patient in (A) (arrow). In (B) the oval-shaped region of interest is depicted (arrow) and (C) and (D) show the volume analysed in the sagittal and coronal images from MDCT acquisition.

Quantitative Ultrasound

Quantitative ultrasound (QUS) is a low-cost technique performed with dedicated devices acquiring data, mostly at the calcaneus. Using a water bath or ultrasound jelly, an emitter and receiver probe are brought in close proximity to the soft tissue surrounding the bone (e.g. calcaneus). The propagation of ultrasound waves through the bone is measured, which is characterised by the velocity of transmission and the amplitude of the ultrasound signal. Velocity is measured as m/s (metre/second) and defined as speed of sound (SoS), which is independent of ultrasound wave attenuation. SoS decreases in osteoporotic bone. In addition, broadband ultrasound attenuation (BUA) is calculated in dB/MHz (decibel/megahertz), which increases in osteoporotic bone. Recent meta-analyses confirmed that both DXA and calcaneal quantitative ultrasonography predicted fractures in an older patient population but that the correlation between the two techniques was low.[70] However, the limitations of QUS are that (i) neither the WHO definition of osteoporosis nor the FRAX 10-year fracture risk calculator are applicable to QUS, (ii) the measures are temperature dependent and (iii) there is no cross-calibration phantom available. Also the method has been applied to a large number of different anatomical sites (fingers, forearm, tibia) without clear recommendations on the preferred site. Consequently, QUS remains largely a research technique.

Radiogrammetry

Radiogrammetry involves cortical thickness measurements on radiographs of various long bones. The bone most frequently used is the second metacarpal of the non-dominant hand, but the method has also been applied to other bones (clavicle, radius, humerus, femur and tibia). In the metacarpal the diameter of the bone in its mid portion (from each periosteal surface) and the medullary width (distance between endosteal surfaces) are measured using callipers.[71,72] A variety of indices have been described, including cortical thickness, metacarpal index and parameters of cortical area. The technique is simple to perform, uses a low radiation dose, and has been widely applied. However, the reproducibility is limited (coefficient of variation (CV) up to 11%). This is because the endosteal surface becomes irregular and more difficult to identify with bone resorption. Now modern computer vision methods (active shape models, ASM) have been applied and improve precision to better than 1% (digital X-ray radiogrammetry, DXR).[73]

Vertebral Morphometry

Over the past decade efforts have been made to standardise the subjective visual assessment of vertebral fracture, and to quantitate alterations in vertebral height and shape. These developments have been stimulated not only by the need for comparable methods to be used in epidemiological studies but also by the fact that the prevalence and incidence of vertebral fractures are used as inclusion criteria and treatment outcome measures in therapeutic trials in which the efficacy of new drugs for the treatment of osteoporosis is being assessed.[50,74]

The technique for spinal radiography should be standardised, with a fixed film focus distance (FFD), and the spine parallel to the radiographic table for the lateral projection. Any scoliosis or tilting of the spine due to poor positioning will cause apparent, but false, biconcavity of the end-plates ('bean-can effect'). Centring is at T7 spinous process for the lateral thoracic spine and L3 spinous process for the lateral lumbar spine projections. Assessments for vertebral fractures are usually made from T4 to L4 on the lateral spinal projections. Vertebral fractures are defined as end-plate, wedge or crush. Changes in shape of the vertebrae (deforming events) are generally defined by the 6-point method, in which the anterior, mid and posterior points of the superior and inferior end-plates of the vertebral body are identified to measure anterior, mid and posterior heights. Vertebral deformity is defined by relating the anterior or mid vertical heights to the posterior height, expressed as a percentage or by specified standard deviations from normal reference data for vertebral size. A vertebral fracture can be defined by grading from 0 (normal) to grade 3 (obvious fracture) in a semiquantitative scheme, which has now largely replaced 6-point morphometry.[16]

The introduction of fan beam technology and improvements in spatial resolution in DXA enabled good-quality (dual and single energy modes) images (postero-anterior and lateral projections) of the thoracic and lumbar spine, from which vertebral fracture assessment (VFA) and morphometric measurements can be made (MXA).[75,76] It may be feasible for this process to be automated by computer techniques.[77] The advantages of VFA over conventional spinal radiography are a lower radiation dose (1/100th),[52] less end-plate distortion since the X-ray beam is parallel to the end-plate at each vertebral level, and the entire spine is visualised on a single image, and BMD measurement can be made on the same equipment.[78]

Other Research Methods

High-resolution multidetector computed tomography (HR-MDCT)[79,80] and high-resolution magnetic resonance imaging (HR-MRI)[81,82] have been used to analyse trabecular bone structure in vivo. One of the most important developments to assess bone architecture over the past 10 years has been the introduction of high-resolution peripheral CT (HR-pQCT)[83–87] (Fig. 6-20). The dedicated in vivo extremity imaging system is

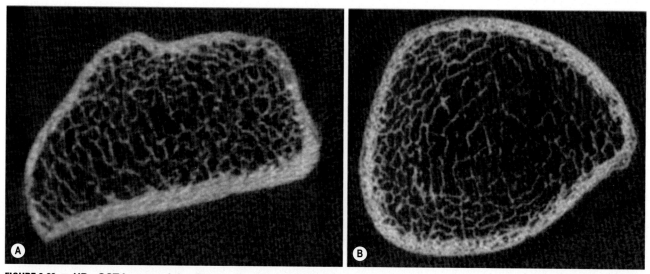

FIGURE 6-20 ■ **HR-pQCT images of the distal radius (A) and tibia (B).** These high-resolution images demonstrate the trabecular bone structure and the cortical bone architecture, including the cortical porosity. These images can be used to quantify a number of trabecular and cortical structure parameters in addition to biomechanical surrogate markers of bone strength through finite element modelling (FEM).

designed for imaging trabecular and cortical bone architecture and has the advantage of significantly higher signal-to-noise ratio (SNR) and spatial resolution (nominal isotropic voxel dimension of 82 μm) compared to multidetector CT (MDCT) and MRI.[87] In comparison MDCT has a maximum in-plane spatial resolution of 250–300 μm and MRI of 150–200 μm, with slice thicknesses of 0.5–0.7 and 0.3–0.5 mm, respectively. Furthermore, the effective radiation dose is substantially lower compared to whole-body MDCT and does not involve critical, radiosensitive organs (effective dose <3 μSv). The aquisition time for HR-pQCT is long, at approximately 3 min each for the tibia and radius, so motion artefact can be problematic. There are several disadvantages to this technology, most notably that it is limited to peripheral skeletal sites and therefore can provide no direct insight into bone quality in the lumbar spine or proximal femur—common sites for osteoporotic insufficiency fractures.[87]

PARATHYROID DISORDERS

Most parathyroid tumours are functionally active and result in the clinical syndrome of primary hyperparathyroidism. This is the most common endocrine disorder after diabetes and thyroid disease, with an incidence within the population of about 1 in 1000 (0.1%). The incidence is higher in the elderly and is most common in women aged 60 or older. Over the past 50 years the diagnosed prevalence of the condition has increased some tenfold, due principally to the detection by chance of hypercalcaemia in patients, many of whom are asymptomatic.

Hyperparathyroidism

Primary Hyperparathyroidism

The majority (80%) of patients with primary hyperparathyroidism have a single adenoma. Multiple parathyroid adenomas may occur in 4% of cases. Hyperplasia of all glands occurs in 15–20% of patients. Genetic factors are relevant in a proportion of these patients (familial hyperplasia, multiple endocrine neoplasia (MEN) syndromes).

Carcinoma of the parathyroid is an infrequent cause of primary hyperparathyroidism (1%);[88] the malignant tumour is slow growing but locally invasive. Cure may be obtained by adequate surgical excision and there is a 50% or greater 5-year survival rate. Persistent or recurrent disease occurs in more than 50% of patients with parathyroid carcinoma.[88] Surgical resection is also the primary mode of therapy for recurrence since it can offer significant palliation for the metabolic derangement caused by hyperparathyroidism and allows hypercalcaemia to become more medically manageable. However, reoperation is rarely curative and eventual relapse is likely. Chemotherapy and external beam radiation treatments have been generally ineffective in the treatment of parathyroid carcinoma.

Secondary Hyperparathyroidism

Secondary hyperparathyroidism is induced by any condition, or circumstance, which causes the serum calcium to fall. This occurs in vitamin D deficiency, intestinal malabsorption of calcium (e.g. coeliac disease), chronic kidney disease (CKD) (azotaemic osteodystrophy)—through lack of the active metabolite of vitamin D, $1,25(OH)_2D$, and retention of phosphorus. In long-standing secondary hyperparathyroidism an autonomous adenoma may develop in the hyperplastic parathyroid glands, a condition referred to as tertiary hyperparathyroidism. This is usually associated with CKD but it has also been observed in patients with long-standing vitamin D deficiency and osteomalacia from other causes.

Clinical Presentation

Most patients with primary hyperparathyroidism have mild disease and commonly have no symptoms, the diagnosis being made by the finding of asymptomatic hypercalcaemia. The most common clinical presentations, particularly in younger patients, are related to renal stones and nephrocalcinosis (25–35%), high blood pressure (40–60%), acute arthropathy (pseudogout) caused by calcium pyrophosphate dihydrate deposition (chondrocalcinosis), osteoporosis, bone and muscle pain, proximal muscle weakness, peptic ulcer and acute pancreatitis, depression, confusional states and mild non-specific symptoms such as lethargy, arthralgia and difficulties with mental concentration.

Treatment

Surgical removal of the overactive parathyroid tissue in primary hyperparathyroidism is generally recommended.[89] In experienced hands surgical excision is successful in curing the condition in over 90% of patients.[90] The decision to operate, particularly in the elderly and those with asymptomatic disease, requires careful assessment. For patients who do not undergo parathyroidectomy, annual monitoring of serum calcium and creatinine levels and assessment of bone mineral density every 1 or 2 years is recommended, but at present, there is no definitive medical therapy for primary hyperparathyroidism,[90] although a calcimimetic, cinacalcet, which acts through the calcium sensing receptor, has been used in various causes of hypercalcaemia, including primary and secondary hyperparathyroidism.

In secondary hyperparathyroidism treatment should include a combination of dietary phosphorus restriction, phosphate binders, vitamin D sterols, and calcimimetics; parathyroidectomy is effective in suitable candidates refractory to medical therapy.[91]

Radiological Findings

With increased numbers of patients with primary hyperparathyroidism being diagnosed with asymptomatic hypercalcaemia, the majority (95%) of patients will have no radiological abnormalities. In more advanced stages typical radiographic abnormalities are found, that include

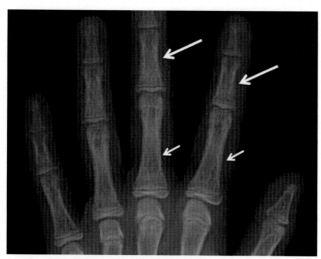

FIGURE 6-21 ■ **Primary hyperparathyroidism.** Radiograph of the left hand demonstrating subperiosteal erosions, particularly in the radial aspect of the middle phalanges of the index and middle fingers (large arrows). Also as a result of increased osteoclastic resorption, cortical 'tunnelling' (areas of resorption within the bone cortex) is evident in the proximal phalanges (small arrows).

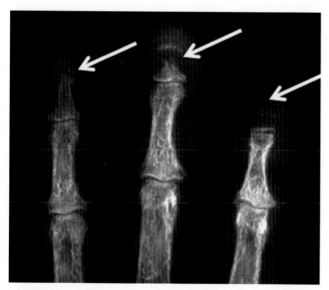

FIGURE 6-22 ■ **Primary hyperparathyroidism.** Radiograph of the left hand showing advanced subperiosteal erosions and acro-osteolysis of the second to fourth digits (arrows).

subperiosteal erosions, chondrocalcinosis, brown tumours and soft-tissue metastatic calcifications, the latter occurring only in secondary hyperparathyroidism associated with CKD in which there is phosphate retention.

Subperiosteal Erosions. Subperiosteal erosion of cortical bone, particularly in the phalanges, is pathognomonic of hyperparathyroidism[92] (Fig. 6-21). The most sensitive site in which to identify this early subperiosteal erosion is along the radial aspects of the middle phalanges of the index and middle fingers. Typically also the tufts of the distal phalanges may be affected. Other sites may be involved, including the distal phalanges (acro-osteolysis) (Fig. 6-22), the outer ends of the clavicle, the symphysis

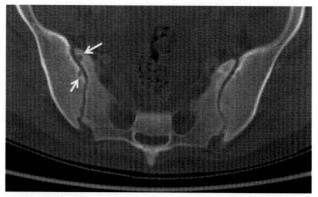

FIGURE 6-23 ■ **Primary hyperparathyroidism.** CT of the sacroiliac joints with subchondral erosions (arrows) mimicking inflammatory sacroiliitis.

pubis, the sacroiliac joints (Fig. 6-23), the proximal medial cortex of the tibia, the proximal humeral shaft, ribs and femur. However, if no subperiosteal erosions are identified in the phalanges, they are unlikely to be identified radiographically elsewhere in the skeleton. Subperiosteal erosions in sites other than the phalanges indicate more severe and long-standing hyperparathyroidism, such as may be found secondary to CKD. It should be noted that erosions can also affect the joints such as the metacarpophalangeal joints or the sacroiliac joints and, simply based on radiographic findings, differential diagnosis from inflammatory arthropathies, such as rheumatoid arthritis and ankylosing spondylitis, can be challenging.

Intracortical Bone Resorption. This results from increased osteoclastic activity in Haversian canals. Radiographically it causes linear translucencies within the cortex (cortical 'tunnelling') (Fig. 6-21). This feature is not specific for hyperparathyroidism and may be found in other conditions in which bone turnover is increased (e.g. normal childhood, Paget's disease of bone).

Chondrocalcinosis. The deposition of calcium pyrophosphate dihydrate (CPPD) causes articular cartilage and fibrocartilage to become visible on radiographs (Fig. 6-24). Chondrocalcinosis is found in 6–11% of patients with primary hyperparathyroidism.[93] This is most likely to be identified on radiographs of the hand (triangular ligament), the knees (articular cartilage and menisci) and symphysis pubis. Other joints less commonly involved are the shoulder and the hip. Clinically the patients may present with acute pain resembling gout, but on joint aspiration pyrophosphate crystals, rather than urate crystals, are found. However, this is relatively rare and was reported in 25% of patients with CPPD and primary hyperparathyroidism.[93] Affected joints may be asymptomatic, and chondrocalcinosis noted radiographically might bring the diagnosis of hyperparathyroidism to light in an asymptomatic patient. The combination of chondrocalcinosis in the symphysis pubis and nephrocalcinosis on an abdominal radiograph is diagnostic of hyperparathyroidism. Chondrocalcinosis is a feature of primary disease, rather than that secondary to CKD.

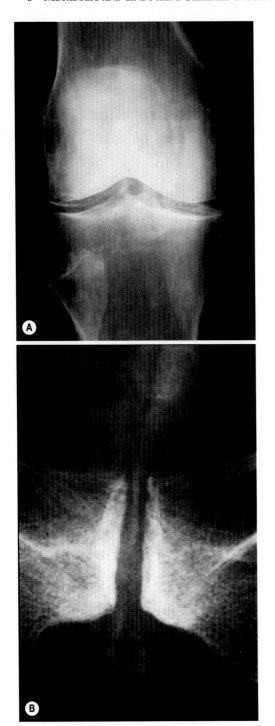

FIGURE 6-24 ■ Primary hyperparathyroidism. With chondrocalcinosis (calcification of cartilage) at the knee (A) and the symphysis pubis (B). Other sites where this may be present are the triangular fibrocartilage complex of the wrist and the large joints (hip and shoulder).

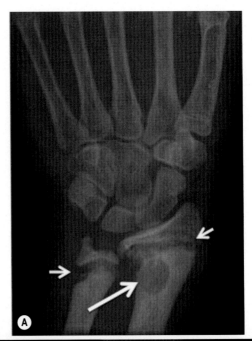

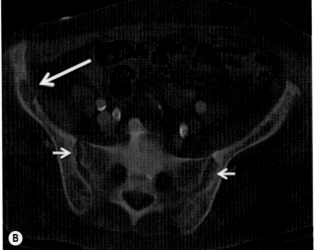

FIGURE 6-25 ■ Secondary hyperparathyroidism related to chronic kidney disease. Radiograph of the left hand (A) and CT of the pelvis (B). Brown tumours (osteitis fibrosa cystica) can occur in any site, seen here in the distal radius and the right ilium (arrows). Additionally, resorptive changes are evident at the growth plates and bilateral sacroiliac joints (small arrows).

Brown Tumours (Osteitis Fibrosa Cystica). Brown tumours are cystic lesions within bone in which there has been excessive osteoclastic resorption (Fig. 6-25). Histologically the cavities are filled with fibrous tissue and osteoclasts, with necrosis and haemorrhagic liquefaction. Radiographically, brown tumours appear as low-density, multiloculated cysts that can occur in any skeletal site and may cause expansion of bones. If the clinical history in these patients is not known, brown tumours may be easily interpreted as neoplastic lesions.

Osteosclerosis. Osteosclerosis occurs uncommonly in primary hyperparathyroidism but is a common feature of disease secondary to CKD. In primary disease with normal renal function it results from an exaggerated osteoblastic response following bone resorption. In secondary causes of hyperparathyroidism it results from excessive accumulation of poorly mineralised osteoid, which appears more dense radiographically than normal bone. The increase in bone density affects particularly the axial skeleton. In the vertebral bodies the end-plates

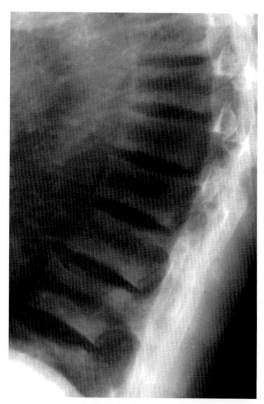

FIGURE 6-26 ■ **Secondary hyperparathyroidism.** Lateral radiograph of the thoracic spine demonstrating increased sclerosis along the end-plates and increased lucency of the central part, giving a 'rugger jersey' spine appearance. Also note deformity of the vertebral bodies, with loss of height and increased diameter, in addition to wedge-shaped deformities at the upper thoracic spine related to decreased stability and weakness of the abnormal bone.

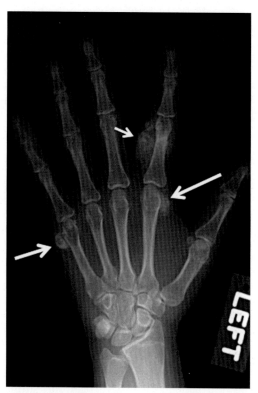

FIGURE 6-27 ■ **Secondary hyperparathyroidism related to chronic kidney disease.** Phosphate retention leads to increase in the phosphate × calcium product and precipitation of amorphous calcium phosphate in the arteries and soft tissues. AP radiograph of the left hand shows metastatic calcifications around the second and fifth metacarpophalangeal joints (large arrows) and along the second proximal phalanx (small arrow). More typically these calcifications are seen around the large joints.

are preferentially involved, giving bands of dense bones adjacent to the end-plates with a central band of lower normal bone density. These alternating bands of normal and sclerotic bone give a striped pattern described as a 'rugger jersey' spine (Fig. 6-26).

Osteoporosis. With excessive bone resorption, the bones may appear reduced in radiodensity in some patients. This particularly occurs in postmenopausal women and the elderly, in whom bone resorption exceeds new bone formation, with a net reduction in bone mass. This can be confirmed by bone densitometry, which is an integral component in the evaluation of hyperparathyroidism. In primary hyperparathyroidism there is a pattern of skeletal involvement that preferentially affects the cortical, as opposed to the trabecular, bone. BMD measurements made in sites in which cortical bone predominates, e.g. in the distal forearm, may show the most marked reduction.[94] Bone density increases after parathyroidectomy in primary hyperparathyroidism.

Metastatic Calcification. Metastatic calcifications are typically found in secondary hyperparathyroidism; soft-tissue calcification, other than in articular cartilage and fibrocartilage, does not occur in primary hyperparathyroidism unless there is associated reduced glomerular

function resulting in phosphate retention. The latter results in an increase in the calcium × phosphate product, and as a consequence amorphous calcium phosphate is precipitated in organs, blood vessels and soft tissues (Fig. 6-27). If there are features of hyperparathyroidism, i.e. subperiosteal erosions and additionally extensive vascular or soft-tissue calcifications, e.g. around joints and in tendons, this implies impaired renal function in association with hyperparathyroidism.

Hypoparathyroidism
Aetiology

Hypoparathyroidism can result from reduced or absent parathyroid hormone production or from end-organ (kidney, bone or both) resistance. This may be the result of the parathyroid glands failing to develop, the glands being damaged or removed, the function of the glands being reduced by altered regulation, or the action of parathyroid hormone (PTH) being impaired. The resulting biochemical abnormality is hypocalcaemia; this can clinically cause neuromuscular symptoms and signs such as tetany and fits.[95] Acquired hypoparathyroidism results from either surgical removal of the parathyroid glands or from autoimmune disorders. Post-surgical hypoparathyroidism is more common and occurs in approximately 13% of patients following thyroid or parathyroid surgery. Idiopathic hypoparathyroidism usually presents during childhood, is more common in girls and is rare in black races. It may be associated with pernicious anaemia and Addison's disease. There may be antibodies to a number of endocrine glands as part of a generalised autoimmune disorder.

Radiological Abnormalities

There may be localised (23%) or generalised (9%) osteosclerosis in affected patients.[96] This particularly affects the skull where the vault is thickened. At an early age of onset, the dentition is hypoplastic. Metastatic calcification may be present in the basal ganglia or in the subcutaneous tissue, particularly around the hips and shoulders (Fig. 6-28). A rare but recognised complication of hypoparathyroidism is an enthesopathy with extraskeletal ossification in a paraspinal distribution and elsewhere.[97] In the spine this skeletal hyperostosis resembles most closely that described by Forestier as 'senile' hyperostosis.[97,98] Differentiating features from ankylosing spondylitis are that there is no erosive arthropathy and the sacroiliac joints appear normal. Clinically the patients may have pain and stiffness in the back with limitation of movement. Extraskeletal ossification may be present around the pelvis, hip and in the interosseous membranes and tendinous insertions elsewhere.

Pseudohypoparathyroidism (PHP)

Pseudohypoparathyroidism describes a group of genetic disorders characterised by hypocalcaemia, hyperphosphataemia, raised PTH and target tissue unresponsiveness to PTH, first described by Albright et al in 1942.[99–101] The condition results from mutations of the *GNAS1* gene.[101] Affected patients are short in stature, have reduced intellect, rounded faces and shortened metacarpals, particularly the fourth and fifth (Fig. 6-29). Metastatic calcification, bowing of long bones and exostoses can occur. Clinical features include tetany, cataracts and nail dystrophy. Some of the clinical and radiological features of PHP may resemble those in other hereditary syndromes, including Turner's syndrome, acrodysostosis, Prader–Willi syndrome, fibrodysplasia ossificans progressiva and multiple hereditary exostosis. In PHP there is end-organ unresponsiveness to PTH since the parathyroid glands are normal and produce PTH. This usually involves unresponsiveness of both bone and kidneys. However, there is a rare variation of PHP in which the kidneys are unresponsive to PTH but the osseous response to the hormone is normal.[102] The condition is referred to as pseudohypohyperparathyroidism, and the histological and radiological features resemble those of azotaemic osteodystrophy.

Radiographic Abnormalities

Abnormalities may not be evident at birth but subsequently patients develop premature epiphyseal fusion,

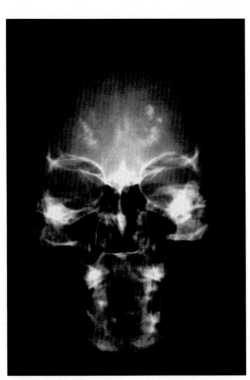

FIGURE 6-28 ■ **Hypoparathyroidism.** In hypoparathyroidism soft-tissue calcifications are a typical finding, seen in the basal ganglia in this AP radiograph of the skull.

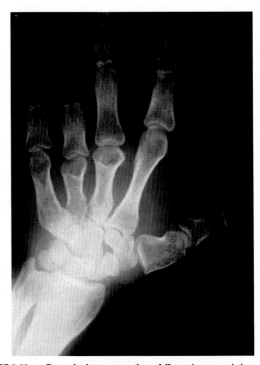

FIGURE 6-29 ■ **Pseudo-hypoparathyroidism.** In pseudohyperparathyroidism (PHP osteodystrophy of Albright) affected individuals are short in stature, and there are dysplastic features, including shortened metacarpals (brachydactyly), particularly the fourth and fifth, as shown in this AP radiograph of the left hand.

calvarial thickening, bone exostoses and calcification in the basal ganglia and the soft tissue (Fig. 6-28). Metacarpal shortening is present, particularly affecting the fourth and fifth digits (Fig. 6-29). This may result in a positive metacarpal sign; normally a line drawn tangential to the heads of the fourth and fifth metacarpals should not intersect the third metacarpal, but shorting of the fourth metacarpal means that it will. This feature is not specific for PHP and can occur in other congenital (Beckwith–Wiedemann and basal cell naevus syndromes, multiple epiphyseal dysplasia) and acquired (juvenile chronic arthritis, sickle-cell disease with infarction) conditions. Soft-tissue calcification occurs in a plaque-like distribution in the subcutaneous area. Rarely, soft-tissue ossification can occur in a periarticular distribution, usually involving the hands and feet.

Pseudo-Pseudohypoparathyroidism (PPHP)

In these affected individuals the dysplastic and other features are the same as PHP, but there are no associated parathyroid or other biochemical abnormalities. The abnormalities include metacarpal and metatarsal shortening, calvarial thickening and exostoses; soft-tissue calcification and ossification are best identified on radiographs. CT of the brain is more sensitive at identifying basal ganglia calcification than radiographs. BMD may be normal, reduced or increased.

RICKETS AND OSTEOMALACIA

Mineralisation of bone matrix depends on the presence of adequate supplies of 1,25-dihydroxy vitamin D (1,25(OH)$_2$D), calcium, phosphorus and alkaline phosphatase, and on a normal body pH. If there is a deficiency of any of these, or severe systemic acidosis, the mineralisation of bone will be defective. This results in a qualitative abnormality of bone, with a reduction in the mineral-to-osteoid ratio, resulting in rickets in children and osteomalacia in adults. Rickets and osteomalacia are therefore synonymous and represent the same disease process, but manifest in either the growing or the mature skeleton.

In the immature skeleton the radiographic abnormalities predominate at the growing ends of the bones where enchondral ossification is taking place, giving the classic appearance of rickets. At skeletal maturity, when the process of enchondral ossification has ceased, the defective mineralisation of osteoid is evident radiographically as Looser's zones, which are pathognomonic of osteomalacia.[103]

The pro-hormone forms of vitamin D require two hydroxylation stages to form the active metabolite, through which the hormone exerts its physiological action. There are two pro-hormonal forms of 1,25-dihydroxy vitamin D in humans: vitamin D$_2$ and vitamin D$_3$. Vitamin D$_2$ is prepared by irradiation of ergosterol obtained from yeast or fungi, and is used for food supplementation and pharmaceutical preparations. Vitamin D$_3$ occurs naturally through the interaction of

ultraviolet light on 7-dehydrocholesterol in the deep layers of the skin. Vitamin D$_2$ and D$_3$ are initially hydroxylated at the 25 position to form 25(OH)D$_2$ and 25(OH)D$_3$, the latter predominating and circulating bound to a specific protein. This hydroxylation occurs predominantly in the liver. A further hydroxylation in the 1 position in the kidney produces 1,25(OH)$_2$D, which is the active form of the hormone.

Vitamin D Deficiency

Deficiency may occur as a consequence of simple nutritional lack (diet, lack of sunlight), malabsorption states (vitamin D is fat soluble and absorbed in the small bowel), chronic liver disease (which affects hydroxylation at the 25 position) and chronic renal disease (in which the active metabolite 1,25(OH)$_2$D is not produced). Consequently, a wide variety of diseases may result in vitamin D deficiency; the radiological features will be similar, being those of rickets or osteomalacia. This similarity of radiological features, but variation in response to treatment, contributed to some of the early confusion. Rickets due to nutritional deprivation was cured by ultraviolet light or physiological doses of vitamin D (400 IU per day), but that associated with chronic renal disease was not, except when very large pharmacological doses (up to 300,000 IU per day) were used. This led to the terms 'refractory rickets' and 'vitamin D resistant rickets' being used for these conditions. Within these terms were included the diseases that cause the clinical and radiological features of rickets, but were related to phosphate, not vitamin D, deficiency, such as X-linked hypophosphataemia, and genetic disorders involving defects in 1α-hydroxylase and the vitamin D receptor.

Genetic Disorders of Vitamin D Metabolism

Prader et al. in 1961 described the condition in which rickets occurred within the first year of life, was characterised by severe hypocalcaemia and dental enamel hypoplasia, and responded to large amounts of vitamin D. The term 'vitamin D dependency' was used for this syndrome. It is now recognised that this disease is due to an inborn error of metabolism in which there is defective hydroxylation of 25(OH)D in the kidney due to defective activity of the renal 25(OH)D 1α-hydroxylase. This results in insufficient synthesis of 1,25(OH)$_2$D. The preferred term for this condition is pseudo vitamin D deficiency rickets (PDDR) and it is inherited as an autosomal recessive trait.[104]

Another inborn error of vitamin D metabolism was described in 1978.[105] Clinically it resembled pseudo vitamin D deficiency rickets but with high circulating concentrations of 1,25(OH)$_2$D. This condition results from a spectrum of mutations which affect the vitamin D receptor (VDR) in target tissues, causing resistance to the action of 1,25(OH)$_2$D (end-organ resistance). Affected patients have complete alopecia.

Oncogenic Osteomalacia

Oncogenic osteomalacia, also termed tumour-induced osteomalacia (TIO), is a rare paraneoplastic syndrome in

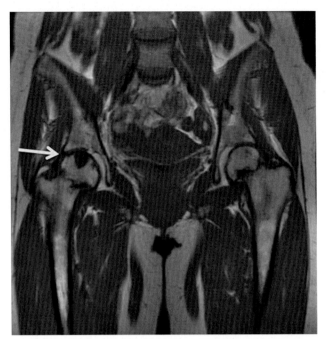

FIGURE 6-30 ■ **Oncogenic osteomalacia.** T1-weighted fast spin-echo coronal MR image of the pelvis showing incomplete bilateral femoral neck fractures and a tumour in the right femoral head (arrow); histologically, this was found to be a mesenchymal tumour which was responsible for oncogenic osteomalacia.

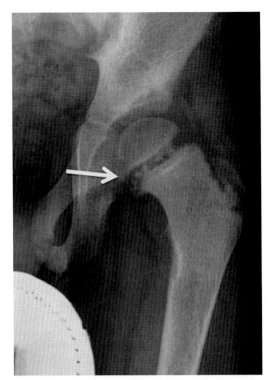

FIGURE 6-31 ■ **Rickets in the immature skeleton.** Evidence of defective mineralisation is evident in sites of endochondral ossification. The growth plate is widened and shows irregular calcification as demonstrated at the hip joint in this AP radiograph of the left hip (arrow).

which patients present with bone pain, fractures, and muscle weakness (Fig. 6-30).[106,107] The cause is a high blood level of the recently identified phosphate and vitamin D-regulating hormone, fibroblast growth factor 23 (FGF23).[108] In oncogenic osteomalacia, FGF23 is secreted by mesenchymal tumours that are usually benign, but are typically very small and difficult to locate. FGF23 acts primarily at the renal tubule and impairs phosphate reabsorption and 1α-hydroxylation of 25(OH)D, leading to hypophosphataemia and low levels of 1,25-dihydroxy vitamin D. Removal of the tumour cures the condition and imaging plays an important role in tumour localisation. A step-wise approach utilising functional imaging (F-18 fluorodeoxyglucose positron emission tomography and octreotide scintigraphy) followed by anatomical imaging (CT and/or MRI), and, if needed, selective venous sampling with measurement of FGF23, is usually successful in locating the tumours.[108]

Radiological Appearances

Rickets. In the immature skeleton the effect of vitamin D deficiency and the consequent defective mineralisation of osteoid is seen principally at the growing ends of bones.[103,109–111] In the early stage there is apparent widening of the growth plate (Fig. 6-31). More severe change produces 'cupping' of the metaphysis, with irregular and poor mineralisation (Fig. 6-32). Some expansion in width of the metaphysis results in the swelling around the ends of the long bones affected. This expansion of the anterior ends of the ribs is referred to as a 'rachitic rosary'. There may be a thin 'ghostlike' rim of mineralisation at the

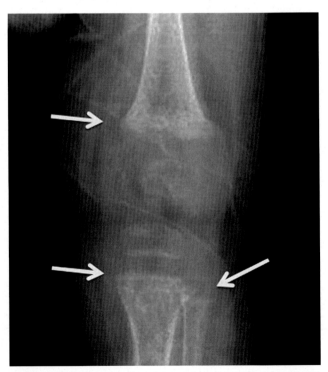

FIGURE 6-32 ■ **Rickets.** Severe osteopenia, widening of the growth plate and cupping of the metaphyses (arrows) in this AP radiograph of the knee.

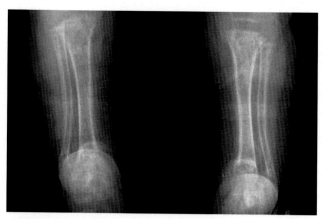

FIGURE 6-33 ■ **Rickets.** Severe osteopenia with medial bowing of bilateral tibia and fibula and cupping of the metaphyses in this AP radiograph of bilateral distal lower extremities.

periphery of the metaphysis, as this mineralisation occurs by membranous ossification at the periosteum. The margin of the epiphysis appears indistinct as enchondral ossification at this site is also defective. These changes predominate at the sites of bones which are growing most actively, in particular around the knee (Fig. 6-32), the wrist (particularly the ulna), the anterior ends of the middle ribs, the proximal femur (Fig. 6-31) and the distal tibia, and depend on the age of the child. MRI may show abnormalities of the physeal cartilage.[109]

Rachitic bone is soft and bends, and this results in genu valgum or genu varum, deformity of the hips (coxa valga or more commonly coxa vara), deformity of the long bones with bowing (Fig. 6-33), in-drawing of the ribs at the insertion of the diaphragm (Harrison's sulcus) and protrusio acetabuli and triradiate deformity of the pelvis, which can cause problems with subsequent parturition. Involvement of the bones in the thorax and respiratory tract (larynx and trachea) occasionally results in stridor and respiratory distress. In very severe rickets, when little skeletal growth is taking place (i.e. owing to nutritional deprivation or chronic ill health), paradoxically the radiological features of rickets may not be evident at the growth plate. In rickets of prematurity, little abnormality may be present at the metaphysis since no skeletal growth is taking place in the premature infant. However, the bones are osteopenic and prone to fractures. In mild vitamin D deficiency the radiographic features of rickets may only become apparent at puberty during the growth spurt, and the metaphyseal abnormalities predominate at the knee.

With appropriate treatment of vitamin D deficiency, the radiographic features of healing (after 3–4 months) lag behind the improvement in biochemical parameters (after 2 weeks) and clinical symptoms. With treatment, the zone of provisional calcification will mineralise. This mineralised zone is initially separated by translucent osteoid from the shaft of the bone, and may be mistaken for a metaphyseal fracture of child abuse.[112] Reduced bone density and poor definition of epiphyses are helpful distinguishing features for rickets. The section of abnormal bone following healing of rickets may be visible for a period of time, and give some indication as to the age

of onset and duration of the period of rickets. Eventually this zone will become indistinguishable from normal bone with remodelling over a period of 3–4 months. The zone of provisional calcification which was present at the onset of the disturbance to enchondral ossification may remain (Harris growth arrest line) as a marker of the age of skeletal maturity at which the rickets occurred. However, this is not specific for rickets and may occur in any condition (e.g. period of ill health, lead poisoning) that inhibits normal enchondral ossification. There will be evidence of retarded growth and development in rickets; this tends to be more marked when the vitamin D deficiency is associated with chronic diseases that reduce calorie intake, general well-being and activity (i.e. malabsorption, chronic renal disease) than with simple nutritional vitamin D deficiency.

Vitamin D deficiency is associated with hypocalcaemia. In an attempt to maintain calcium homeostasis, the parathyroid glands are stimulated to secrete PTH. This results in another important feature of vitamin D deficiency rickets. Evidence of secondary hyperparathyroidism, with increased osteoclastic resorption, is always shown histologically, although not always radiographically.

Metaphyseal chondrodysplasias may mimic rickets and in a variety of inherited bone dysplasias there are metaphyseal abnormalities which may range from mild (Schmid type) to severe (Jansen).[113] Normal serum biochemistry serves to differentiate these dysplasias from other rachitic disorders, which the radiographic abnormalities at the metaphyses may simulate.

Osteomalacia. At skeletal maturity the epiphysis fuses to the metaphysis with obliteration of the growth plate and cessation of longitudinal bone growth. Vitamin D deficiency in the adult skeleton results in osteomalacia, the pathognomonic radiographic feature of which is the Looser's zone[114] (Fig. 6-34). Looser's zones (pseudofractures, Milkman's fractures) are translucent areas in the bone that are composed of unmineralised osteoid. They are typically (but not always) bilateral and symmetrical. Radiographically they appear as radiolucent lines that are perpendicular to the bone cortex, do not usually extend across the entire bone shaft, and characteristically have a slightly sclerotic margin. Looser's zones can occur in any bone but most typically are found in the medial aspect of the femoral neck (Fig. 6-34), the pubic rami, the lateral border of the scapula and the ribs. They may involve the first and second ribs, in which traumatic fractures are uncommon, being usually associated with severe trauma. Other less common sites for Looser's zones are the metatarsals and metacarpals, the base of the acromion and the ilium. They may not always be visible on radiographs; radionuclide bone scintigraphy and MRI may be more sensitive in identifying radiographic occult Looser's zones.

Looser's zones must be differentiated from insufficiency fractures that may occur in osteoporotic bone, particularly in the pubic rami, sacrum and calcaneus. Such insufficiency fractures consist of multiple microfractures in brittle osteoporotic bone and often show florid callus formation, serving to differentiate them from

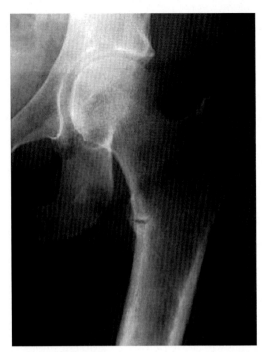

FIGURE 6-34 ■ Osteomalacia. In the mature skeleton following fusion of the growth plates, the pathognomonic radiographic feature is the Looser's zone. These are radiolucent, unmineralised linear areas which are perpendicular to the cortex and which may have a sclerotic margin. They occur most frequently in the medial aspects of the femoral necks (arrow in this AP radiograph of the proximal femur), symphysis pubis, ribs and lateral borders of the scapulae.

Looser's zones.[30,115] Incremental fractures occur in Paget's disease of bone and resemble Looser's zones in appearance, but tend to occur on the convexity of the cortex of the bone involved,[116] rather than medially on the concave side, as in osteomalacia. The other typical features of Paget's disease serve as distinguishing radiological features.[116]

Complete fractures can occur through Looser's zones, but with no evidence of callus formation until the osteomalacia is treated with vitamin D. Then there will be quite florid callus formation around fractures with healing of the fractures and Looser's zones with little residual deformity. As in rickets, osteomalacic bone is soft and bends. This is evident radiographically by protrusio acetabuli, in which the femoral head deforms the acetabular margin so that the normal medial 'teardrop' outline is lost. There may be bowing of the long bones of the legs and a triradiate deformity of the pelvis, particularly if the cause of the vitamin D deficiency has persisted since childhood and has been inadequately treated or untreated.

In osteomalacia, as in rickets, hypocalcaemia acts as stimulus to *secondary hyperparathyroidism*. This may be manifested radiographically as subperiosteal erosion, particularly in the phalanges but other sites (sacroiliac joints, symphysis pubis, proximal tibia, outer ends of the clavicle, skull vault—'pepperpot' skull) may be involved, depending on the intensity of the hyperparathyroidism and how long it has been present. There may also be cortical tunnelling and a hazy trabecular pattern. Generalised osteopenia may occur and vertebral bodies may have biconcave end-plates, due to deformation of the malacic bone by the cartilaginous intervertebral disc ('cod fish' deformity).

Azotaemic Osteodystrophy

The bone disease associated with CKD is complex and multifactorial, and has changed over past decades.[117–119] Whereas originally features of vitamin D deficiency (rickets/osteomalacia) and secondary hyperparathyroidism (erosions, osteosclerosis, brown cysts) (Fig. 6-26) predominated, improvements in management and therapy have resulted in such radiographic features being present in only a minority of patients. Soft-tissue and extensive vascular metastatic calcification (Fig. 6-27) and 'adynamic' bone develop as a complication of disease (phosphate retention) and treatment (phosphate binders). New complications (amyloid deposition, non-infective spondyloarthropathy, osteonecrosis) are now seen in long-term haemodialysis and/or renal transplantation. Radiographs remain the most important imaging technique, but occasionally other imaging and quantitative techniques (CT, MRI, bone densitometry) are relevant to diagnosis and management.

In extreme cases of soft-tissue calcification there may be ischaemic necrosis of the skin, muscle and subcutaneous tissue, referred to as 'calciphylaxis'. This condition can occur in patients with advanced renal disease, in those on regular dialysis, and also those with functioning renal allografts.[120]

Renal Tubular Defects

Glucose, inorganic phosphate and amino acids are absorbed in the proximal renal tubule. Concentration and acidification of urine in exchange for a fixed base occur in the distal renal tubule. Renal tubular disorders may involve either the proximal or the distal tubule, or both. Such disorders result in a spectrum of biochemical disturbances that may result in loss of phosphate, glucose, or amino acids alone, or in combination, with additional defects in urine acidification and concentration. Such defects of tubular function may be inherited and present from birth (Toni– Fanconi syndrome, cystinosis, X-linked hypophosphataemia) or may be acquired later in life (e.g. tubular function being compromised by deposition of copper in Wilson's disease, hereditary tyrosinaemia). Renal tubular dysfunction may also be acquired, with dysfunction being induced by the effects of toxins or therapies (Paraquat, Lysol burns, toluene 'glue sniffing' inhalation, ifosfamide, gentamicin, streptozotocin, valproic acid), deposition of heavy metals or other substances (multiple myeloma, cadmium, lead, mercury), related to immunological disorders (interstitial nephritis, renal transplantation), or with the production of a humoral substance in oncogenic osteomalacia, also termed tumour induced osteomalacia.[108] In these renal tubular-disorders, rickets or osteomalacia can be caused by multiple factors, including hyperphosphaturia, hypophosphataemia and reduced 1α-hydroxylation of 25(OH)D. As the serum calcium is generally normal in these disorders, secondary hyperparathyroidism does not occur.

X-linked Hypophosphataemia (XLH). This genetic disorder is transmitted as an X-linked dominant trait.[121] Sporadic cases also occur through spontaneous mutations. The incidence is approximately 1 in 25,000, and XLH is now the most common cause of genetically induced rickets. The disease is characterised by phosphaturia throughout life, hypophosphataemia, rickets and osteomalacia. Clinically affected individuals may be short in stature, principally due to defective growth in the legs, which are bowed; the trunk is usually normal.[122] Rickets becomes clinically evident at about 6–12 months of age or older. Treatment with phosphate supplements and large pharmacological doses of vitamin D (hence the term 'vitamin D-resistant rickets') can heal the radiological features of rickets and also improve longitudinal growth. The radiological features of XLH are characteristic.[123] There is defective mineralisation of the metaphysis and widening of the growth plate (rickets). The metaphyseal margin tends to be less indistinct than in nutritional rickets and the affected metaphysis is not as wide. Changes are most marked at the knee, wrist, ankle and proximal femur. Healing can be induced with appropriate treatment (phosphate supplements, $1,25(OH)_2D$). The growth plates fuse normally at skeletal maturation. The bones are often short and under-tubulated (shaft wide in relation to bone length) with bowing of the femur and tibia, which may be marked. Following skeletal maturation, Looser's zones appear and persist in patients with XLH (Fig. 6-35A). They tend to be in different sites to those which occur in nutritional osteomalacia, and often affect the outer cortex of the bowed femur, although they also occur along the medial cortex of the shaft. Looser's zones in the ribs and pelvis are rare. Although Looser's zones may heal with appropriate treatment, those that have been present for many years persist radiographically and are presumably filled with fibrous tissue.

Although there is defective mineralisation of osteoid in XLH, the bones are commonly and characteristically increased in radiodensity with a coarse and prominent trabecular pattern. This is a feature of the disease, and is not related to treatment with vitamin D and phosphate supplements, as it is present in those who have not received treatment. This bone sclerosis can involve the petrous bone and structures of the inner ear, and may be responsible for the hydropic cochlea pattern of deafness that these patients may develop in later life.[124] X-linked hypophosphataemia is characterised by an enthesopathy, in which there is inflammation in the junctional area between bone and tendon insertion that heals by ossification at affected sites[125] (Fig. 6-35B). As a result, ectopic bone forms around the pelvis and spine. This may result in complete ankylosis of the spine, resembling ankylosing spondylitis, and clinically limiting mobility. However, the absence of inflammatory arthritis, with normal sacroiliac joints, serves to differentiate XLH from ankylosing spondylitis.

Ossification may occur in the interosseous membrane of the forearm and in the leg between the tibia and the fibula. Separate, small ossicles may be present around the joints of the hands and ossification of tendon insertions in the hands causes 'whiskering' of bone margins.

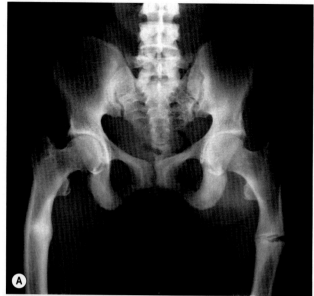

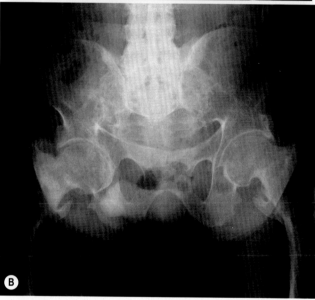

FIGURE 6-35 ■ **X-linked hypophosphataemic osteomalacia.** This is the most common of the genetic causes of rickets and osteomalacia. The bones may be radiodense with a coarse trabecular pattern. In affected children there will be evidence of rickets. (A) In adults chronic Looser's zones may be present, as in the outer cortex of both femora. (B) There may be evidence of an enthesopathy in older patients with ossification of ligamentous insertion to bone, as present in the pelvis at the psoas insertion to the lesser trochanters. The paraspinal ossification resembles ankylosing spondylitis, but the sacroiliac joints are not eroded, which differentiates the two conditions.

A rare, but recognised, important complication of XLH is spinal cord compression caused by a combination of ossification of the ligamentum flavum, thickening of the laminae and hyperostosis around the apophyseal joints.[126] Ossification of the ligamentum flavum causes the most significant narrowing of the spinal canal and occurs most commonly in the thoracic spine, generally involving two or three adjacent segments. Affected patients may be asymptomatic, even when there is severe spinal canal narrowing. Acute spinal cord compression can be precipitated by quite minor trauma. It is important to be aware of this rare complication of the disease since surgical decompression by laminectomy is curative and is best performed as an elective procedure by an experienced surgeon rather than as an emergency. The extent of intraspinal ossification cannot be predicted by the degree of paraspinal or extraskeletal ossification at other sites. CT is a useful imaging technique for demonstrating the extent of intraspinal ossification.

Extraskeletal ossification is uncommon in patients with XLH before the age of 40 years. The extent to which radiographic abnormalities of rickets and osteomalacia, osteosclerosis, abnormalities of bone modelling and extraskeletal ossification are present varies between affected individuals.[127] In some patients, all the features are present and so are diagnostic of the condition. In others, there may only be minor abnormalities and the diagnosis of X-linked hypophosphataemic rickets may be overlooked.[128]

Other Causes of Rickets and Osteomalacia (Not Related to Vitamin D Deficiency or Hypophosphataemia)

Hypophosphatasia

This rare disorder is generally transmitted as an autosomal recessive trait, but autosomal dominant inheritance has also been reported. The disease is characterised by reduced levels of serum alkaline phosphatase (both bone and liver isoenzymes), with raised levels of phosphoethanolamine in both the blood and the urine. Serum calcium and phosphorus levels are not reduced; in perinatal and infantile disease there can be hypercalciuria and hypercalcaemia attributed to the imbalance between calcium absorption from the gut and defective growth and mineralisation of the skeleton. The latter results in rickets in childhood and osteomalacia in adults. The severity of the condition varies greatly, being diagnosed either in the perinatal period, in infancy or childhood, but in some patients only becoming apparent in adult life.[129] The condition can wax and wane and tends to be more severe in children than when it becomes apparent in later life.

OTHER METABOLIC BONE DISORDERS

A number of congenital and familial disorders can be associated with increased bone density (osteosclerosis) and abnormal bone modelling. These include osteopetrosis, pyknodysostosis, metaphyseal dysplasia (Pyle's disease), craniometaphyseal dysplasia, frontometaphyseal dysplasia, osteodysplasty (Melnick–Needles syndrome), progressive diaphyseal dysplasia (Camurati–Engelmann disease), hereditary multiple diaphyseal sclerosis (Ribbing's disease), craniodiaphyseal dysplasia, endosteal hyperostosis (Worth and Van Buchem types), dysosteosclerosis, tubular stenosis, and oculodento-osseous dysplasia. All are rare and have different natural histories, genetic transmission, complications and radiographic

features. Many are dysplasias rather than metabolic bone disorders.

Osteopetrosis

In osteopetrosis there is defective osteoclastic resorption of the primary spongiosa of bone. Osteoclasts in affected bone are usually devoid of the ruffled borders by which osteoclasts adhere to the bone surface and through which their resorptive activity is expressed. In the presence of continued bone formation, there is generalised osteosclerosis and abnormalities of metaphyseal modelling[130,131] (Fig. 6-36). There have been reports of reversal of the osteosclerosis following successful bone marrow transplantation.

Osteopetrosis was first described by Albers-Schönberg in 1904, and is sometimes referred to as marble bone disease, osteosclerosis fragilis generalisata and osteopetrosis generalisata. There are two main clinical forms:
1. The lethal form of osteopetrosis with precocious manifestations and an autosomal recessive transmission.
2. Benign osteopetrosis with late manifestations, inherited by autosomal dominant transmission.

There is also a rarer autosomal recessive (intermediate) form, which presents during childhood with the signs and symptoms of the lethal form but the outcome on life expectancy is not known. The syndrome previously described as osteopetrosis with renal tubular acidosis and cerebral calcification is now recognised as an inborn error of metabolism, carbonic anhydrase II deficiency. Neuronal storage disease with malignant osteopetrosis has been described, as has the rare lethal, transient infantile and postinfectious form of the disorder.

Autosomal Recessive Lethal Type of Osteopetrosis

In affected individuals there is obliteration of the marrow cavity leading to anaemia, thrombocytopenia and recurrent infection. Clinically there is hepatosplenomegaly, hydrocephalus and cranial nerve involvement resulting in blindness and deafness. Radiographically all the bones are dense with lack of corticomedullary differentiation. Modelling of affected bones is abnormal with expansion of the metaphyseal region and under-tubulation of bone. This is most evident in the long bones, particularly the distal femur and proximal humerus. Although the bones are dense, they are brittle, and horizontal pathological fractures are common. The entire skull, particularly the base, is involved and the paranasal and mastoid air cells are poorly developed. Sclerosis of end-plates of the vertebral bodies produces a 'sandwich' appearance. MR imaging may assist in monitoring those with severe disease who undergo marrow transplantation, since success will be indicated by expansion of the marrow cavity. Findings on MR and CT of the brain have been described.

There is an intermediate recessive form of the disease, which is milder than that seen in infants and distinct from the less severe autosomal dominant disease. Affected individuals suffer pathological fracture and anaemia and are of short stature, with hepatomegaly. The radiographic

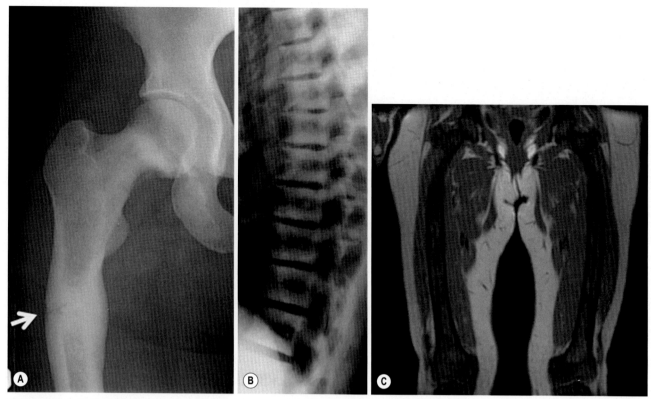

FIGURE 6-36 ■ **Osteopetrosis.** Osteoclastic function is defective, resulting in dense sclerotic bones which are brittle and prone to fracture. There is evidence of abnormal modelling of the long bones due to the failure of normal osteoclastic periosteal bone resorption which remodels the distal shafts of bones as they grow in length by endochondral ossification. In (A) the AP radiograph of the hip and femur shows increased density of the proximal femur with a remote diaphysis fracture (arrow) and cortical thickening. The lateral thoracic spine radiograph in (B) demonstrates increased sclerosis along the end-plates with a 'sandwich' appearance and the coronal T1-weighted MRI of bilateral femora in (C) shows partial obliteration of the marrow space due extensive sclerosis.

features include diffuse osteosclerosis with involvement of the skull base and facial bones, abnormal bone modelling and a 'bone within a bone' appearance.

Benign, Autosomal Dominant Type of Osteopetrosis (Albers-Schönberg Disease)

This is often asymptomatic, and the diagnosis may come to light either incidentally or through the occurrence of a pathological fracture (Fig. 6-36A). Other presentations include anaemia and facial palsy or deafness from cranial nerve compression. Problems may occur after tooth extraction, and there is an increased incidence of osteomyelitis, particularly of the mandible. Radiographic features are similar to those of the autosomal recessive form of the disease, but are less severe. The bones are diffusely sclerotic, with thickened cortices and defective modelling. There may be alternating sclerotic and radiolucent bands at the ends of diaphyses, a 'bone within a bone' appearance and the vertebral end-plates appear sclerotic (Fig. 6-36B). In 1987, Andersen and Bollerslev classified this form of the disease into two distinct radiological types. In type I fractures are unusual, in contrast to type II in which fractures are common. Transverse bands in the metaphyses are more commonly a feature in type II disease, as is a raised serum acid phosphatase.

Hyperphosphatasia

Hyperphosphatasia is a rare genetic disorder resulting from mutations in osteoprotegerin (OPG), and is characterised by markedly elevated serum alkaline phosphatase levels.[132] Affected children have episodes of fever, bone pain and progressive enlargement of the skull, with bowing of the long bones and associated pathological fractures. Radiographically the features resemble Paget's disease of bone, and it is sometimes referred to as 'juvenile' Paget's disease, osteitis deformans in children or hyperostosis corticalis (Fig. 6-37). There is an increased rate of bone turnover, with woven bone failing to mature into lamellar bone.

Radiographically, this increased rate of bone turnover is evidenced by decreased bone radiodensity with coarsening and disorganisation of the trabecular pattern. In the skull the diploic space is widened and there is patchy sclerosis. The diaphyses of the long bones become expanded with cortical thickening along their concave aspects. The long bones may be bowed, resulting in coxa vara and protrusio acetabulae. The vertebral bodies are reduced in radiodensity, reduced in height with biconcave end-plates. The bowing of the limbs causes affected individuals to be short in height. There is often premature loss of dentition due to resorption of dentine with replacement of the pulp by osteoid.

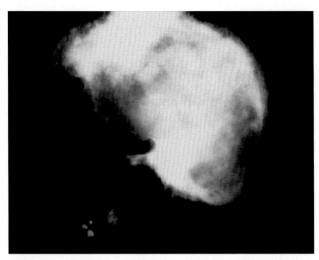

FIGURE 6-37 ■ **Hyperphosphatasia (juvenile Paget's disease).** There is increased bone turnover, resulting in immature woven bone being formed instead of mature lamellar bone. Bones are under-tubulated with a disorganised trabecular pattern, resembling the radiographic features of Paget's disease. In the lateral skull radiograph there is sclerosis, thickening of the skull vault and evidence of bone softening with basilar invagination. Platyspondyly may also be present.

The radiographic features closely resemble those of Paget's disease but are diagnostic as they involve the whole skeleton (as opposed to the monostotic or asymmetrical polyostotic involvement in Paget's disease) and affect children from the age of 2 years. On radionuclide imaging there is generalised increase in uptake, giving a 'super scan' due to excessive osteoblastic activity with absence of evidence of renal uptake.

MISCELLANEOUS

Vitamin D Intoxication

In the past, vitamin D was advocated in the treatment of a variety of conditions, including sarcoidosis, tuberculosis (especially lupus vulgaris), rheumatoid arthritis, hay fever, chilblains and asthma. The treatment had no beneficial effect in these conditions and its use was eventually abandoned. However, this was not before cases of vitamin D intoxication had been described. Vitamin D intoxication has become less common with the introduction of $1,25(OH)_2D$ (calcitriol) and other active metabolites. However, the more recent use of vitamin D to treat cancer, psoriasis and immunological disease may result in a resurgence of interest in vitamin D intoxication. The clinical symptoms include fatigue, malaise, weakness, thirst and polyuria, anorexia, nausea and vomiting due to hypercalcaemia. The latter results in hypercalciuria, nephrocalcinosis, impaired renal function and hypertension. Radiographically, metastatic calcification may be present in tendons, ligaments, fascial planes and arteries, and in the periosteum, resembling periostitis and causing bone sclerosis.

Hypervitaminosis A

Hypervitaminosis A can occur in those who are receiving vitamin A or one of its synthetic derivatives (retinoic acids) for treatment of skin disorders (refractory cystic acne, keratinising dermatoses, psoriasis). The skeletal manifestations include large bone outgrowths from the spine, particularly in the cervical region. In the peripheral skeleton there is evidence of a mild enthesopathy. In affected children there can occur cupping and splaying of the metaphyses, diaphyseal periostitis, particularly in the metatarsals and ulnae, and widening of the cranial sutures.

Fluorosis

Fluorosis results from the long-term ingestion of excessive amounts of fluoride. In some parts of the world fluorosis is endemic (e.g. India). The radiological features that result include osteosclerosis, particularly in the axial skeleton, and an enthesopathy with ossification of ligaments and large spinal osteophytes.[133] The paraspinal ossification may cause compression myelopathy.

Other Endocrine Diseases

Cushing's Disease

Cushing's disease is caused by a basophil pituitary adenoma, usually a micro adenoma (smaller than 10 mm); Cushing's syndrome is caused by a tumour of the adrenal glands (adenoma, carcinoma), ectopic ACTH production by a tumour (e.g. bronchial carcinoma), or iatrogenically by treatment with glucocorticoids. The cardinal skeletal manifestation is osteoporosis, which affects sites rich in trabecular bone (axial skeleton). Low-trauma fractures can occur, and these may heal with exuberant callus formation. Avascular necrosis and bone infarction is also a typical finding.

Thyroid Disease

There may be over- or underactivity of the gland (thyrotoxicosis and myxoedema, respectively). Thyroid disease in adults may be a cause of osteoporosis. Congenital or childhood onset of hypothyroidism (cretinism) results in retarded skeletal maturation, fragmented epiphyses, 'slipper-shaped' vertebrae and Wormian bones in the skull.[134] Thyroid acropachy is the triad of pretibial myxoedema, thyroid eye disease (exophthalmos) and clubbing of the fingers. Radiologically there may be diaphyseal periostitis, predominantly involving the tubular bones of the hand.[135] Patients may be thyrotoxic, euthyroid or hypothyroid.

Acromegaly

Acromegaly is the result of an eosinophilic adenoma of the pituitary gland, usually a macro adenoma (greater than 10 mm in size); if it occurs in children, gigantism results. There is overgrowth of all tissues and organs. The hypertrophied cartilage may initially cause widening of the joints, seen best in the hand radiograph in the metacarpophalangeal (MCP) joints. However, the hypertrophied cartilage is poor in tensile strength and liable to fissures. This results in premature osteoarthritis with relative widening of the joint space (acromegalic arthropathy).[136,137] When the joints in the spine are involved, cord compression can occur. Acromegaly can also result in generalised osteoporosis.

REFERENCES

1. Greulich W, Pyle S. Radiographic Atlas of Skeletal Development of the Hand and Wrist. 2nd ed. Stanford, CA: Stanford University Press; 1959.
2. Tanner JM, Whitehouse RH, Cameron N, et al. Assessment of Skeletal Maturity and Prediction of Adult Height (TW2 Method). 2nd ed. London: Academic Press; 1983.
3. Sambrook P, Cooper C. Osteoporosis. Lancet 2006;367(9527):2010–18.
4. Services DoHaH. Bone health and osteoporosis: a report of the Surgeon-General. In: US Department of Health and Human Services OotSG, ed. 2010/10/15 ed. Rockville. 2004.
5. NIH Consensus Development Panel on Osteoporosis Prevention Diagnosis, and Therapy. Osteoporosis prevention, diagnosis, and therapy. JAMA 2001;285:785–95.
6. WHO. Technical Report: Assessment of fracture risk and its application to screening for postmenopausal osteoporosis: a report of a WHO study group. Paper presented at World Health Organization, Geneva, Switzerland. 1994.
7. Kanis JA. Diagnosis of osteoporosis and assessment of fracture risk. Lancet 2002;359(9321):1929–36.
8. Baim S, Binkley N, Bilezikian JP, et al. Official positions of the International Society for Clinical Densitometry and executive summary of the 2007 ISCD Position Development Conference. J Clin Densitom 2008;11(1):75–91.
9. Lewiecki EM, Baim S, Langman CB, Bilezikian JP. The official positions of the International Society for Clinical Densitometry: perceptions and commentary. J Clin Densitom 2009;12(3):267–71.
10. Lewiecki EM, Gordon CM, Baim S, et al. Special report on the 2007 adult and pediatric Position Development Conferences of the International Society for Clinical Densitometry. Osteoporos Int 2008;19(10):1369–78.
11. Lachmann E, Whelan M. The roentgen diagnosis of osteoporosis and its limitations. Radiology 1936;26:165–77.
12. Compston J. Recent advances in the management of osteoporosis. Clin Med 2009;9(6):565–9.
13. Compston J. Clinical and therapeutic aspects of osteoporosis. Eur J Radiol 2009;71(3):388–91.
14. Resnick D, Niwayama G. Osteoporosis. In: Resnick D, editor. Diagnosis of Bone and Joint Disorders. 3rd ed. Philadelphia: W B Saunders; 1995. pp. 1783–853.
15. Ferrar L, Jiang G, Adams J, Eastell R. Identification of vertebral fractures: an update. Osteoporos Int 2005;16(7):717–28.
16. Genant HK, Wu CY, van Kuijk C, Nevitt MC. Vertebral fracture assessment using a semiquantitative technique. J Bone Miner Res 1993;8:1137–48.
17. Delmas PD, van de Langerijt L, Watts NB, et al. Underdiagnosis of vertebral fractures is a worldwide problem: the IMPACT study. J Bone Miner Res 2005;20(4):557–63.
18. Delmas PD, Watts N, Eastell R. Underdiagnosis of vertebral fractures is a world wide problem. J Bone Miner Res 2001;16(Suppl.):S139.
19. Gehlbach S, Bigelow C, Heimisdottir M, et al. Recognition of vertebral fracture in a clinical setting. Osteoporos Int 2000;11:577–82.
20. Kobayashi K, Shimoyama K, Nakamura K, Murata K. Percutaneous vertebroplasty immediately relieves pain of osteoporotic vertebral compression fractures and prevents prolonged immobilization of patients. Eur Radiol 2005;15(2):360–7.
21. Ohlin A, Johnell O. Vertebroplasty and kyphoplasty in the fractured osteoporotic spine. Clin Calcium 2004;14(1):65–9.
22. Papanastassiou ID, Phillips FM, Van Meirhaeghe J, et al. Comparing effects of kyphoplasty, vertebroplasty, and non-surgical management in a systematic review of randomized and non-randomized controlled studies. Eur Spine J 2012;21(9):1826–43.
23. Buchbinder R, Osborne RH, Ebeling PR, et al. A randomized trial of vertebroplasty for painful osteoporotic vertebral fractures. N Engl J Med 2009;361(6):557–68.
24. Kallmes DF, Comstock BA, Heagerty PJ, et al. A randomized trial of vertebroplasty for osteoporotic spinal fractures. N Engl J Med 2009;361(6):569–79.
25. Klazen CA, Lohle PN, de Vries J, et al. Vertebroplasty versus conservative treatment in acute osteoporotic vertebral compression fractures (Vertos II): an open-label randomised trial. Lancet 2010;376(9746):1085–92.
26. McGraw JK, Lippert JA, Minkus KD, et al. Prospective evaluation of pain relief in 100 patients undergoing percutaneous vertebroplasty: results and follow-up. J Vasc Interv Radiol 2002;13(9 Pt 1):883–6.
27. Li X, Yang H, Tang T, et al. Comparison of kyphoplasty and vertebroplasty for treatment of painful osteoporotic vertebral compression fractures: twelve-month follow-up in a prospective nonrandomized comparative study. J Spinal Disord Tech 2012;25(3):142–9.
28. Gangi A, Guth S, Imbert JP, et al. Percutaneous vertebroplasty: indications, technique, and results. Radiographics 2003;23(2):e10.
29. Blake SP, Connors AM. Sacral insufficiency fracture. Br J Radiol 2004;77(922):891–6.
30. Cabarrus MC, Ambekar A, Lu Y, Link TM. MRI and CT of insufficiency fractures of the pelvis and the proximal femur. AJR Am J Roentgenol 2008;191(4):995–1001.
31. Lin J, Lachmann E, Nagler W. Sacral insufficiency fractures: a report of two cases and a review of the literature. J Womens Health Gend Based Med 2001;10(7):699–705.
32. Kattapuram TM, Kattapuram SV. Spontaneous osteonecrosis of the knee. Eur J Radiol 2008;67(1):42–8.
33. Yamamoto T, Bullough PG. Spontaneous osteonecrosis of the knee: the result of subchondral insufficiency fracture. J Bone Joint Surg Am 2000;82(6):858–66.
34. Yamamoto T, Iwamoto Y, Schneider R, Bullough PG. Histopathological prevalence of subchondral insufficiency fracture of the femoral head. Ann Rheum Dis 2008;67(2):150–3.
35. Yamamoto T, Schneider R, Bullough PG. Subchondral insufficiency fracture of the femoral head: histopathologic correlation with MRI. Skeletal Radiol 2001;30(5):247–54.
36. Black DM, Kelly MP, Genant HK, et al. Bisphosphonates and fractures of the subtrochanteric or diaphyseal femur. N Engl J Med 2010;362(19):1761–71.
37. Chan SS, Rosenberg ZS, Chan K, Capeci C. Subtrochanteric femoral fractures in patients receiving long-term alendronate therapy: imaging features. AJR Am J Roentgenol 2010;194(6):1581–6.
38. Shane E, Burr D, Ebeling PR, et al. Atypical subtrochanteric and diaphyseal femoral fractures: report of a task force of the American Society for Bone and Mineral Research. J Bone Miner Res 2010;25(11):2267–94.
39. Jones G. Radiological appearances of disuse osteoporosis. Clin Radiol 1969;20(4):345–53.
40. de Abreu MR, Wessely M, Chung CB, Resnick D. Bone marrow MR imaging findings in disuse osteoporosis. Skeletal Radiol 2011;40(5):571–5.
41. Sintzoff S, Sintzoff S Jr, Stallenberg B, Matos C. Imaging in reflex sympathetic dystrophy. Hand Clin 1997;13(3):431–42.
42. Karantanas AH. Acute bone marrow edema of the hip: role of MR imaging. Eur Radiol 2007;17(9):2225–36.
43. Korompilias AV, Karantanas AH, Lykissas MG, Beris AE. Bone marrow edema syndrome. Skeletal Radiol 2009;38(5):425–36.
44. Dent CE, Friedman M. Idiopathic juvenile osteoporosis. Q J Med 1965;34:177–210.
45. Smith R. Idiopathic osteoporosis in the young. J Bone Joint Surg Br 1980;62-B(4):417–27.
46. Riggs BL, Melton LJ 3rd. Involutional osteoporosis. N Engl J Med 1986;314(26):1676–86.
47. Rauch F, Glorieux FH. Osteogenesis imperfecta. Lancet 2004;363(9418):1377–85.
48. Sillence D. Osteogenesis imperfecta: an expanding panorama of variants. Clin Orthop Relat Res 1981;(159):11–25.
49. Gahagan S, Rimsza ME. Child abuse or osteogenesis imperfecta: how can we tell? Pediatrics 1991;88(5):987–92.

50. Guglielmi G, Diacinti D, van Kuijk C, et al. Vertebral morphometry: current methods and recent advances. Eur Radiol 2008;18(7):1484–96.

51. Gluer CC. Monitoring skeletal changes by radiological techniques. J Bone Miner Res 1999;14(11):1952–62.

52. Damilakis J, Adams JE, Guglielmi G, Link TM. Radiation exposure in X-ray-based imaging techniques used in osteoporosis. Eur Radiol 2011;20(11):2707–14.

53. Kanis JA, Johansson H, Oden A, McCloskey EV. Assessment of fracture risk. Eur J Radiol 2009;71(3):392–7.

54. Kanis JA, Oden A, Johnell O, et al. The use of clinical risk factors enhances the performance of BMD in the prediction of hip and osteoporotic fractures in men and women. Osteoporos Int 2007;18(8):1033–46.

55. Compston J, Cooper A, Cooper C, et al. Guidelines for the diagnosis and management of osteoporosis in postmenopausal women and men from the age of 50 years in the UK. Maturitas 2009;62(2):105–8.

56. Kanis JA, McCloskey EV, Johansson H, et al. Case finding for the management of osteoporosis with FRAX—assessment and intervention thresholds for the UK. Osteoporos Int 2008;19(10):1395–408.

57. Johansson H, Kanis JA, Oden A, et al. A comparison of case-finding strategies in the UK for the management of hip fractures. Osteoporos Int 2012;23(3):907–15.

58. Black DM, Greenspan SL, Ensrud KE, et al. The effects of parathyroid hormone and alendronate alone or in combination in postmenopausal osteoporosis. N Engl J Med 2003;349(13):1207–15.

59. Bergot C, Laval-Jeantet A, Hutchinson K, et al. A comparison of spinal quantitative computed tomography with dual energy X-ray absorptiometry in European women with vertebral and nonvertebral fractures. Calcif Tissue Int 2001;68:74–82.

60. Yu W, Gluer C, Grampp S, et al. Spinal bone mineral assessment in postmenopausal women: a comparison between dual X-ray absorptiometry and quantitative computed tomography. Osteoporos Int 1995;5:433–9.

61. Binkley N, Krueger D, Vallarta-Ast N. An overlying fat panniculus affects femur bone mass measurement. J Clin Densitom 2003;6(3):199–204.

62. Tothill P, Hannan WJ, Cowen S, Freeman CP. Anomalies in the measurement of changes in total-body bone mineral by dual-energy X-ray absorptiometry during weight change. J Bone Miner Res 1997;12(11):1908–21.

63. Weigert J, Cann C. DXA in obese patients: are normal values really normal? J Women's Imaging 1999;1:11–17.

64. Bousson V, Le Bras A, Roqueplan F, et al. Volumetric quantitative computed tomography of the proximal femur: relationships linking geometric and densitometric variables to bone strength. Role for compact bone. Osteoporos Int 2006;17(6):855–64.

65. Farhat GN, Cauley JA, Matthews KA, et al. Volumetric BMD and vascular calcification in middle-aged women: the Study of Women's Health Across the Nation. J Bone Miner Res 2006;21(12):1839–46.

66. Farhat GN, Strotmeyer ES, Newman AB, et al. Volumetric and areal bone mineral density measures are associated with cardiovascular disease in older men and women: the health, aging, and body composition study. Calcif Tissue Int 2006;79(2):102–11.

67. Lang T, Li J, Harris S, Genant H. Assessment of vertebral bone mineral density using volumetric quantitative CT. J Comput Assist Tomogr 1999;23:130–7.

68. Radiology ACo. ACR Practice Guideline for the Performance of Quantitative Computed Tomography (QCT) Bone Densitometry. 2008.

69. Diederichs G, Engelken F, Marshall LM, et al. Diffuse idiopathic skeletal hyperostosis (DISH): relation to vertebral fractures and bone density. Osteoporos Int 2011;22(6):1789–97.

70. Nelson HD, Haney EM, Dana T, et al. Screening for osteoporosis: an update for the U.S. Preventive Services Task Force. Ann Intern Med 2010;153(2):99–111.

71. Barnett E, Nordin B. The radiological diagnosis of osteoporosis: a new approach. Clin Radiol 1960;11:166–74.

72. Horsman A, Simpson M. The measurement of sequential changes in cortical bone geometry. Br J Radiol 1975;48(570):471–6.

73. Adams JE. Radiogrammetry and radiographic absorptiometry. Radiol Clin North Am 2010;48(3):531–40.

74. Link TM, Guglielmi G, van Kuijk C, Adams JE. Radiologic assessment of osteoporotic vertebral fractures: diagnostic and prognostic implications. Eur Radiol 2005;15(8):1521–32.

75. Jiang G, Eastell R, Barrington NA, Ferrar L. Comparison of methods for the visual identification of prevalent vertebral fracture in osteoporosis. Osteoporos Int 2004;15(11):887–96.

76. Rea JA, Steiger P, Blake GM, Fogelman I. Optimizing data acquisition and analysis of morphometric X-ray absorptiometry. Osteoporos Int 1998;8(2):177–83.

77. Smyth PP, Taylor CJ, Adams JE. Vertebral shape: automatic measurement with active shape models. Radiology 1999;211(2):571–8.

78. Vokes T, Bachman D, Baim S, et al. Vertebral fracture assessment: the 2005 ISCD Official Positions. J Clin Densitom 2006;9(1):37–46.

79. Graeff C, Timm W, Nickelsen TN, et al. Monitoring teriparatide-associated changes in vertebral microstructure by high-resolution CT in vivo: results from the EUROFORS study. J Bone Miner Res 2007;22(9):1426–33.

80. Ito M, Ikeda K, Nishiguchi M, et al. Multi-detector row CT imaging of vertebral microstructure for evaluation of fracture risk. J Bone Miner Res 2005;20(10):1828–36.

81. Chesnut CH 3rd, Majumdar S, Newitt DC, et al. Effects of salmon calcitonin on trabecular microarchitecture as determined by magnetic resonance imaging: results from the QUEST study. J Bone Miner Res 2005;20(9):1548–61.

82. Link TM, Lotter A, Beyer F, et al. Changes in calcaneal trabecular bone structure after heart transplantation: an MR imaging study. Radiology 2000;217(3):855–62.

83. Boutroy S, Bouxsein ML, Munoz F, Delmas PD. In vivo assessment of trabecular bone microarchitecture by high-resolution peripheral quantitative computed tomography. J Clin Endocrinol Metab 2005;90(12):6508–15.

84. Burghardt AJ, Dais KA, Masharani U, et al. In vivo quantification of intra-cortical porosity in human cortical bone using hr-pQCT in patients with type II diabetes. J Bone Miner Res 2008;23:S450.

85. Burghardt AJ, Kazakia GJ, Sode M, et al. A longitudinal HR-pQCT study of alendronate treatment in post-menopausal women with low bone density: Relations between density, cortical and trabecular micro-architecture, biomechanics, and bone turnover. J Bone Miner Res 2010;25:2282–95.

86. Burrows M, Liu D, McKay H. High-resolution peripheral QCT imaging of bone micro-structure in adolescents. Osteoporos Int 2009;21(3):515–20.

87. Krug R, Burghardt AJ, Majumdar S, Link TM. High-resolution imaging techniques for the assessment of osteoporosis. Radiol Clin North Am 2010;48(3):601–21.

88. Wei CH, Harari A. Parathyroid carcinoma: update and guidelines for management. Curr Treat Options Oncol 2012;13(1):11–23.

89. American Association of Clinical Endocrinologists and the American Association of Endocrine Surgeons position statement on the diagnosis and management of primary hyperparathyroidism. Endocr Pract 2005;11(1):49–54.

90. Marcocci C, Cetani F. Clinical practice. Primary hyperparathyroidism. N Engl J Med 2012;365(25):2389–97.

91. Cunningham J, Locatelli F, Rodriguez M. Secondary hyperparathyroidism: pathogenesis, disease progression, and therapeutic options. Clin J Am Soc Nephrol 2012;6(4):913–21.

92. Hayes CW, Conway WF. Hyperparathyroidism. Radiol Clin North Am 1991;29(1):85–96.

93. Yashiro T, Okamoto T, Tanaka R, et al. Prevalence of chondrocalcinosis in patients with primary hyperparathyroidism in Japan. Endocrinol Jpn 1991;38(5):457–64.

94. Wishart J, Horowitz M, Need A, Nordin BE. Relationship between forearm and vertebral mineral density in postmenopausal women with primary hyperparathyroidism. Arch Intern Med 1990;150(6):1329–31.

95. Wen HY, Schumacher HR Jr, Zhang LY. Parathyroid disease. Rheum Dis Clin North Am 2011;36(4):647–64.

96. Steinbach H, Waldron BR. Idiopathic hypoparathyroidism: analysis of 52 cases, including report of new case. Medicine 1952;31:133–54.

97. Lambert RG, Becker EJ. Diffuse skeletal hyperostosis in idiopathic hypoparathyroidism. Clin Radiol 1989;40(2):212–15.

98. Adams JE, Davies M. Paravertebral and peripheral ligamentous ossification: an unusual association of hypoparathyroidism. Postgrad Med J 1977;53(617):167–72.

99. Albright F, Burnett CH, Smith PH, Parson W. Pseudohypoparathyroidism—An example of Seabright-Bantam syndrome. Report of 3 cases. Endocrinol 1942;30:922–32.

100. Steinbach HL, Young DA. The roentgen appearance of pseudo-hypoparathyroidism (PH) and pseudo-pseudohypoparathyroidism (PPH). Differentiation from other syndromes associated with short metacarpals, metatarsals, and phalanges. Am J Roentgenol Radium Ther Nucl Med 1966;97(1):49–66.

101. Wilson LC, Hall CM. Albright's hereditary osteodystrophy and pseudohypoparathyroidism. Semin Musculoskelet Radiol 2002; 6(4):273–83.

102. Kolb FO, Steinbach HL. Pseudohypoparathyroidism with secondary hyperparathyroidism and osteitis fibrosa. J Clin Endocrinol Metab 1962;22:59–70.

103. Adams J. Radiology of rickets and osteomalacia. In: Feldman D, Glorieux FH, Pike JW, editors. Vitamin D. 2nd ed. San Diego: Elsevier Academic Press; 2005. pp. 967–94.

104. Glorieux FH, St-Arnaud R. Vitamin D Pseudodeficiency. San Diego: Academic Press; 1997.

105. Brooks MH, Bell NH, Love L, et al. Vitamin-D-dependent rickets type II. Resistance of target organs to 1,25-dihydroxyvitamin D. N Engl J Med 1978;298(18):996–9.

106. Edmister KA, Sundaram M. Oncogenic osteomalacia. Semin Musculoskelet Radiol 2002;6(3):191–6.

107. Sundaram M, McCarthy EF. Oncogenic osteomalacia. Skeletal Radiol 2000;29(3):117–24.

108. Chong WH, Molinolo AA, Chen CC, Collins MT. Tumor-induced osteomalacia. Endocr Relat Cancer 2012;18(3):R53–77.

109. Ecklund K, Doria AS, Jaramillo D. Rickets on MR images. Pediatr Radiol 1999;29(9):673–5.

110. States LJ. Imaging of metabolic bone disease and marrow disorders in children. Radiol Clin North Am 2001;39(4):749–72.

111. States LJ. Imaging of rachitic bone. Endocr Dev 2003;6:80–92.

112. Dwek JR. The radiographic approach to child abuse. Clin Orthop Relat Res 2011;469(3):776–89.

113. Taybi H, Lachman R. Radiology of Syndromes, Metabolic Disorders and Skeletal Dysplasias. 4th ed. St. Louis: Mosby Year Book; 1996.

114. Looser E. Ueber Spaetrachitis und Osteomalazie; Klinische roentgenologische und pathologisch-anatomische Untersuchungen. Drsch Z Chir 1920;152:210–357.

115. McKenna MJ, Kleerekoper M, Ellis BI, et al. Atypical insufficiency fractures confused with Looser zones of osteomalacia. Bone 1987;8(2):71–8.

116. Whitehouse RW. Paget's disease of bone. Semin Musculoskelet Radiol 2002;6(4):313–22.

117. Adams JE. Dialysis bone disease. Semin Dial 2002;15(4):277–89.

118. Adams JE. Imaging in metabolic bone disease. Semin Musculoskelet Radiol 2002;6(3):171–2.

119. Sundaram M. Renal osteodystrophy. Skeletal Radiol 1989;18(6): 415–26.

120. Bhambri A, Del Rosso JQ. Calciphylaxis: a review. J Clin Aesthet Dermatol 2008;1(2):38–41.

121. Weisman Y, Hochberg Z. Genetic rickets and osteomalacia. Curr Ther Endocrinol Metab 1997;6:527–9.

122. Steendijk R, Hauspie RC. The pattern of growth and growth retardation of patients with hypophosphataemic vitamin D-resistant rickets: a longitudinal study. Eur J Pediatr 1992; 151(6):422–7.

123. Milgram JW, Compere CL. Hypophosphatemic vitamin D refractory osteomalacia with bilateral femoral pseudofractures. Clin Orthop Relat Res 1981;(160):78–85.

124. O'Malley SP, Adams JE, Davies M, Ramsden RT. The petrous temporal bone and deafness in X-linked hypophosphataemic osteomalacia. Clin Radiol 1988;39(5):528–30.

125. Polisson RP, Martinez S, Khoury M, et al. Calcification of entheses associated with X-linked hypophosphatemic osteomalacia. N Engl J Med 1985;313(1):1–6.

126. Adams JE, Davies M. Intra-spinal new bone formation and spinal cord compression in familial hypophosphataemic vitamin D resistant osteomalacia. Q J Med 1986;61(236):1117–29.

127. Hardy DC, Murphy WA, Siegel BA, et al. X-linked hypophosphatemia in adults: prevalence of skeletal radiographic and scintigraphic features. Radiology 1989;171(2):403–14.

128. Econs MJ, Samsa GP, Monger M, et al. X-Linked hypophosphatemic rickets: a disease often unknown to affected patients. Bone Miner 1994;24(1):17–24.

129. Weinstein RS, Whyte MP. Heterogeneity of adult hypophosphatasia. Report of severe and mild cases. Arch Intern Med 1981;141(6):727–31.

130. Ihde LL, Forrester DM, Gottsegen CJ, et al. Sclerosing bone dysplasias: review and differentiation from other causes of osteosclerosis. Radiographics 2011;31(7):1865–82.

131. Stoker DJ. Osteopetrosis. Semin Musculoskelet Radiol 2002; 6(4):299–305.

132. Cundy T. Idiopathic hyperphosphatasia. Semin Musculoskelet Radiol 2002;6(4):307–12.

133. Nemeth L, Zsogon E. Occupational skeletal fluorosis. Bailliere's Clin Rheumatol 1989;3(1):81–8.

134. Mann DC. Endocrine disorders and orthopedic problems in children. Curr Opin Pediatr 1996;8(1):68–70.

135. Winkler A, Wilson D. Thyroid acropachy. Case report and literature review. Mo Med 1985;82(12):756–61.

136. Bluestone R, Bywaters EG, Hartog M, et al. Acromegalic arthropathy. Ann Rheum Dis 1971;30(3):243–58.

137. Colao A, Pivonello R, Scarpa R, et al. The acromegalic arthropathy. J Endocrinol Invest 2005;28(Suppl. 8):24–31.

CHAPTER 7

ARTHRITIS

Andrew J. Grainger • Philip O'Connor

CHAPTER OUTLINE

IMAGING OF JOINT DISEASE

OSTEOARTHRITIS

THE INFLAMMATORY ARTHRITIDES

IMAGING OF JOINT DISEASE

The imaging of joint disease is complex, with the radiologist required to combine imaging findings and clinical information to accurately characterise arthritis. This chapter details the general principles of the plain radiographic assessment of arthritis and the key features of common arthritic conditions encountered.

Plain Radiographic Interpretation; General Principles

A systematic approach to the review of radiographs for arthritis is required. Important features to identify are:

- Soft-tissue swelling,
- Alteration in joint space,
- Bone changes
  - erosion
  - osteopenia
  - enthesitis.
- Joint alignment.

Finally, the distribution of joint disease provides important information when forming a differential diagnosis.

Soft-Tissue Swelling

Soft-tissue swelling is usually the earliest sign on CR of an inflammatory arthritis, representing synovial hypertrophy, soft-tissue oedema and joint effusion. When seen at the small joints the swelling has a symmetrical spindle shape about the joint. This pattern contrasts with soft-tissue swelling seen in gout, which tends to show a more irregular asymmetrical 'lumpy' appearance. Diffuse swelling of the soft-tissues of a digit is the characteristic finding in the dactylitis seen in hand involvement of the sero-negative inflammatory arthritides (Fig. 7-1). Radiographic soft-tissue abnormality around large joints tends to be limited to the detection of intra-articular effusion or synovitis.

Alteration in Joint Space

Loss of joint space as a result of cartilage destruction is a characteristic feature of many joint diseases. In inflammatory arthritis joint space loss is typically uniform, across the joint. In many joints this is helpful in distinguishing inflammatory arthritis from osteoarthritis (OA), which typically shows non-uniform joint space loss. However, in small joints, both forms of arthritis can show uniform joint space loss (Fig. 7-2).

Preserved joint space in a joint otherwise showing evidence of significant arthropathic change is important and may help with the differential diagnosis. In particular gout and psoriatic arthropathy typically show joint space preservation until late in the disease.

In severe arthritic change bony ankylosis may occur. This is most commonly seen in the sero-negative arthritides and in juvenile arthritis and represents end-stage disease.

Bone Changes

Osteopenia. Periarticular osteopenia is a well-recognised feature of some arthritides but is difficult to reliably identify. It may be more obvious in cases of mono- or pauci-articular joint involvement, where other joints are visible for comparison. An overexposed radiograph can mimic periarticular osteopenia, as can generalised osteoporosis. Often it is easier to identify that there is no evidence of osteopenia, which in itself is a useful observation when forming a differential diagnosis. Sero-negative disease, OA and gout typically preserve or increase bone density (Fig. 7-3).

Erosion. Bone erosion is the hallmark of inflammatory arthritis. Erosions can be described by their relationship to the joint and can be categorised as central, marginal or juxta-articular. Marginal erosions occur at the edge of the joint line involving exposed bone between the edge of the articular cartilage and the joint capsule. They are a classical feature of rheumatoid arthritis (RA). Central erosions occur into bone normally covered by the articular cartilage. They are less common and are typical of inflammatory (erosive) OA. Juxta-articular erosions occur further away from the joint and are characteristic of gout.

Rheumatoid erosions characteristically have no associated bone proliferation when untreated (Fig. 7-4A),

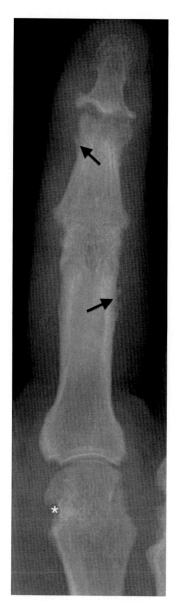

FIGURE 7-1 ■ **Diffuse soft-tissue swelling in the 'sausage' finger of a patient with sero-negative arthritis.** An erosion with bone proliferation (*) and periosteal new bone formation (arrows) is also present.

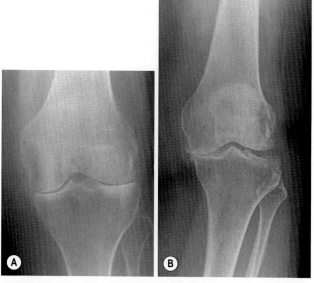

FIGURE 7-2 ■ (A) Rheumatoid arthritis. There is diffuse symmetrical panarticular joint space loss typical for inflammatory arthritis. (B) Osteoarthritis. Joint space loss is confined to the medial compartment; such asymmetrical joint space loss is typical for osteoarthritis. Note also the osteophytes in the medial joint line and subchondral sclerosis in the medial compartment.

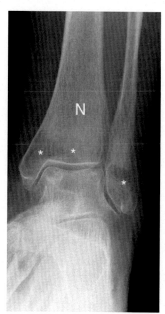

FIGURE 7-3 ■ **AP ankle radiograph demonstrating periarticular osteopenia (*); the distal tibial metaphysis demonstrates normal bone density (N).**

whereas sero-negative erosions typically show proliferative bone formation in or around the erosion (Fig. 7-4B), a useful distinguishing feature. Gout erosions have characteristic overhanging sharply demarcated margins giving them a punched-out appearance (Fig. 7-4C).

Entheseal Disease. Enthesitis is a feature of the sero-negative arthritides. Entheses represent the bony attachment sites of ligaments, tendons or capsule. On radiographs the important bone changes that can be visualised in enthesitis are enthesophyte formation and erosion (Fig. 7-5). Enthesophytes develop at, or immediately adjacent to, the site of an enthesis. They generally have a coarse appearance, with both cortical and medullary bone involved.

Bone Alignment

Joint malalignment is a feature of many arthropathic processes and results from a variety of causes, including tendon or ligament dysfunction and cartilage or bone loss. In most case this represents late changes of arthropathy though joint malalignment can be seen in several conditions without established bone or soft-tissue

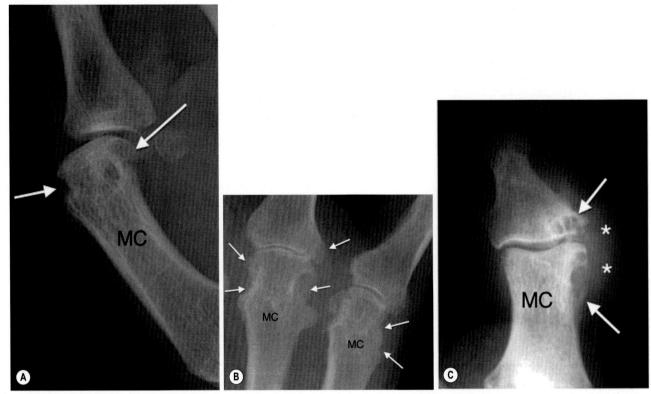

FIGURE 7-4 ■ (A) Rheumatoid arthritis. The metacarpal head (MC) marginal erosions are characteristic of rheumatoid arthritis. There is cortical loss without any associated new bone formation (arrows). (B) Sero-negative arthritis. Again, erosions are seen in the metacarpal head, but in addition to the bone destruction there is associated new bone formation typical for sero-negative arthritis (arrows). (C) Gout. There is asymmetrical dense soft-tissue swelling (*) and well-defined, punched-out periarticular erosion with overhanging margins (arrows).

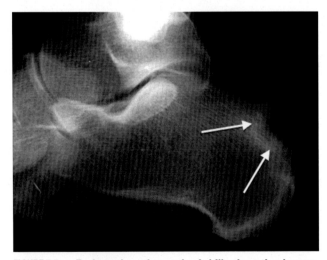

FIGURE 7-5 ■ **Entheseal erosion at the Achilles insertion in sero-negative disease.** There is cortical loss, with reactive new bone formation and sclerosis around the erosion (arrows).

arthropathy. The best known of these is systemic lupus erythematosus (SLE) where subluxations and ulnar deviation of the fingers and toes are seen in patients without bone erosion or cartilage loss (Fig. 7-6).

Distribution of Joint Involvement

An important aid to diagnosis is the distribution of polyarthritic disease when involving the hand and wrist.

Symmetrical proximal disease involving the carpal bones and metacarpophalangeal (MCP) joints is typical in rheumatoid arthritis. Distal disease of the interphalangeal joints is characteristic of sero-negative disease and osteoarthritis.

OSTEOARTHRITIS

Osteoarthritis (OA) is a ubiquitous disease and the most common articular disease. It affects the majority of the population at some time and is seen in other vertebrates.

Unsurprisingly, considerable research continues to be centred on understanding the pathogenesis of this condition and developing new ways to treat it. However, it is becoming clear that the disease has a complex aetiology which includes genetic and mechanical factors.[1] Fundamentally, the condition results from an alteration in the normal transmission of forces across a joint. This may occur due to an abnormality in the quality of the tissues at the joint, for instance ligamentous laxity as a result of a connective tissue disorder such as Ehlers–Danlos syndrome, or a change in the biomechanics at the joint such as might arise following trauma. However, it is recognised that there are strong influences on the aetiology of osteoarthritis that occur at a personal level such as genetics, race and ethnicity, diet, obesity, age and gender. It will be appreciated that some of these, such as obesity, will also act to alter joint biomechanics, but in general the understanding of how these and particularly

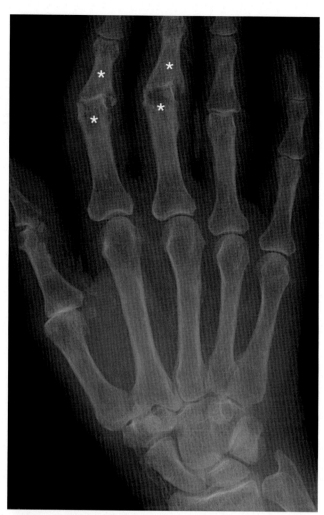

TABLE 7-1 Secondary Causes of Osteoarthritis

Trauma
• Acute
• Chronic repetitive
Systemic metabolic
• Hemochromatosis
• Wilson's disease
• Ochronosis
Endocrine
• Acromegaly
• Hypothyroidism
• Hyperparathyroidism
• Diabetes mellitus
Crystal deposition diseases
• CPPD
• Gout
Other
• Rheumatoid arthritis
• Paget's disease
• Bone/joint dysplasias

FIGURE 7-6 ■ SLE arthropathy with subluxation and malalignment of the PIP joint of the index and middle finger (*) without erosive change.

is not identified. Only a single joint may be involved (for instance, when trauma has occurred), or in generalised conditions there may be multiple joint involvement. The radiological findings are identical to those of primary osteoarthritis.

Radiographic Findings

Typically, the changes of osteoarthritis seen at the joint represent a combination of destruction and repair, although the balance between these two processes varies.

1. Joint space loss: in common with other arthropathic processes, cartilage thinning is a feature of osteoarthritis, which is seen directly on MRI and identified on conventional radiographs as joint space narrowing. In osteoarthritis, cartilage loss occurs in a more asymmetric distribution across the joint, generally occurring in areas of stress (Figs. 7-2B and 7-7). This results in an uneven pattern of joint space loss, a useful distinguishing feature from other causes of arthropathy.

2. Osteophyte formation: osteophytes are an important diagnostic feature for osteoarthritis, representing the hypertrophic aspect of the disease. They represent new bone formation, generally at the joint margins, although subchondral osteophyte may develop within the joint line itself. They comprise trabeculated bone and may be seen on one or both sides of the joint (Fig. 7-7).

3. Subchondral bone change: the bone deep to the cartilage shows characteristic changes in osteoarthritis. Increased osteoblastic activity brings about sclerosis, while subchondral cysts and bony collapse may also be seen (Figs. 7-7 and 7-8). Cyst formation is thought to be the result of synovial fluid passing into the bone through the damaged cartilage.

4. Loose bodies: as fragments of cartilage and bone are shed into the joint, they may be resorbed but often persist as loose bodies (Fig. 7-8). They may become revascularised and actually grow in situ.

genotypes affect the joint structures to bring about osteoarthritis remains unclear and is an important field for research.

The term primary generalised osteoarthritis is used to refer to osteoarthritis occurring without an apparent underlying cause. Secondary osteoarthritis refers to cases where an underlying cause is identified. A wide range of secondary causes exists, but characteristically they tend to result in either altered structure in the constituent parts of the joint, altered loading across the joint or a combination of both (Table 7-1).

Primary Osteoarthritis

Primary osteoarthritis is more common in women than men and has a strong genetic predisposition. It occurs in a typical distribution, characteristically affecting the hands, thumb bases, the hips, knees and first metatarsophalangeal joint in the foot.

Secondary Osteoarthritis

Many conditions, including trauma, may result in secondary osteoarthritis (Table 7-1). In many cases the cause

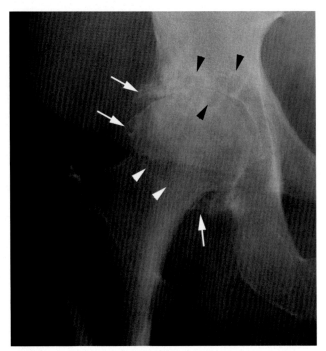

FIGURE 7-7 ■ **Severe osteoarthritis of the hip.** There is joint space narrowing which has occurred asymmetrically within the joint, in this case affecting the superior joint (the most common pattern of hip involvement). Note also subchondral cyst formation (black arrowheads) and osteophytosis (arrows). The osteophytes form a rim around the femoral head/neck junction and are superimposed over the neck visible as a sclerotic line (white arrowheads), which should not be mistaken for a fracture.

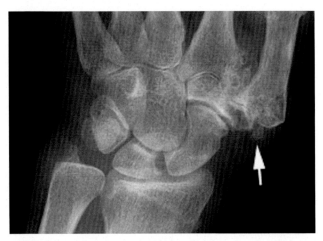

FIGURE 7-8 ■ **Severe osteoarthritis affecting the thumb base.** There is loss of joint space and subchondral sclerosis along with osteophyte formation affecting the thumb carpometacarpal joint. An osteochondral loose body is present (arrow) and there is joint subluxation. Early involvement of the STT joint is also seen as subchondral sclerosis.

This means it may not be possible to identify the source of a loose body.
5. Joint deformity and subluxation: the diseased joint will commonly show ligamentous laxity, allowing deformity (which may be contributed to by bony collapse and cartilage loss) and subluxation (Fig. 7-8). Further factors leading to deformity relate to

reduced proprioception and reduced muscle tone in the elderly.

It has long been recognised that pain experienced by the patient is poorly related to the changes of osteoarthritis seen in a joint on conventional radiographs. One patient may be severely incapacitated, despite only minor changes being evident on the radiograph, while another patient may have very little in the way of symptoms despite radiographically severe changes of osteoarthritis. This has led to investigation of osteoarthritis with more advanced imaging techniques, particularly ultrasound and MRI, in an effort to identify likely pain generators within the osteoarthritic joint. MRI and ultrasound will demonstrate other features such as synovitis, effusion and ligamentous change in addition to the features already described. MRI also demonstrates oedema-like marrow signal in the subchondral bone. Despite this new information, the source of pain in the joint remains unclear, although some evidence suggests that it may be associated with synovitis or bone marrow abnormalities.

Radiographic Changes at Specific Joints

Knee

Osteoarthritis of the knee may show any or all the above features on conventional radiographs. As already noted, joint space loss is usually asymmetrical within a joint in osteoarthritis. The knee demonstrates this observation well as varying degrees of joint space loss are typically seen in the three compartments, often with relative preservation of a compartment despite severe joint space loss elsewhere.[2] The most commonly seen pattern of osteoarthritis involves joint space loss in the medial compartment, often leading to varus deformity (Fig. 7-2B), but on occasion patellofemoral or lateral compartment disease will predominate (Fig. 7-9). Weight-bearing radiographs are more sensitive in identifying joint space loss in the medial and lateral compartments. Semi-flexed views also increase sensitivity to the detection of joint space loss compared to views obtained in extension[3] (Fig. 7-9). 'Skyline' views of the patellofemoral joint are best suited to demonstrate the differential involvement of the medial and lateral facet.

Hip

Again, joint space loss is typically asymmetrical across the joint. The most common pattern involves the superior aspect of the joint with superior migration of the femoral head and narrowing of the superior joint space. As disease progresses, sclerosis and cyst formation may be seen along with flattening of the femoral head (Fig. 7-7). Less commonly, medial joint space loss will predominate (Fig. 7-10). This pattern of joint space loss is more common in women than men. On occasions, central osteophyte forming within the hip joint will displace the femur laterally, giving apparent preservation of joint space. Osteophytes around the femoral head/neck margin will be appreciated as areas of sclerosis on the femoral neck as the anterior and posterior osteophyte overlies the femoral neck. A particular characteristic pattern of

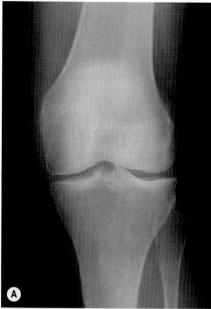

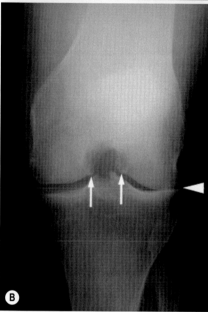

FIGURE 7-9 ■ **Knee osteoarthritis showing the effect of weight-bearing on joint space narrowing.** (A) Non-weight-bearing radiograph shows some subchondral bone irregularity reflecting the knee osteoarthritis, but the medial and lateral compartment joint spaces look to be relatively well preserved. (B) Radiograph with the patient standing with 30° flexion. Severe loss of lateral compartment joint space is now appreciated (arrowhead). The knee flexion also demonstrates osteophyte in the intercondylar notch (arrows).

osseous hypertrophy is seen along the femoral neck, typically on the medial side, and is known as buttressing.[4] It is appreciated as thickening of the medial femoral neck cortex (Fig. 7-10).

Hands and Wrists

Changes in the hands are characteristically associated with the development of firm nodules, which are

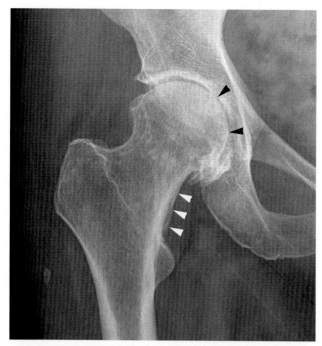

FIGURE 7-10 ■ **Severe osteoarthritis of the hip.** AP radiograph: In this case joint space loss is in a less common medial distribution (black arrowheads). The study also shows osseous hypertrophy along the medial neck of the femur (buttressing) (white arrowheads). Note also the marginal osteophytes which can also be seen projected over the femoral neck (cf. Fig. 7-7).

generally the result of osteophyte formation or synovial hypertrophy. These are known as Heberden's (distal interphalangeal joint) and Bouchard's (proximal) nodes. The interphalangeal joints (proximal and distal) are typically involved in primary osteoarthritis. However, the pattern of involvement is usually asymmetrical, with different joints on the two hands affected. Metacarpophalangeal joint disease is less frequently seen. At the wrists the disease usually affects the thumb base, involving the thumb carpometacarpal joint and/or the scaphotrapeziotrapezoid (STT) joint (Fig. 7-8).

Spine

Degenerative changes, representing osteoarthritis of the spine, are also discussed elsewhere. This most commonly occurs in the cervical and lower lumbar spine where degeneration in the intervertebral disc is seen as loss of disc height. Large osteophytes may be seen arising from the vertebral bodies, along with sclerotic change in the vertebral endplates. On occasion, osteophytes will bridge the intervertebral disc space. Typical osteoarthritic change may also be seen in the facet joints where osseous hypertrophy may contribute to spinal stenosis.

Abnormalities of vertebral alignment may also occur as a result of ligamentous laxity and degenerative changes in the disc and facet joints; typically, anterior displacement of the vertebra superior to a degenerative disc is seen with respect to its more caudal neighbour. This can be distinguished from the spondylolisthesis seen in association with pars defects (spondylolysis) because the

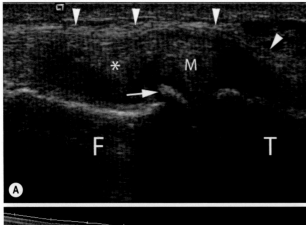

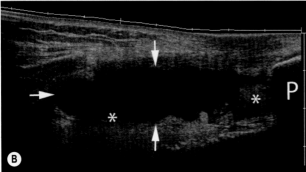

FIGURE 7-11 ■ **Knee osteoarthritis.** (A) Longitudinal ultrasound image of the medial knee joint. F = femur, T = tibia. There is osteophyte formation (arrow). Note the synovitis (*) surrounded by anechoic joint effusion bulging the overlying medial collateral ligament (arrowheads). The medial meniscus (M) is partially extruded from the joint line. (B) Longitudinal ultrasound image through the suprapatellar pouch. P = patella. There is an anechoic joint effusion distending the pouch (arrows) with synovitis seen along the walls (*).

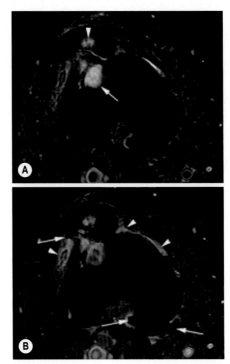

FIGURE 7-12 ■ **Patellofemoral osteoarthritis.** (A) T2-weighted axial fat-suppressed image. A large subchondral cyst is seen in the trochlea subchondral bone (arrow), along with a subchondral marrow lesion in the patella (arrowhead). The different nature of the two areas of subchondral signal change is difficult to appreciate on the T2-weighted image. (B) T1-weighted axial fat-suppressed image with gadolinium contrast enhancement. The cystic lesion shows enhancement of its periphery with gadolinium contrast with a low signal (cystic) centre. The contrast medium enhances the synovitis (arrowheads). Osteophytes are also appreciated (arrows).

posterior elements of the vertebral body will also slip forward along with the vertebral bodies, as there is no separation of the anterior and posterior spinal elements.

Advanced Imaging

For the most part the advanced imaging of OA remains the preserve of the research environment. However, given the ubiquitous nature of the disease it is not uncommon to identify features of OA on studies undertaken for other purposes or suspected diagnoses.

In recent years it had become recognised that OA is not just a disease of cartilage but affects multiple components of the joint. These include the synovium, ligaments, subchondral bone, articular fibrocartilage (for instance, the menisci in the knee and TFC in the wrist) and the periarticular tendons.

Both MRI and ultrasound readily identify synovitis in OA and this can be marked in osteoarthritis (Figs. 7-11 and 7-12). Osteophytes are also demonstrated by both techniques, ultrasound having been shown to be more sensitive to their detection in the wrist than conventional radiography.[5] While ultrasound is unable to demonstrate the changes in the subchondral bone, MRI will show cystic change and sclerosis but in addition may show

oedema-like signal (Fig. 7-12). Research studies suggest this is not due to true oedema within the bone marrow, and thus the term 'bone marrow lesion' is increasingly used in this context.

Erosive (Inflammatory) Osteoarthritis

Erosive osteoarthritis represents a subset of osteoarthritis with more inflammatory and destructive changes. It is usually seen as a polyarthritis classically involving the distal and proximal interphalangeal joints in the hands, although large joint involvement has been described. It is more common in women and has been shown to have a worse outcome than non-erosive OA.[6] While clinical clues may exist as to the inflammatory pattern of disease, the distinction from non-erosive OA is made on the radiographic appearances and the demonstration of erosions. Controversy still exists as to whether this condition represents a separate subgroup of patients with osteoarthritis or represents one end of a spectrum of increasing inflammatory change in osteoarthritis.

The pattern of erosion seen in erosive osteoarthritis is characteristically described as being central in location (occurring in the subchondral bone) and gives rise to the characteristic 'seagull wing' pattern of erosion[7]

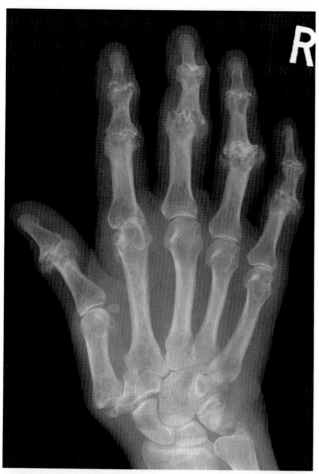

FIGURE 7-13 ■ **Erosive osteoarthritis.** DP radiograph: in addition to the typical osteoarthritis changes seen in multiple joints, including the thumb base carpometacarpal joint, there is erosive change seen at many of the interphalangeal joints. The majority of these are central in location (subchondral) and give rise to the characteristic 'seagull wing' appearance of the distal articular surface (seen for example at the index, middle and ring distal interphalangeal joints).

(Fig. 7-13). Marginal erosions may also be seen but appear to be much less common. Reparative change may occur and can lead to bony ankylosis, not a typical feature of non-erosive OA.[8]

THE INFLAMMATORY ARTHRITIDES

The inflammatory arthritides are characterised by multiple joint involvement with inflammatory change either within the joint, the enthesis or periarticular soft tissues. The management of inflammatory arthritis has changed dramatically in recent years with the advent of powerful biological therapies that, if instigated early, can induce disease remission and prevent the severe joint destruction previously seen. This has led to a greater emphasis on early diagnosis. While CR shows characteristic features of inflammatory arthritis, these represent late findings in the disease process and the use of advanced imaging techniques such as magnetic resonance or ultrasound is becoming more common. These allow early diagnosis

and treatment before irreversible joint damage has occurred. Nevertheless, radiography continues to play an important role in the diagnosis and characterisation of inflammatory arthritis and usually forms the initial imaging study.

Rheumatoid Arthritis

Rheumatoid arthritis (RA) is a chronic multisystem autoimmune disorder of unknown aetiology. In Europe it has an incidence of approximately 1%. It is more common in women and is characterised initially by a polyarticular symmetrical synovitis.[9] The later stages of the disease involve joint destruction as a result of bone erosion and cartilage loss. Synovitis is considered to be a strong predictor of bone erosion.[10,11] The hands and wrists are most commonly involved although any synovial joint in the body can be affected. Soft-tissue involvement is seen with the development of tenosynovitis and rheumatoid nodules, which can precede joint changes.

The clinical, and consequently radiological, picture of RA has changed over recent years due to dramatic advances in the way RA is treated. The use of powerful biological agents early in the disease process to arrest joint damage and induce disease remission has resulted in a change in the radiographic assessment of RA, with the detection of early or subtle change increasingly important.[12]

Radiographic Features

The classical plain film appearance of RA is of a symmetrical polyarthritis of the hands and wrists with a proximal distribution typically involving the carpal, MCP and proximal interphalangeal (PIP) joints. Characteristically the distal interphalangeal (DIP) joints are spared, providing an important distinguishing feature from OA and psoriatic arthritis.

The earliest plain film changes are soft-tissue swelling and periarticular osteopenia. At the MCP and PIP joints the soft-tissue swelling is appreciated as spindle-shaped thickening of the soft tissues developing symmetrically about the joint. Periarticular osteopenia can be a difficult radiographic sign to evaluate, particularly when there is symmetrical polyarticular involvement. Joint space loss in RA is usually panarticular, with diffuse joint space loss. Marginal erosions are characteristic of rheumatoid arthritis, and are seen most frequently in the joints of the hands, wrists and feet, erosions being more commonly seen in small joints than large joints. The earliest sites of erosion are typically the radial aspect of the index and middle metacarpal heads and the ulnar aspect of the wrist (Fig. 7-14). Cortical bone loss is first seen as subtle breaks in the bone giving the cortex a 'dot-dash' appearance; subsequently, frank bone erosion is seen (Fig. 7-4A). A form of the disease featuring large cystic areas, typically occurring in active men, has been termed robust rheumatoid and is thought to occur as a result of continued physical activity despite active inflammatory arthropathy.[13]

Ankylosis may occur in the later stages of the disease. Typically this involves the wrist with intercarpal and carpometacarpal fusions.

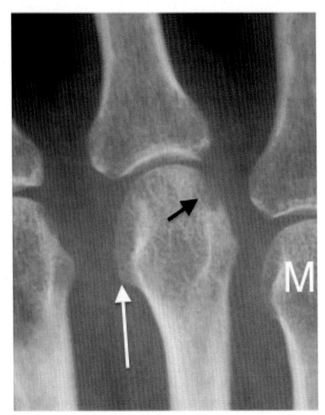

FIGURE 7-14 ■ **Rheumatoid arthritis with the earliest feature of erosive change seen along the radial border of this middle metacarpal head.** There is localised osteopenia with a 'dot-dash' pattern of deossification (white arrow). Note also the symmetrical soft-tissue swelling and frank erosion of the ulna border (black arrow).

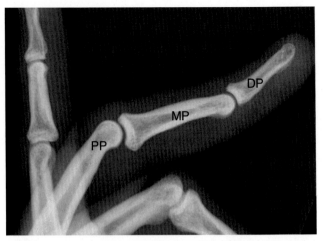

FIGURE 7-15 ■ **Boutonnière deformity of the finger with hyperextension of the DIP joint and flexion of the PIP joint.** PP, proximal phalanx; MP, middle phalanx; DP, distal phalanx.

Tendon and ligamentous dysfunction along with bone erosion results in deformity and malalignment in the later stages of the disease. Ulnar deviation of the fingers and the radial deviation of the wrist giving a 'zigzag' deformity to the hand is also typical for RA.[14] In the fingers, deformity involving flexion of the PIP joint and extension of the DIP joint (Boutonnière) (Fig. 7-15) or flexion of the DIP joint and extension of the PIP joint (swan neck) are common.

Subcutaneous rheumatoid nodules over the extensor surfaces of joints and in tendons are a common feature of RA seen in around 20% of patients.

Radiographs in Treated Inflammatory Disease

Preservation of bone density may be seen with successfully treated rheumatoid arthritis. In cases where irreversible joint damage has occurred, secondary osteoarthritic change can develop. It is important to recognise this when present, as it can lead to persisting symptoms and inappropriate continuation of biological therapy. The proximal distribution of these secondary osteoarthritic changes and the superimposition of proliferative bone changes on rheumatoid erosions are the key observations in making this diagnosis (Fig. 7-16).

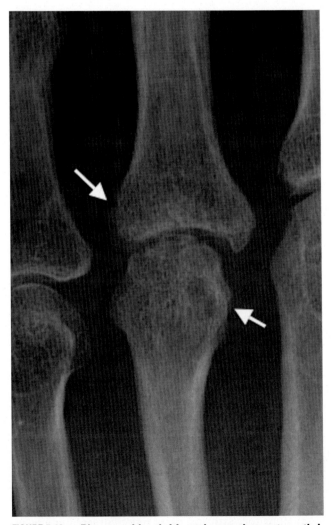

FIGURE 7-16 ■ **Rheumatoid arthritis and secondary osteoarthritis.** There is rheumatoid erosion and joint space loss with superadded sclerosis and proliferative new bone formation (arrows) indicating the development of secondary OA.

Sero-Negative Arthritis

The sero-negative arthropathies comprise a group of interrelated inflammatory arthritides sharing common features. Chief among these is the characteristic involvement of the entheses with inflammation classically seen at the bony insertions of tendons and ligaments. Other important features are:

- An absence of rheumatoid factors.
- A strong association with the HLA-B27 histocompatibility antigen (although it is important to realise this is not necessary for the development of these diseases, or required for the diagnosis).
- A tendency for axial skeletal involvement (spondyloarthritis).

Four main conditions are considered under this heading: ankylosing spondylitis, psoriatic arthritis, reactive arthritis (formally known as Reiter's disease) and enteropathic spondyloarthritis.

Ankylosing Spondylitis

Ankylosing spondylitis (AS) is a multisystem inflammatory spondyloarthopathy primarily affecting the axial skeleton. It is most common in HLA-B27-positive adolescents and young adults, who present with inflammatory back pain. Sacroiliitis and enthesitis of the axial skeleton is the hallmark of AS. Peripheral joint involvement is seen in up to 30% of patients.[15]

Sacroiliitis. Sacroiliac disease in AS is usually bilateral and symmetrical, with conventional radiographs and CT showing erosive change and subchondral sclerosis progressing if untreated to ankylosis. However, these represent later changes and the earliest feature of sacroiliitis is detected with MRI as subchondral bone marrow oedema. In the past skeletal scintigraphy had a role in the early detection of sacroiliitis but it is generally accepted MRI has greater sensitivity and specificity than CR, scintigraphy and CT (Fig. 7-17).

Spinal Disease. Spinal involvement is frequent, with changes seen around the discovertebral unit, costovertebral joints and in the posterior elements of the spine. Occasionally it may precede sacroiliac joint involvement. The changes seen represent enthesitis. Around the discovertebral unit inflammatory change is first seen at the insertion of the peripheral fibres of the annulus fibrosus, Sharpey's fibres. The earliest CR changes of spine disease are seen as sclerosis at these insertion points, identified on the lateral view as sclerotic 'shiny' corners to the vertebral bodies, known as Romanus lesions. Erosive change at these sites is harder to detect radiographically but, along with ossification in the anterior longitudinal ligament, contributes to a characteristic squared appearance to the vertebral bodies (Fig. 7-18).

The MRI equivalent of the Romanus lesions is bone oedema in the corners of vertebral bodies and this will be detected before the sclerosis becomes apparent on CR. Entheseal bone and soft-tissue oedema may also be found on MRI at other sites in the spine before CR changes are found, such as in association with the spinous processes,

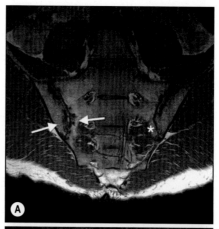

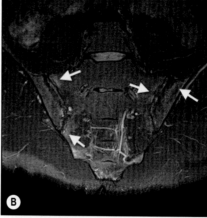

FIGURE 7-17 ■ T1-weighted (A) and T2 fat-supressed (B) coronal MR images of the sacroiliac joints (SIJ) in ankylosing spondylitis. The T1-weighted image readily demonstrates erosion (arrows) in the right SIJ with joint space loss on the left (*), all indicative of damage. Note how poor the T2-weighted image is at demonstrating erosion; however, it shows subchondral oedema (arrows) more reflective of disease activity.

facet joints and costovertebral joints. With time, erosive change may also become apparent on MRI.

Bone marrow oedema in the corners of vertebrae can also be seen in degenerative disease; AS-related oedema is normally greater in craniocaudal size than transverse diameter and is not usually associated with disc dehydration or loss of disc height.

Proliferative new bone formation occurs later in the disease and can be imaged with CT and radiography. Syndesmophytes, seen initially as thin bone outgrowths, develop typically at the site of Romanus lesions. As is the case with the inflammatory MR changes, they characteristically have a vertical orientation. These are useful features distinguishing them from osteophytes or the more coarse syndesmophytes of psoriatic and reactive arthritis.

If the condition is untreated, progression to fusion is typical, affecting the facet joints as well as the anterior vertebral bodies. The classical spine radiograph is that of the bamboo spine with complete fusion of the vertebral bodies and sacroiliac joints. Fusion between the spinous processes may also be seen. Fusion of the posterior elements of the spine can occur before fusion of the

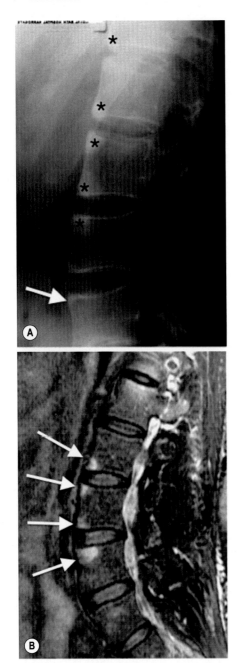

FIGURE 7-18 ■ (A) Ankylosing spondylitis (AS) with sclerosis of the vertebral corners (Romanus lesions). The radiograph shows advanced lesions (*) and an early lesion (arrow). (B) STIR sagittal MR image of a different AS patient with oedema of the vertebral corners (arrows) termed MR Romanus lesions.

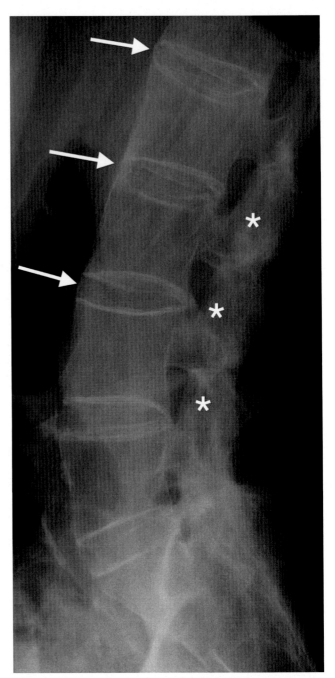

FIGURE 7-19 ■ **Ankylosing spondylitis with bamboo spine.** Bridging vertical syndesmophytes are seen around the intervertebral discs (arrows). Note no facet joint spaces are visualised, indicating fusion of the posterior joints between L3 and S1 (*).

vertebral bodies and can be difficult to appreciate on plain radiographs (Fig. 7-19).

Spinal fracture is relatively common in AS, despite appearances of sclerosis patients are generally osteopenic and the rigid spine is particularly prone to injury. A transverse fracture through a fused section of spine is highly unstable and is frequently a catastrophic event (Fig. 7-20).

In a largely fused spine, movement may only occur at certain unfused levels. The inflammatory Andersson's lesion may develop where movement occurs and the irregularity and sclerosis present around can be mistaken for infection by the unwary.

Peripheral Joint Involvement. The hip joint is the second most common joint involved after the sacroiliac joint.[16] Patients develop a cuff of entheseal new bone around the femoral head leading to a somewhat flattened appearance to the femoral head that can be misinterpreted as the cam deformity seen in femoroacetabular

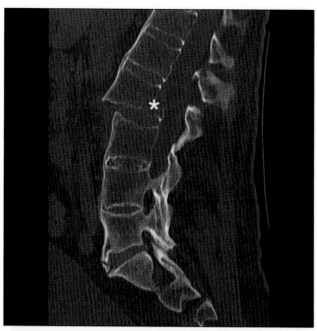

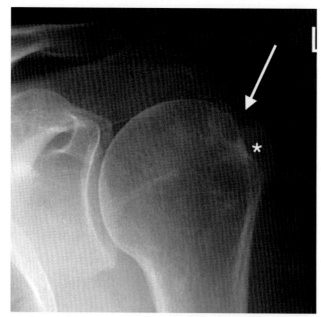

FIGURE 7-20 ■ **Spine fracture in ankylosing spondylitis.** Sagittal CT reconstruction shows spinal fusion and osteopenia. There is an unstable fracture of the L2 vertebral body (*) with anterior displacement of L2 on L3.

FIGURE 7-22 ■ **Patient with ankylosing spondylitis shoulder disease.** There is erosion of the rotator cuff insertion on the greater tuberosity (arrow) associated with surrounding proliferative new bone formation (*).

large and readily visualised radiographically. Erosion of the greater tuberosity at the insertion of the rotator cuff with proliferative new bone formation is a common radiographic feature of shoulder disease in AS (Fig. 7-22).

The hands and feet are involved in 15% of patients with AS, who typically present with diffuse swelling of the finger (dactylitis) and characteristic appearances of preserved bone density, proliferative new bone formation entheseal and peripheral joint erosion.

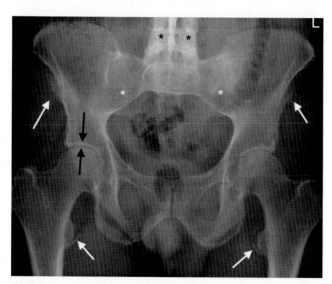

FIGURE 7-21 ■ **Patient with ankylosing spondylitis with spinal fusion (black *) and SIJ fusion (white *).** There is hip arthropathy with diffuse loss of joint space (black arrows) and flattened configuration of the femoral heads. Widespread entheseal new bone formation is noted around the pelvis (white arrows).

impingement. Joint space loss is diffuse with preservation of bone density. Entheseal new bone is not a prominent feature of AS hip disease per se but is often present in the adjacent hamstring and other pelvic ring entheses (Fig. 7-21).

The shoulder is involved in up to 30% of patients, again showing panarticular joint space loss with preservation of bone density. The entheses of the shoulder are

Psoriatic Arthritis

The link between psoriasis and arthritis is complex. Patients with inflammatory arthritis have an increased incidence of psoriasis and vice versa, but there is also an increased incidence of rheumatoid arthritis in psoriatic patients. If sero-positive rheumatoid patients are not included, the link between psoriasis and inflammatory arthritis is strengthened, with 20% of patients with sero-negative inflammatory arthritis having psoriasis.[17]

Five clinical subgroups of psoriatic arthritis (PsA) are recognised:
- Asymmetrical distal interphalangeal arthritis often associated with dactylitis.
- Arthritis mutilans, a severe destructive arthropathy mainly involving the small joints of the hands and feet.
- A pattern of arthritis indistinguishable from RA, which usually has a more benign course.
- Oligoarthritis distributed asymmetrically and involving any synovial joint.
- A pattern of spinal and large joint disease similar to ankylosing spondylitis.

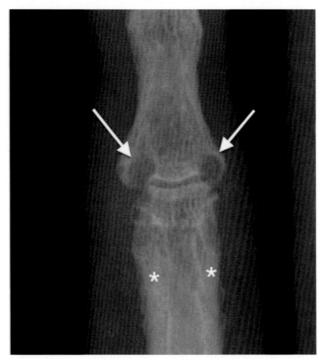

FIGURE 7-23 ■ **Psoriatic arthritis.** There is erosion of the distal phalanx (arrows) with prominent fluffy enthesophyte formation seen both proximal and distal to the distal interphalangeal joint (*).

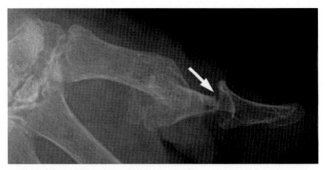

FIGURE 7-24 ■ **Psoriatic arthritis.** There is a severe deforming arthritis of the thumb and the 'pencil in cup' pattern of erosive change is appreciated at the interphalangeal joint (arrow).

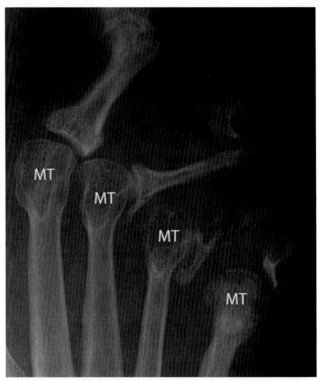

FIGURE 7-25 ■ **Psoriatic arthritis.** There is arthritis mutilans present with subluxation and erosion of the metacarpophalangeal joints and marked bone loss with a peg-like appearance to the phalanges. MT, metatarsal heads.

The disease classically involves enthesitis and it is suggested that inflammation in the multiple closely related entheseal sites in a digit is the cause of dactylitis.[18] The presence of nail dystrophy among psoriasis sufferers is a significant risk factor for the development of psoriatic arthritis.

Joints of the Hands and Feet. Soft-tissue joint swelling is seen as an early but non-specific radiographic feature of psoriatic arthritis. Global swelling of a digit in the form of dactylitis 'sausage digit' is typical (Fig. 7-1). Periarticular osteopenia is not a feature of psoriatic arthritis and can be useful in distinguishing it from RA. Bone erosion is seen most commonly at the joint margins and shows an entheseal pattern with new bone formation at and adjacent to the erosion site (Fig. 7-23). In the digits, erosions on the distal side of the joint classically merge together to produce a 'pencil-in-cup' appearance considered by some to be pathognomonic of the disease[19] (Fig. 7-24).

Bone loss is not limited to periarticular erosion in psoriatic arthritis and acro-osteolysis (distal tuft resorption) is a well-recognised feature. It can help distinguish psoriatic arthritis from erosive OA. Progressive osteolysis of the terminal phalanges may give them a 'peg-like' appearance, although osteolysis may progress to involve the majority of the phalanx (Fig. 7-25).

Bony ankylosis is a late feature of psoriatic arthritis and commences as a result of fibrous tissue forming within the joint; this can initially give the impression of a widened joint space.

Spinal and Large Joint Disease. Psoriatic spondylitis develops in 20% of patients with peripheral PsA. The clinical presentation is very similar to AS with inflammatory changes developing in the sacroiliac joints and at enthesis sites in the spine. In contrast to AS, psoriatic spondylitis typically shows asymmetrical involvement of sacroiliac joints and spinal syndesmophytes are coarse and more horizontal in orientation. They are also more asymmetrically distributed about the spine (Fig. 7-26). In contrast to AS, costovertebral disease is rare in PsA.

In large joints entheseal disease is less well visualised radiographically. The commonest presentation is one of

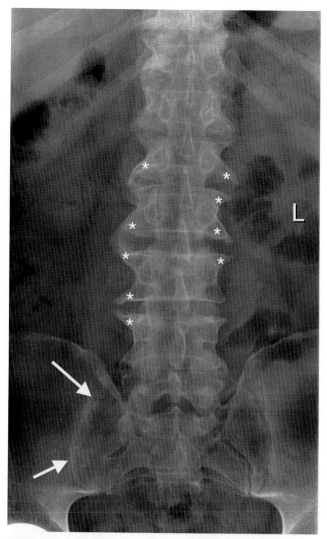

FIGURE 7-26 ■ **Psoriatic arthritis spinal involvement.** There is asymmetric sacroiliitis with loss of joint space (arrows). There are spinal enthesophytes (*), which are more horizontally orientated than those seen in ankylosing spondylitis.

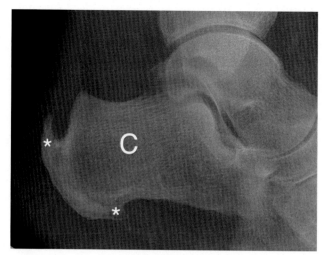

FIGURE 7-27 ■ **Reactive arthritis with prominent new bone formation at the calcaneal entheses (*).** C, calcaneus.

mild large joint oligoarthritis characterised by low-grade diffuse synovitis and recurrent effusions.

Reactive Arthritis

Reactive arthritis is a sterile inflammatory arthritis precipitated by extra-articular infection. It results from a combination of host susceptibility and an environmental trigger and affects a wide variety of joints. It usually occurs 2 to 4 weeks after infection, with gastrointestinal and genitourinary infection the most common triggers. Classically, reactive arthritis involves the small and large joints of the lower limb, with upper limb involvement unusual. As with psoriatic arthritis, joint involvement tends to the asymmetrical. The changes seen in the feet are similar to those seen in psoriatic arthritis, with soft-tissue swelling, joint space narrowing, proliferative marginal erosions and entheseal new bone formation. There may also be sesamoid enlargement as a result of the periostitis. New bone formation at the entheses of the feet is a prominent feature (Fig. 7-27).

Enteropathy-Associated Arthritis

Arthritis associated with inflammatory bowel disease is very similar to that seen in AS. While axial involvement predominates, 15 to 20% of patients with inflammatory bowel disease exhibit a peripheral arthritis, more frequently seen with Crohn's disease than ulcerative colitis.[20] The sacroiliac involvement is that of relatively asymmetrical involvement with bone oedema progressing to erosion, joint space loss to joint fusion. Peripheral joint involvement commonly involves the wrists, knees, ankles and elbows, with patients presenting with a transient arthritis characterised by effusion and diffuse synovitis. This is frequently asymmetric and occurrences tend to parallel the inflammatory bowel disease activity. The arthritis is characteristically non-destructive and while CR may show soft-tissue swelling and periarticular osteopenia, erosions and joint space loss are unusual.

The Crystal Arthritides

The crystal arthropathies all involve crystal deposition, either in or adjacent to an affected joint. This is a heterogeneous group of diseases resulting in a variety of radiographic findings. Common crystals implicated are monosodium urate (producing gout), calcium pyrophosphate dihydrate and hydroxyapatite.

Gout

Gout is a potentially destructive inflammatory disorder occurring in the setting of hyperuricaemia. Urate crystals are deposited into the soft tissues or joint where they can produce either an acute neutrophil-mediated inflammatory reaction or a more chronic macrophage-mediated response. The variation in response is the result of differing crystal sizes, with larger crystals failing to cause acute inflammatory reactions. Smaller proinflammatory crystals tend to be produced when there are rapid changes in a patient's serum urate levels. Asymptomatic hyperuricaemia is common, occurring in approximately 19%

of individuals in the USA and the UK. Studies show that this hyperuricaemic state can persist for decades, with studies showing only 1 in 8 of patients with urate levels between 7 and 8 mg/dL developing clinical gout over a 14-year period.[21] Factors that increase the likelihood of developing clinical gout are blood urate level > 9 mg/dL and co-morbidities such as renal failure, cardiovascular disease, obesity and diabetes. Gout is much more common in men (95%) than women, men normally developing gout in their fourth to sixth decades with female gout occurring postmenopause. Gout initially presents as an acute intermittent arthritis, but in time may progress to chronic tophaceous gout.

Acute Intermittent Gout. Acute gout presents with severe pain, erythema and swelling in the affected joint, which is usually in the lower limb. In 50% of cases this occurs in the first metatarsophalangeal joint, but the midfoot, ankle and knee are also commonly involved. In imaging terms, the patients have effusion and synovitis in the affected joint. On ultrasound, fine hyperechoic foci may be seen either within the effusion, synovium or on the cartilage surface.[22] These changes can also be seen in the tendon sheaths, especially around the hand and wrist. Frequently, aspiration to exclude infection is required, with microscopy required to confirm or refute the presence of infection and crystals. As the name suggests, the patient is asymptomatic between attacks of acute intermittent gout.

Chronic Tophaceous Gout. When affected joints are no longer pain free between attacks, the patient has developed chronic gouty arthritis. Chronic crystal deposition occurs in both the joints and soft tissues. Joint changes involve effusion, synovitis and erosion, with the small joints of the hands and feet most commonly affected. Large joint disease does occur, with a predilection for the ankle and knee. Crystal deposition within synovium and on the cartilage surface is a prominent feature seen on ultrasound, but also leads to increased effusion and synovitis density on radiographs (Fig. 7-4C). The erosions seen in chronic gout are characteristically periarticular, with a broad base and sharply demarcated overhanging sclerotic margins (Fig. 7-28).

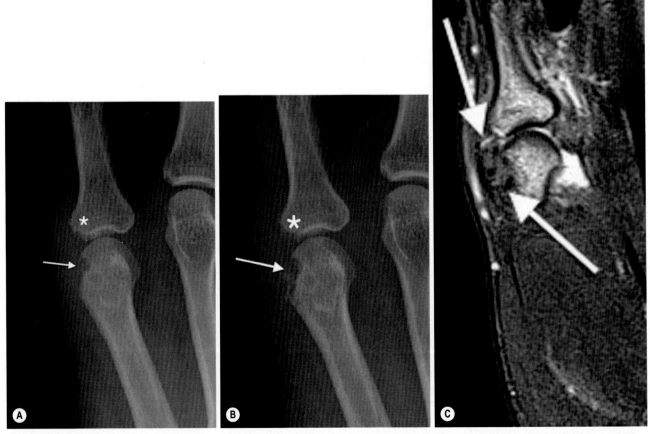

FIGURE 7-28 ■ Gout. There is progressive formation of a periarticular gout erosion. (A) There is asymmetrical soft-tissue swelling with cortical loss in the metacarpal head (arrow) and cortical irregularity in the adjacent phalangeal base (*). (B) With time the changes progress to a typical punched-out erosion (arrow) with erosion developing at the phalangeal base (*). (C) Coronal STIR MR. There is asymmetrical soft-tissue thickening, demonstrating characteristic heterogeneous intermediate and low signal (arrows).

Tophi, representing soft-tissue crystal deposition, are a sentinel feature of chronic gout seen as soft-tissue mass lesions occurring most commonly in the hands and wrist (ulnar aspect) and on the extensor surface of the knees and elbows. The asymmetrical soft-tissue swelling is radiographically and sonographically dense due to crystal deposition within deposits (Fig. 7-4C). Tendon crystal deposition is also common in tophaceous gout.

Calcium Pyrophosphate Dihydrate (CPPD) Crystal Deposition Disease

The nomenclature surrounding calcium pyrophosphate deposition disease is confusing and controversial.

- **Chondrocalcinosis**: the presence of cartilage calcification identified radiologically or pathologically. It can be due to a variety or combination of calcium crystals including calcium pyrophosphate dihydrate.
- **CPPD deposition disease**: a specific term indicating a disorder characterised by CPPD crystals in or around joints.
- **Pseudogout**: a clinical condition produced by acute CPPD crystals shedding into joints, resulting in acute attacks of gout-like symptoms. The diagnosis is clinical and cannot be made radiologically.
- **Pyrophosphate arthropathy**: a pattern of joint damage occurring in CPPD deposition disease resembling OA but with some distinct features. Chondrocalcinosis may or may not be present on radiographs demonstrating pyrophosphate arthropathy.

It is important to distinguish between CPPD deposition in cartilage (chondrocalcinosis) or synovium and pyrophosphate arthropathy. Chondrocalcinosis is common in older patients and occurs in association with other conditions such as haemochromatosis, osteoarthritis or Wilson's disease. Pyrophosphate arthropathy has a somewhat variable presentation with an ability to mimic other arthritides.[23] Patients with pyrophosphate arthropathy generally present with an OA-like pattern, although an acute inflammatory component may be seen. Intermittent attacks of pseudogout are said to occur in 10 to 20% of symptomatic patients.[23]

Imaging Findings. Chondrocalcinosis classically occurs in the hyaline and fibrocartilage structures of the knee and wrist but crystal deposition may also occur in virtually any joint. Synovial crystal deposition is also a common feature and is best appreciated radiographically in the suprapatellar pouch of the knee (Fig. 7-29). Chondral pyrophosphate crystals can also be seen on ultrasound examination, having virtually identical features to urate crystals but lying within rather than on the surface of the articular cartilage.[24]

Pyrophosphate Arthropathy. Pyrophosphate arthropathy most commonly shows similar changes to OA with joint space narrowing along with subchondral sclerosis and prominent cyst formation. However, the distribution of these changes is different to primary OA, with a predilection for the patellofemoral compartment in the knee

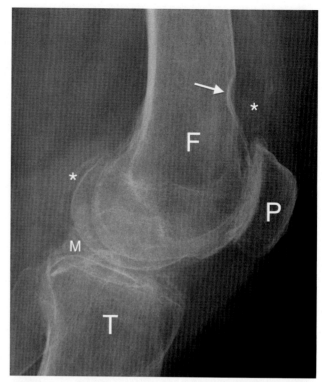

FIGURE 7-29 ■ **Pyrophosphate arthropathy with loss of patellofemoral joint space and characteristic remodelling of the distal femoral metaphysis (arrow).** There is synovial crystal deposition (*) and meniscal (M) chondrocalcinosis present. P, patella; F, femur; T, tibia.

and the radiocarpal compartment in the wrist. Erosion is not a feature of pyrophosphate arthropathy, though remodelling of the femoral aspect of the patellofemoral joint is well recognised (Fig. 7-29). Ligamentous dysfunction resulting in scapholunate and triquetrolunate diastasis is common.

Calcium Hydroxyapatite Crystal Deposition Disease

Hydroxyapatite (HA) deposition disease is a condition of unknown aetiology, which has both an acute and chronic presentation. Crystal deposition may occur both in the periarticular tissues, most commonly tendons and ligaments, or within the joint itself.[25]

Periarticular HA Deposition Disease. This occurs in both large and small joints. Deposition around large joints is commonest in the hip and shoulder, with small joint involvement most frequently seen in the hands and feet. In the shoulder and hip, HA deposition is within the tendons where is produces an increase in size of the tendon and inflammatory change in the tendon surrounding the deposit. This produces a combination of inflammatory and mechanical symptoms such as secondary external impingement of the shoulder. In small joints HA deposition is usually pericapsular or peritendinous and is associated with acute inflammatory symptoms. HA deposition disease is normally self-limiting, with the vast

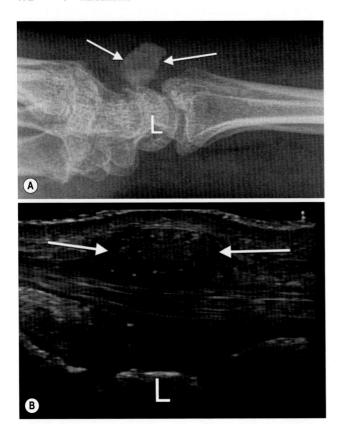

FIGURE 7-30 ■ **Hydroxyapatite deposition in the wrist.** The lateral wrist radiograph (A) demonstrates a large amorphous calcific deposit (arrows) with no internal architecture typical of an HA deposit. The ultrasound of the same patient (B) shows the deposit has a somewhat heterogeneous echotexture containing bright foci without acoustic shadowing (arrows). L, Lunate.

majority of patients recovering without the need for intervention.

The imaging findings are those of an amorphous calcific deposit, which, unlike soft-tissue ossification, contains no internal structure (Fig. 7-30A). Ultrasonically acute deposits are hyperechoic and cast no acoustic shadow (Fig. 7-30B). As deposits mature, they become denser, leading to acoustic shadowing, and become fragmented. Complications can result for HA deposition, with a small number of patients continuing with persisting symptoms normally as a result of secondary dysfunction and secondary impingement. When deposition occurs in the shoulder or hip close to the enthesis, interosseous extension of the HA deposit can occur which can produce marked intraosseous inflammatory change.

Intra-articular HA Deposition Disease. Intra-articular HA deposition can occur, but the influence this has on the development of arthropathy is poorly understood. The best-described articular condition linked to intra-articular HA deposition is Milwaukee shoulder, characterised by cranial migration of the humeral head as a result of rotator cuff tearing, rapid bone loss in the humeral head with remodelling of the undersurface of the acromion. This has also been termed rotator cuff arthropathy with some authors proposing cuff

derangement as the primary aetiological factor with HA deposition a secondary finding.

Connective Tissue Disease

The connective tissue disorders include scleroderma, systemic lupus erythematosus (SLE), dermatomyositis and polymyositis and have certain common features, including arthropathy.

Scleroderma

Systemic sclerosis is commonly associated with joint disease and patients will frequently present with joint pain. CREST syndrome is a common variation of scleroderma seen as the association of *c*alcinosis, *R*aynaud's disease, *oe*sophageal dysmotility, *s*clerodactyly and *t*elangiectasia.

Scleroderma is characterised by excessive deposition of collagen in soft tissues and is associated with fibrosis seen in the skin and internal organs. In the soft tissues flexion contractures and soft-tissue atrophy over the distal phalanges are common findings. However, soft-tissue calcification (calcinosis) is perhaps the most obvious soft-tissue finding of the disease. The calcification is amorphous in appearance and is most commonly seen in the digits, although it may be seen anywhere, including intra-articular locations, characteristically with absence of joint destruction (Fig. 7-31).

Bony resorption is a well-recognised feature of the disease, typically in the tufts of the terminal phalanges, acro-osteolysis. This is much more common in the fingers than the toes. Bony resorption may also be seen at the angle of the mandible, the posterior ribs and diffusely around the wrist.[26] Arthropathy is commonly associated with osteopenia, but joint erosions are uncommon.

Dermatomyositis and Polymyositis

The most common radiographic change of dermatomyositis is the finding of calcification within the subcutaneous soft tissues along muscle or fascial planes (Fig. 7-32). Typically, calcification involves both the skin and skeletal muscles, with the thigh being the most common site of involvement. Joint disease may also occur clinically but radiographs are usually unremarkable or may demonstrate subtle changes such as periarticular osteopenia and soft-tissue swelling. MRI may show other changes within the muscle, which, depending on the stage of the disease, include oedema, fatty infiltration and wasting. Polymyositis has similar radiographic findings but only involves the skeletal muscle.

Systemic Lupus Erythematosus

SLE is a connective tissue disorder predominantly affecting women of childbearing age. Clinical manifestations include systemic malaise and fever, skin rash and articular symptoms. In the later stages of the disease more severe multisystem involvement may be seen.

Articular symptoms are common and have been reported in 76% of patients with this condition.[27] The

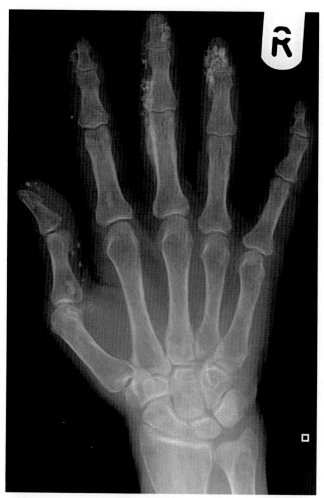

FIGURE 7-31 ■ Scleroderma (CREST syndrome). There is extensive soft-tissue calcinosis in the fingers. Soft-tissue atrophy is also evident, particularly over the fingertips.

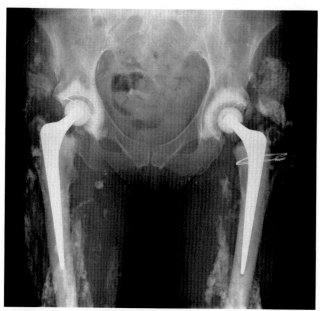

FIGURE 7-32 ■ Dermatomyositis. There is extensive soft-tissue calcium deposition. Note how this is associated with the muscle groups and can be seen tracking along these groups and in the associated fascial planes.

hands and wrists are most often affected, although the feet are also sometimes involved. The most frequent finding is synovitis, which will be demonstrated on ultrasound or MRI. Conventional radiographs are often normal, but may show soft-tissue swelling and/or osteopenia.

The most distinctive feature of SLE is a deforming non-erosive arthropathy (Fig. 7-6). This is more frequently seen later in the course of the disease, but may develop as an early feature of the disease.[28,29] In distinction to rheumatoid arthritis, erosions are not typical, having only occasionally been reported.[29] It is suggested that these patients actually represent a group of patients with both SLE and RA.

Deformities are secondary to ligamentous laxity and include ulnar subluxation of the MCP joints and hyperextension at the thumb interphalangeal joint. An important feature of the deformities is their reversibility. This may lead to normal-appearing radiographs despite obvious clinical deformity as the dislocations and subluxations may be reduced by the act of positioning the patient for the radiograph.

Osteonecrosis is a well-recognised feature in SLE and may occur in the femoral head, humeral head, knee and MCP heads. Soft-tissue calcification is a less common radiographic feature in some patients and is usually seen in a periarticular distribution.

Rheumatic Fever (Jaccoud's Arthropathy)

Jaccoud's arthropathy is a rare sequel of rheumatic fever and is initially radiologically indistinguishable from the deforming non-erosive arthropathy of SLE. During an acute attack joint involvement may be manifest as synovitis and effusion, appreciated as soft-tissue swelling on conventional radiographs. With repeated acute attacks, Jaccoud's arthropathy may develop. Late in the disease, erosions, bone projections and contractures may develop as the deformities become irreversible.

Mixed Connective Tissue Disease (MCTD)

Mixed connective tissue disease is recognised as a specific syndrome, which as its name suggests combines overlapping features of the connective tissue diseases and RA. Arthritis is a very common feature of the disease and a wide range of articular and soft-tissue abnormalities may be seen. In the hands these include osteopenia, joint erosions, flexion deformities, ulnar deviation of the phalanges, soft-tissue calcification and atrophy, and resorption of the terminal phalanges. Articular changes are most commonly seen in a proximal distribution similar to that seen in RA, involving PIP and MCP joints and the wrist. Large joint involvement is rare.

Miscellaneous Joint Disease

Diffuse Idiopathic Skeletal Hyperostosis (DISH)

DISH, also known as Forestier's disease, is a common condition found in the late middle-aged/elderly with an unknown aetiology. It is characterised by marked hyperostosis seen at multiple sites, but classically

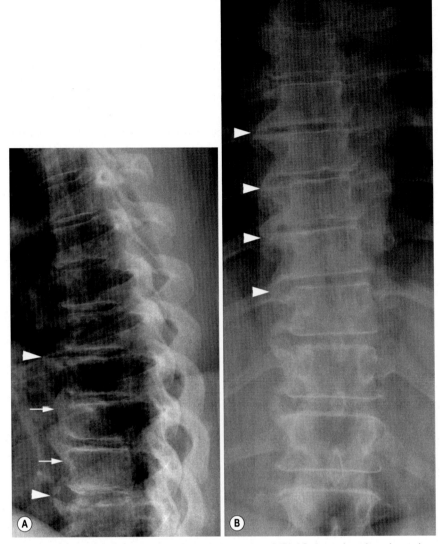

FIGURE 7-33 ■ Diffuse idiopathic skeletal hyperostosis (DISH). (A) Lateral and (B) AP thoracic spine views demonstrate marked bony hyperostosis along the line of the anterior longitudinal ligament (arrows) with large claw-like osteophytes (arrowheads), Note the relative preservation of disc space (in contrast to degenerative disc disease) and characteristic sparing of the left side of the spine shown on the AP view.

involving the spine. Sites of involvement typically occur at enthesis sites where tendons and ligaments attach to bone. Characteristically there is multilevel spinal involvement with flowing ligamentous ossification. Compared with degenerative disc disease, there is relative preservation of disc height. Certain diagnostic criteria are recognised for the diagnosis of spinal DISH and these help in distinguishing it from other causes of diffuse spinal hyperostosis such as ankylosing spondylitis and osteoarthritis.[30] These are:

- the presence of ossification along the anterolateral aspect of at least four contiguous vertebral bodies;
- relative preservation of disc height at the involved levels and absence of other OA features; and
- the absence of facet joint ankylosis or sacroiliac joint erosion or fusion.

The most common site for spinal involvement of DISH is typically T7 to T12, although cervical and lumbar involvement is also frequently seen. Here hyperostosis along the anterolateral aspect of the vertebral bodies is seen, with bridging across the intervertebral disc spaces. A feature of the condition is the tendency to see hyperostosis more commonly along the anterior-right side of the vertebral column (Fig. 7-33). This is thought to be due to inhibition of ossification on the left as a result of aortic pulsation. Compared with the changes seen in spondyloarthritis, the spinal hyperostosis of DISH tends to be more irregular with a wavy surface contour.

DISH is not confined to the spine, with hyperostosis also seen elsewhere in the skeleton, typically associated with the attachments of ligaments to bone. Characteristic sites include enthesis sites about the pelvis, the calcaneus and other tarsal bones, the elbow, hands and the patella.[31]

DISH is fundamentally a radiological diagnosis and generally the symptoms are mild in comparison to the radiographic changes. In addition to stiffness and back discomfort, there may be symptoms of tendinopathy at the enthesis sites and the hyperostosis can cause mechanical symptoms restricting the range of movement at a joint. Hyperostosis in the cervical and upper thoracic spine may give rise to dysphagia. Features resembling DISH may also be seen with retinoid therapy.

Haemophilic Arthropathy

Haemophilia refers to a group of disorders characterised by a tendency to bleed as a result of deficient clotting factors. These disorders may give rise to skeletal manifestations including soft-tissue and intramuscular bleeds. Of the haemophiliac disorders, haemophilia A (factor XIII deficiency) and haemophilia B or Christmas disease (factor IX deficiency) are most frequently associated with bone and joint complications. Both these conditions are X-linked and because of the recessive nature of the gene only manifested in men, although women may act as carriers.

Haemophilic arthropathy arises as a consequence of recurrent bleeds into joints. Most commonly the knees, elbows and ankles are affected. Blood products in the joint lead to an inflammatory response by the synovium and the release of destructive enzymes. The inflamed synovium itself may be a source of haemorrhage, further damaging the joint. Initially, acute haemarthroses may resolve completely with treatment involving administration of the appropriate clotting factor. With recurrent bleeds, complete recovery no longer occurs and restricted joint motion, contractures and muscle atrophy occur. At this stage radiographic changes become evident.

Haemorrhage and synovial inflammation in the joint lead to periarticular hyperaemia and often striking juxta-articular osteoporosis. Before epiphyseal fusion chronic hyperaemia leads to epithelial overgrowth and premature epiphyseal fusion. The synovium of affected joints initially hypertrophies. The ensuing inflammatory cascade leads to bone erosion and cartilage loss (joint space loss), ultimately producing changes of secondary osteoarthritis including subchondral cyst formation and collapse, osteophyte formation and sclerosis. Subchondral cyst formation may be contributed to by intraosseous haemorrhage. In the knee, widening of the intercondylar notch is a well-recognised feature of haemophilic arthritis and widening of the trochlear notch and olecranon fossa may be seen at the elbow (Fig. 7-34). The associated joint effusions and the synovitis may show increased density on conventional radiographs due to the presence of blood products (Fig. 7-34). Ultimately, the synovium undergoes a process of fibrosis and regression.

As with many forms of arthritis the radiographic changes of haemophilic arthritis are relatively late and advanced forms of imaging are becoming commonplace in the management of this condition. Ultrasound readily identifies acute haemarthrosis, although it cannot reliably distinguish between blood and simple effusion or even pus in a joint, so the correct clinical context is required. It will also identify thickened synovium (which may appear hypervascular). A particular use of ultrasound is to distinguish chronically thickened synovium from acute haemorrhage.[32]

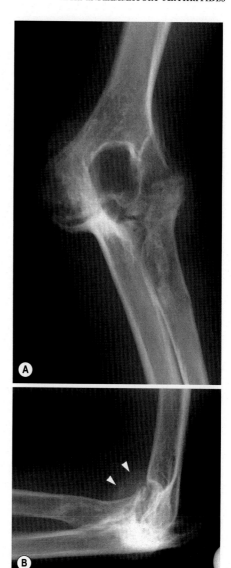

FIGURE 7-34 ■ Chronic haemophilic arthropathy. (A) AP and (B) lateral radiographs of the elbow: there is hypertrophic arthropathy with sclerosis and osteophyte formation. In addition, note the characteristic widening of the trochlea notch and olecranon fossa. On the lateral film, soft-tissue shadowing (arrowheads) representing the hypertrophied synovium is seen and appears dense due to the presence of blood products.

MRI can also assess for the presence of blood in a joint (the signal characteristics will vary depending on the time since the bleed) and for synovial thickening. Fibrosis and haemosiderin in the synovium may give foci of low signal on both T1- and T2-weighted imaging which may show susceptibility artefact on T2* imaging. MRI is also more sensitive than conventional radiographs for the demonstration of bone destruction and cartilage loss (Fig. 7-35).

Other Musculoskeletal Manifestations of Haemophilia. Intramuscular and soft-tissue haemorrhages are frequently seen in patients with haemophilia and may occur spontaneously or following trauma. Commonly involved muscles include the iliopsoas, quadriceps and

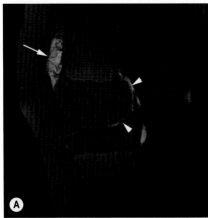

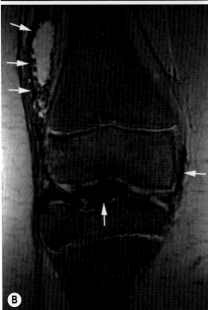

FIGURE 7-35 ■ Haemophilic arthropathy. (A) Sagittal fat-suppressed T2-weighted MRI: there is a joint effusion with synovial hypertrophy in the suprapatellar recess which shows low signal on the T2-weighted image (arrows). Cartilage loss is also evident (arrowheads). (B) Coronal T2* gradient-echo MRI: The t2* weighting emphasises the low signal synovium (arrows) which also shows blooming (susceptibility) artefact.

the gastrocnemius.[33] The resulting haematoma can be readily identified on ultrasound, where the early mixed echogenicity becomes progressively anechoic over 3 to 4 days, and MRI, in which case the signal characteristics will depend on the timing of the bleed. Complications of intramuscular haematoma include the development of fibrous tissue leading to contractures and myositis ossificans.[32]

Pseudotumour is a well-recognised complication of both intraosseous and soft-tissue haemorrhage. This is an encapsulated haematoma, which progressively expands. Osseous involvement may result from subperiosteal or intraosseous haemorrhage. The latter results in a well-defined lytic lesion that may be expansile and cause endosteal scalloping. Subperiosteal pseudotumours lead to elevation of the periosteum and pressure effects causing erosion of the underlying cortex. There may be

TABLE 7-2   Conditions Associated with Neuropathic Arthropathy

Condition	Prevalence of Arthropathy	Joints Most Commonly Affected
Congenital insensitivity to pain	100%	Ankle, tarsal, knee, hip
Syringomyelia	20–50%	Shoulder, elbow, wrist, cervical spine
Neurosyphilis	5–10%	Knee, hip
Diabetes mellitus	1%	Midfoot, forefoot
Alcohol related	Rare	Foot

soft-tissue extension and periosteal reaction leading to a differential diagnosis which includes aggressive lesions such as Ewing's sarcoma and infection.[34]

Neuropathic Arthropathy

This pattern of arthropathy involves both bony hypertrophic change and destructive change in varying proportions. It is associated with a loss of pain sensation and/or proprioception in the joint and as a result occurs in a number of conditions with neurological sequelae, the joint affected depending on the distribution of neurological disease (Table 7-2).

The radiographic findings associated with a neuropathic joint are similar irrespective of the aetiology and two distinct patterns are recognised, atrophic and hypertrophic neuropathic osteoarthropathy. The most common pattern of involvement is hypertrophic and the findings at an affected joint reflect this, consisting of increased bone density and production of bone debris. Periosteal new bone formation may be seen, as may osteophytes, although these tend to be less well defined than those seen in osteoarthritis. However, alongside these hypertrophic changes, the joint becomes increasingly disorganised with dislocations and bone destruction (Fig. 7-36). Early changes may be difficult to differentiate from osteoarthritis, infection or more rarely tumour. Neuropathic changes are much more commonly seen in the lower limbs than in the upper limbs or spine. Fractures associated with neuropathy are common and may be difficult to diagnose due to surrounding destruction and debris.

The less common atrophic pattern of neuropathic arthropathy usually affects the distal ends of tubular bones and comprises a pattern of osteolysis, which may be mistaken for surgical amputation. This form of the arthropathy generally occurs in non-weight-bearing joints.

Synovial (Osteo)-Chondromatosis

This condition is characterised by the formation of multiple synovial cartilage nodules, which may detach and become free intra-articular bodies. While the condition occurs most frequently in joints, it can occur in any synovial-lined structure so it may also be seen in bursae and tendon sheaths. It is most commonly seen in the knee, hip and elbow and is usually a monoarthritic

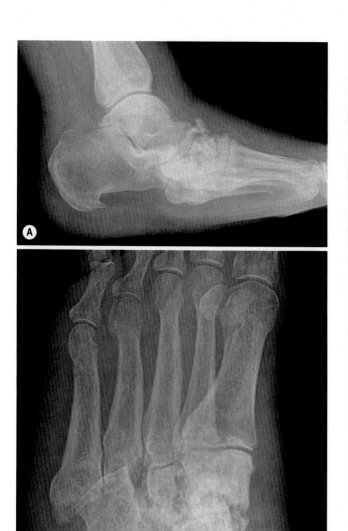

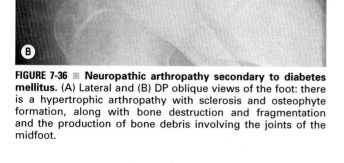

FIGURE 7-36 ■ **Neuropathic arthropathy secondary to diabetes mellitus.** (A) Lateral and (B) DP oblique views of the foot: there is a hypertrophic arthropathy with sclerosis and osteophyte formation, along with bone destruction and fragmentation and the production of bone debris involving the joints of the midfoot.

process. In the majority of cases the chondral bodies become calcified or ossified and at this stage they are evident on conventional radiographs and the term synovial osteochondromatosis is used (Fig. 7-37). In common with other osteochondral bodies, such as those arising through trauma, even after being shed into the joint space the bodies may continue to grow.

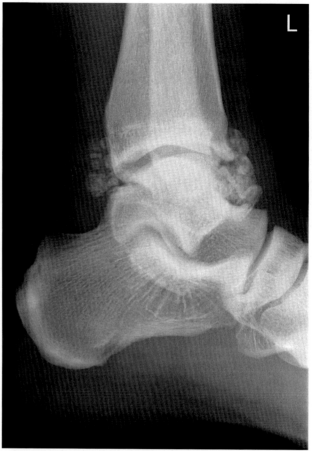

FIGURE 7-37 ■ **Synovial osteochondromatosis.** Lateral ankle radiograph: there are multiple intra-articular osteochondral bodies in this 42-year-old patient. Note the absence of joint space loss or other features of osteoarthritis.

The condition most frequently occurs in young or middle-aged adults and is described as secondary when seen as a consequence of trauma, degenerative disease or inflammation.

Initially, before calcification of the nodules, radiographs may simply show soft-tissue swelling. At this stage the non-calcified bodies and synovial nodules may be visible on MRI or CT arthrography. As the bodies calcify, they will be seen on all imaging techniques as multiple loose bodies, which may demonstrate trabeculation and may be associated with synovial thickening.

Although the presence of numerous similarly sized ossified bodies, in the absence of joint space narrowing, helps to distinguish synovial osteochondromatosis from loose bodies associated with other arthropathic processes such as OA, it is important to recognise that secondary OA may develop on the background of long-standing synovial osteochondromatosis.

Pigmented Villonodular Synovitis (PVNS)

This uncommon condition results from proliferation of the synovium in joints, bursae or tendons. Most

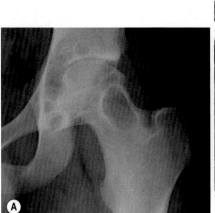
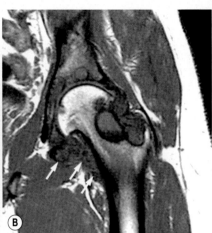
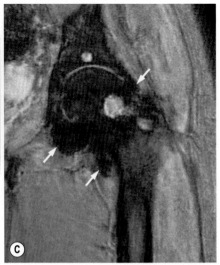

FIGURE 7-38 ■ **Pigmented villonodular synovitis (PVNS) of the hip.** (A) AP hip radiograph: there is extensive well-defined erosive change involving the acetabular fossa and proximal femur. (B) Coronal T1 MRI shows the extent of the erosive change. Note also the synovial hypertrophy, which shows intermediate to low signal, particularly well seen inferiorly (arrows). (C) Coronal T2* GRE MRI shows the synovitis with characteristic low signal and associated blooming artefact (arrows) due to the presence of haemosiderin.

patients are young adults and present with a chronic monoarthropathy, manifest as intermittent pain and swelling, typically in a large joint. The condition may occur in any joint, but it most commonly affects the knee (around 75%), followed by the hip (15%), with other large joints including the ankle, shoulder and elbow less commonly affected.[35] While the condition typically shows diffuse involvement of the entire synovium, a localised form is recognised, presenting as a synovial nodule most often in the anterior knee.[36]

Radiographs are frequently abnormal and may show features of a joint effusion/soft-tissue swelling. Bone erosion is a relatively common finding and is seen on a background of preserved joint space and reduced bone mineral density (Fig. 7-38). The extent of bone erosion is determined by the capacity of the capsule, with large joints such as the knee showing less frequent erosion than joints with smaller capacity, such as the hip. In the hip, erosion may lead to narrowing of the femoral neck, giving an 'apple-core' configuration.

MRI provides the best clue to the diagnosis due to the presence of haemosiderin in the hypertrophied synovium as a result of recurrent haemarthrosis. Compared with most synovial-based masses, the synovium will frequently shown low signal intensity on both T1- and T2-weighted imaging with accentuation of the abnormality on T2* gradient-echo images which may show blooming artefact in areas of haemosiderin deposition (Fig. 7-38C). Bone erosion, subchondral synovial tissue and 'cysts' are also clearly seen on MRI. Similar appearances (haemosiderotic synovitis) can be seen due to recurrent haemarthrosis in haemophilia and synovial haemangioma (Fig. 7-35).

Articular PVNS is histologically identical to nodular PVNS occurring in tendon sheaths, also known as giant cell tumour of tendon sheath, discussed in Chapter 5.

Lipoma Arborescens

This is a rare intra-articular synovial disorder most commonly seen in the knee. It is a benign condition involving synovial metaplasia, leading to delicate branching fronds of synovium. As the name suggests, the hypertrophied fronds of synovium contain fat, giving characteristic high signal on T1-weighted MRI which is reduced with fat suppression (Fig. 7-39).

Amyloid

Amyloid deposition may occur in synovium and in the surrounding periarticular soft tissues. The radiographic features reflect this with asymmetric soft-tissue masses and well-defined erosions and cysts. An important feature of articular amyloid is the preservation of joint space. The appearances may resemble gout or PVNS. MRI will show deposition of abnormal soft tissue, which is of intermediate to low signal intensity on both T1- and T2-weighted imaging.

Sarcoid

Sarcoidosis is a systemic disease with the potential to involve multiple organs including the lungs and skin. Musculoskeletal involvement is well recognised with joint, bone and muscle involvement described. Most commonly an inflammatory arthralgia is seen (in up to 40% of cases). In the majority of cases radiographs are unremarkable, but soft-tissue swelling and occasionally osteopenia may occasionally be seen.[37] Muscle involvement may be nodular or myopathic, the latter showing non-specific MRI features. Nodular sarcoid infiltration of muscle is evident on MRI and the sarcoid nodules may show a characteristic pattern of signal abnormality,

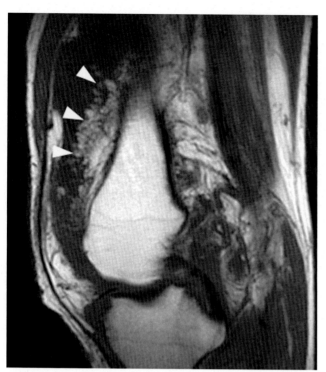

FIGURE 7-39 ■ **Lipoma arborescens of the knee.** Sagittal T1-weighted MRI: there is frond-like synovial hyperplasia evident in the suprapatellar pouch. This shows the characteristic high T1 (fat) signal of lipoma arborescens.

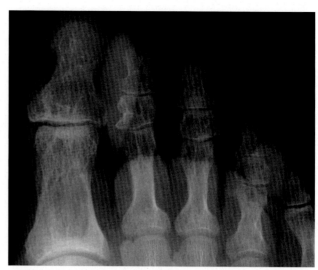

FIGURE 7-40 ■ **Osseous sarcoid.** DP radiograph of toes: the phalanges show abnormal bone texture with a lace-like pattern resulting from coarsening of the trabeculae. Note also the loss of cortical definition in involved areas.

demonstrating a low signal central zone on all sequences, representing fibrosis and peripheral high signal intensity on T2-weighted imaging.[38]

Bone involvement in sarcoid is seen in between 5 and 10% of patients with the phalanges of the hands and feet characteristically affected.[38] The lesions are frequently asymptomatic and are rarely demonstrated in the absence of skin or pulmonary disease. The most common form of osseous involvement involves coarsening of the trabecular pattern and loss of definition between the cortex and the medulla, giving rise to a lace-like or reticular appearance (Fig. 7-40). Localised cystic lesions may also be seen and may be sharply marginated. A rare form of mutilating sarcoidosis is also recognised.

Hypertrophic Pulmonary Osteoarthropathy (HPOA)

This describes a triad of periosteal new bone formation, finger clubbing and synovitis. It is most commonly seen in patients with pulmonary disease, particularly broncho-genic carcinoma but is recognised to also occur in association with other conditions including inflammatory bowel disease and biliary cirrhosis. If synovitis is the presenting feature, the picture may resemble rheumatoid arthritis. Not all patients will manifest all three components of the condition.

Periosteal new bone formation affects the diaphyses and subsequently the metaphyses of tubular bones, most frequently the radius and ulna, and tibia and fibula (Fig. 7-41). The femora, humeri, metacarpals, metatarsals and phalanges are less commonly involved. If the periostitis is long-standing, the bones have thickened cortices.

The triad of findings is not always associated with an underlying disorder. Primary hypertrophic osteoarthropathy, also known as pachydermoperiostosis, occurs most frequently in men of black African descent. It is associated with thickening of the skin and resulting coarsening of the facies, which may resemble acromegaly, although growth hormone levels are normal.

Multicentric Reticulohistiocytosis

This is a rare disease presenting in adult life most frequently affecting women. The soft tissues are infiltrated by multinucleated histiocytes with the formation of cutaneous nodules associated with erosive arthritis. In some patients the polyarthritis is the presenting feature of the disease, with the cutaneous changes occurring later. The interphalangeal joints of the fingers are most frequently affected, with involvement of the wrists generally occurring before metacarpophalangeal joint involvement. Less commonly, large joint involvement and spinal involvement are seen, although atlantoaxial involvement may be severe and occur early.[39] The erosive arthritis begins in the joint margins and is not associated with osteoporosis. Well-circumscribed erosions are typical, and may closely resemble the appearances of gout and progress to an arthritis mutilans.

Haemochromatosis

Haemochromatosis can be a primary or secondary disorder. Primary haemochromatosis results from a genetic error of metabolism, with increased absorption of iron from the gastrointestinal tract. Secondary haemochromatosis results from increased intake and tissue accumulation of iron from a known cause such as excessive dietary

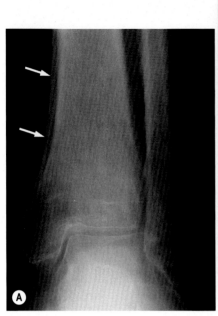

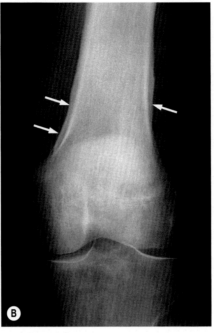

FIGURE 7-41 ■ **Hypertrophic pulmonary osteoarthropathy (HPOA) in a patient with a bronchogenic neoplasm.** (A) AP radiograph of the distal tibia and fibula showing a lamellar pattern of new bone formation along the medial tibial cortex (arrows). (B) AP radiograph of the distal femur: involvement was severe and relatively unusually there was also femoral involvement.

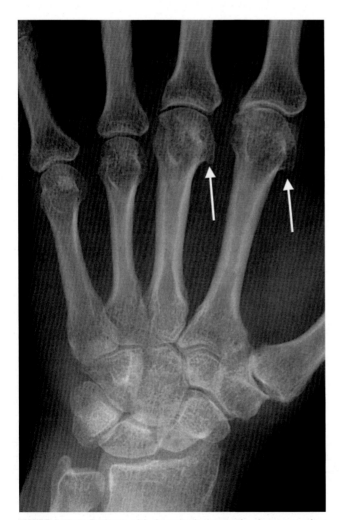

FIGURE 7-42 ■ Patient with haemochromatosis demonstrating classical hook osteophytes arising on the radial aspects of the index and middle finger metacarpal heads (arrows).

intake, cirrhosis, multiple transfusions and refractory anaemia.

Primary haemochromatosis is classically seen in the 40- to 60-year-old male who usually presents with a clinical triad of skin pigmentation, cirrhosis and diabetes, the so-called 'bronze diabetic'. Elevated serum ferritin levels confirm the diagnosis.

Joint disease and chondrocalcinosis are common in haemochromatosis and can be the presenting feature. Appearances resemble OA, but the pattern of joint disease, particularly in the hands, is different, with relative sparing of the interphalangeal joints and predominant involvement of the MCP joints, most frequently those of the index and middle fingers (Fig. 7-42). Another typical feature of the disease is the presence of hook-like osteophytes generally seen on the radial aspect of the metacarpal heads. Chondrocalcinosis is seen in association with the metacarpal changes, usually best appreciated in the wrist. The combination of these findings, although not pathognomonic, should alert the clinician and radiologist to the possibility of haemochromatosis.[23,40]

REFERENCES

1. Arden N, Nevitt MC. Osteoarthritis: epidemiology. Best Pract Res Clin Rheumatol 2006;20(1):3–25.
2. Boegard T, Jonsson K. Radiography in osteoarthritis of the knee. Skeletal Radiol 1999;28(11):605–15.
3. Gossec L, Jordan JM, Mazzuca SA, et al. Comparative evaluation of three semi-quantitative radiographic grading techniques for knee osteoarthritis in terms of validity and reproducibility in 1759 X-rays: report of the OARSI-OMERACT task force. Osteoarthritis Cartilage 2008;16(7):742–8.
4. Dixon T, Benjamin J, Lund P, et al. Femoral neck buttressing: a radiographic and histologic analysis. Skeletal Radiol 2000;29(10):587–92.
5. Keen HI, Wakefield RJ, Grainger AJ, et al. Can ultrasonography improve on radiographic assessment in osteoarthritis of the hands? A comparison between radiographic and ultrasonographic detected pathology. Ann Rheum Dis 2008;67(8):1116–20.

6. Kloppenburg M, Kwok WY. Hand osteoarthritis—a heterogeneous disorder. Nat Rev Rheumatol 2011;8(1):22–31.

7. Greenspan A. Erosive osteoarthritis. Semin Musculoskelet Radiol 2003;7(2):155–9.

8. Punzi L, Frigato M, Frallonardo P, Ramonda R. Inflammatory osteoarthritis of the hand. Best Pract Res Clin Rheumatol 2010; 24(3):301–12.

9. Arend WP. Physiology of cytokine pathways in rheumatoid arthritis. Arthritis Rheum 2001;45(1):101–6.

10. McGonagle D, Conaghan PG, O'Connor P, et al. The relationship between synovitis and bone changes in early untreated rheumatoid arthritis: a controlled magnetic resonance imaging study. Arthritis Rheum 1999;42(8):1706–11.

11. McQueen FM, Stewart N, Crabbe J, et al. Magnetic resonance imaging of the wrist in early rheumatoid arthritis reveals progression of erosions despite clinical improvement. Ann Rheum Dis 1999;58(3):156–63.

12. Villeneuve E, Emery P. Rheumatoid arthritis: what has changed? Skeletal Radiol 2009;38(2):109–12.

13. De Haas WH, De Boer W, Griffioen F, Oosten-Elst P. Rheumatoid arthritis of the robust reaction type. Ann Rheum Dis 1974;33(1): 81–5.

14. Resnick D. Inter-relationship between radiocarpal and metacarpophalangeal joint deformities in rheumatoid arthritis. J Can Assoc Radiol 1976;27(1):29–36.

15. Resnick D. Patterns of peripheral joint disease in ankylosing spondylitis. Radiology 1974;110(3):523–32.

16. Dwosh IL, Resnick D, Becker MA. Hip involvement in ankylosing spondylitis. Arthritis Rheum 1976;19(4):683–92.

17. Baker H. Prevalence of psoriasis in polyarthritic patients and their relatives. Ann Rheum Dis 1966;25(3):229–34.

18. Benjamin M, McGonagle D. The anatomical basis for disease localisation in seronegative spondyloarthropathy at entheses and related sites. J Anat 2001;199(Pt 5):503–26.

19. Arnett FC. Seronegative spondylarthropathies. Bull Rheum Dis 1987;37(1):1–12.

20. Gravallese EM, Kantrowitz FG. Arthritic manifestations of inflammatory bowel disease. Am J Gastroenterol 1988;83(7):703–9.

21. Abbott RD, Brand FN, Kannel WB, Castelli WP. Gout and coronary heart disease: the Framingham Study. J Clin Epidemiol 1988;41(3):237–42.

22. Thiele RG. Role of ultrasound and other advanced imaging in the diagnosis and management of gout. Curr Rheumatol Rep 2011;13(2):146–53.

23. Steinbach LS. Calcium pyrophosphate dihydrate and calcium hydroxyapatite crystal deposition diseases: imaging perspectives. Radiol Clin North Am 2004;42(1):185–205, vii.

24. Filippucci E, Riveros MG, Georgescu D, et al. Hyaline cartilage involvement in patients with gout and calcium pyrophosphate deposition disease. An ultrasound study. Osteoarthritis Cartilage 2009;17(2):178–81.

25. Uri DS, Dalinka MK. Imaging of arthropathies. Crystal disease. Radiol Clin North Am 1996;34(2):359–74, xi.

26. Bassett LW, Blocka KL, Furst DE, et al. Skeletal findings in progressive systemic sclerosis (scleroderma). Am J Roentgenol 1981; 136(6):1121–6.

27. Labowitz R, Schumacher HR Jr. Articular manifestations of systemic lupus erythematosus. Ann Intern Med 1971;74(6):911–21.

28. Resnick D. Systemic lupus erthematosus. In: Resnick D, editor. Diagnosis of Bone and Joint Disorders. 2. Saunders: Philadelphia; 2002. pp. 1171–93.

29. Weissman BN, Rappoport AS, Sosman JL, Schur PH. Radiographic findings in the hands in patients with systemic lupus erythematosus. Radiology 1978;126(2):313–17.

30. Resnick D, Niwayama G. Radiographic and pathologic features of spinal involvement in diffuse idiopathic skeletal hyperostosis (DISH). Radiology 1976;119(3):559–68.

31. Cammisa M, De Serio A, Guglielmi G. Diffuse idiopathic skeletal hyperostosis. Eur J Radiol 1998;27(Suppl. 1):S7–11.

32. Maclachlan J, Gough-Palmer A, Hargunani R, et al. Haemophilia imaging: a review. Skeletal Radiol 2009;38(10):949–57.

33. Hermann G, Gilbert MS, Abdelwahab IF. Hemophilia: evaluation of musculoskeletal involvement with CT, sonography, and MR imaging. Am J Roentgenol 1992;158(1):119–23.

34. Park JS, Ryu KN. Hemophilic pseudotumor involving the musculoskeletal system: spectrum of radiologic findings. Am J Roentgenol 2004;183(1):55–61.

35. Murphey MD, Rhee JH, Lewis RB, et al. Pigmented villonodular synovitis: radiologic-pathologic correlation. Radiographics 2008; 28(5):1493–518.

36. Bravo SM, Winalski CS, Weissman BN. Pigmented villonodular synovitis. Radiol Clin North Am 1996;34(2):311–26, x–xi.

37. Koyama T, Ueda H, Togashi K, et al. Radiologic manifestations of sarcoidosis in various organs. Radiographics 2004;24(1):87–104.

38. Otake S, Ishigaki T. Muscular sarcoidosis. Semin Musculoskelet Radiol 2001;5(2):167–70.

39. Gold RH, Metzger AL, Mirra JM, et al. Multicentric reticulohistiocytosis (lipoid dermato-arthritis). An erosive polyarthritis with distinctive clinical, roentgenographic and pathologic features. Am J Roentgenol 1975;124(4):610–24.

40. Adamson TC 3rd, Resnik CS, Guerra J Jr, et al. Hand and wrist arthropathies of hemochromatosis and calcium pyrophosphate deposition disease: distinct radiographic features. Radiology 1983; 147(2):377–81.

CHAPTER 8

APPENDICULAR AND PELVIC TRAUMA

Nigel Raby • Philip M. Hughes • James Ricketts

CHAPTER OUTLINE

GENERAL CONSIDERATIONS

DESCRIBING FRACTURE TYPES

THE SHOULDER

THE ACROMIO-CLAVICULAR JOINT

THE ELBOW

THE WRIST

PELVIC AND ACETABULAR FRACTURES

THE HIP

THE KNEE

THE ANKLE

FOOT INJURIES

GENERAL CONSIDERATIONS

This chapter will consider skeletal trauma and its consequences. It will be largely confined to appearances on radiographs occasionally supplemented by CT. The soft-tissue aspects of trauma principally imaged with MRI will not be considered in this chapter.

In evaluating any bony injury due to trauma it is essential that two radiographs are obtained, usually at right angles to each other (orthogonal). Many fractures are visible on only one of these radiographs. Inexperienced observers will tend to rely on the anteroposterior (AP) view as this is better understood intuitively. The lateral view, however, will identify at least as many fractures as the AP and may be the only view where the fracture is visible. Time spent becoming familiar with the lateral view will be well rewarded. The old adage 'One view is no view' is particularly relevant when assessing trauma radiographs.

DESCRIBING FRACTURE TYPES

Fractures of bones can be considered to be incomplete or complete. Incomplete fractures are generally confined to injuries in children (Fig. 8-1). There are three types:
1. Plastic bowing injury where the bone is mildly deformed but there is no disruption of the cortex.
2. Torus injury, an impaction fracture with cortical buckling which may be circumferential. There is no true cortical break and the periosteum is intact.
3. Greenstick fracture where there is break of cortex on one side only with buckling of the opposite cortex.

Also seen only in children are fractures related to the epiphyseal growth plate. These have been classified by Salter and Harris into five types (Fig. 8-2).

Complete fractures refer to a fracture which separates one part of bone from the other. The fracture pattern should be described. These fractures can be subdivided by the fracture direction into transverse, oblique, spiral and longitudinal. The presence or absence of angulation, rotation, distraction or shortening with overlap should be stated. The site of the fracture within the bone should be stated. If near a joint, note should be made as to whether the fracture extends to involve the articular surface. This is an important observation as, in general, intra-articular fractures have a poorer prognosis and surgical intervention is more often required.

The term 'comminuted' refers to fractures which have more than two parts of bone at the fracture site, although by convention small bone fragments are often disregarded.

A large triangular bone segment is referred to as a butterfly fragment and a segmental fragment is seen when there is a separate segment of bone between the main fracture components. A compound fracture is one where there is breach of the overlying soft tissue and skin. Although this can sometimes be identified on radiographs it is usually a clinical diagnosis.

It is generally understood that a fracture results in a gap between the bone ends through which the X-ray beam can pass, resulting in a dark or black line on the radiograph. Not so well appreciated is that the presence of a white or sclerotic area of bone is an equally important sign of fracture. In the setting of trauma this finding is due to either impaction or overlap of bone. Both will result in increased bony density. The best-known example

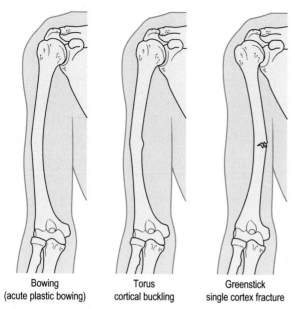

Bowing
(acute plastic bowing)

Torus
cortical buckling

Greenstick
single cortex fracture

FIGURE 8-1 ■ **Children's fractures are often incomplete.**

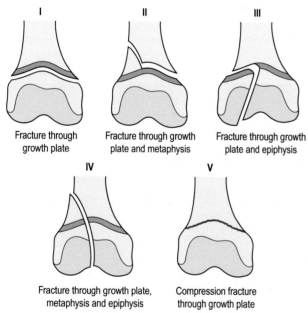

I — Fracture through growth plate

II — Fracture through growth plate and metaphysis

III — Fracture through growth plate and epiphysis

IV — Fracture through growth plate, metaphysis and epiphysis

V — Compression fracture through growth plate

FIGURE 8-2 ■ **The Salter–Harris classification of fractures in children involving the growth plate.** The numbers refer to the prognosis. Type 1 has the best, type 5 the worst.

of this is an impacted fracture of the femoral neck. However, there are many other situations and sites where this can occur. It is a very useful radiological sign which can help detect subtle fractures. Its value will be demonstrated several times in this chapter.

An avulsion fracture occurs at sites of tendon or ligament attachment when a fragment of bone is pulled off the underlying parent bone as a result of traction from either the muscle tendon kinetic chain or a joint ligament. To describe any injury as an avulsion fracture you must be able to identify the mechanism of injury and state what ligament or tendon attaches to the bone fragment. These should not be referred to as flake or chip fractures unless there is a clear mechanism of a direct impact to

the area which would account for the findings; such fractures are rare. Understanding of the above will lead to an appreciation of the severity and significance of the findings. A bone avulsion at the site of tendon attachment occurs due to muscle contraction and will usually be a single-site abnormality (e.g. avulsion of fifth metatarsal base). Ligaments, on the other hand, have no contractile capacity and serve to stabilise joints. For a ligament to avulse a bone fragment there must have been a major distraction or angulation of the joint. This is therefore often associated with other injuries (see discussion of Segond fracture in the section 'The Knee'). A knowledge of major tendon and ligament attachments is essential for correct interpretation of these injuries. The more common examples of this will be described throughout the chapter.

Stress fractures occur when normal bone is subjected to repeated abnormal loading such that microfracturing occurs. Repetition of this loading over a period of time at a rate which exceeds the capacity of reparative processes results in progressive weakening of the bone to the point where a true fracture can occur at the site of stress. A lucent fracture line is, however, often not evident in the early stages of the process. A periosteal reaction and medullary sclerosis may develop at the site of stress and may be the only abnormality on the radiographs. If abnormal loading is continued, a frank fracture will eventually occur. (See examples in the sections 'The Ankle' and 'Foot Injuries'.)

A pathological fracture occurs through an area of abnormally weak bone. The term is usually reserved for fractures occurring at the site of bone involvement by tumour. This may be either primary benign or malignant lesions or secondary malignant deposits. Most commonly pathological fractures occur through the site of a metastatic deposit, including myeloma. Pathological fractures can also occur in weak bone, resulting from osteporosis or metabolic bone disease; these fractures are sometimes referred to as insufficiency fractures.

Dislocation refers to the situation at a joint where the articular surfaces have lost all contact. They may be associated with fractures in addition. Subluxation occurs when the joint surfaces are no longer fully congruous but some articular surface contact is maintained.

THE SHOULDER

The shoulder consists of two separate joints: the glenohumeral and the acromio-clavicular (AC) joint. It is essential that both are carefully evaluated in every patient.

Standard views of the shoulder include an AP radiograph in all cases. A second view is essential but as none are ideal there are local variations. There are three possible additional views: axial, axial oblique and lateral. The authors favour the axial oblique as the patient does not have to move the injured shoulder and it is relatively easy to interpret. Its weakness is that it does not provide a second view of the scapula. A true lateral view can be obtained if a scapular fracture is suspected clinically.

On the AP view it is important to appreciate that the humeral head is an asymmetric structure with more bone

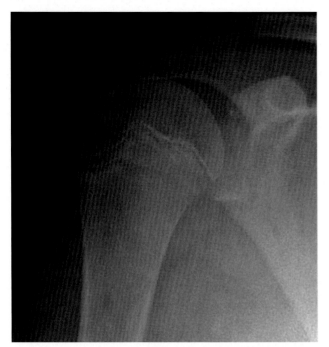

FIGURE 8-3 ■ **Anterior dislocation with a large bone fragment which has been sheared off from the posterior aspect of the humeral head.**

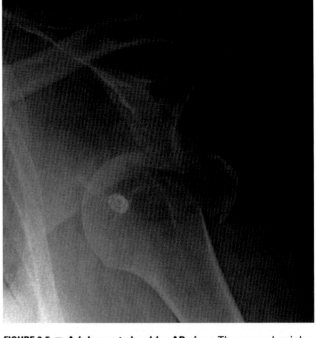

FIGURE 8-5 ■ **Adolescent shoulder AP view.** The normal epiphyseal plate should not be confused with a fracture. The growth plate lies in an oblique plane with the posterior aspect projected inferior to the anterior aspect.

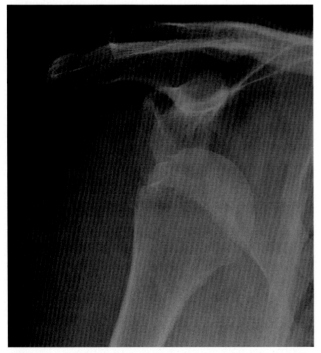

FIGURE 8-4 ■ **Anterior dislocation.** There is loss of the normal joint congruity. The humeral head lies under the coronoid process.

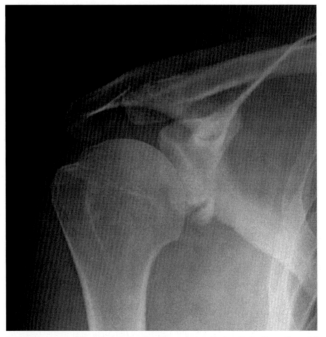

FIGURE 8-6 ■ **AP view showing fracture of the inferior glenoid margin known as a Bankart lesion.**

lying medial than laterally. The humeral head should be congruent with the glenoid fossa. In the adolescent shoulder the appearance of the unfused epiphysis should not be mistaken for a fracture (Fig. 8-3).

Anterior dislocation is common, accounting for 95% of all dislocations[1] and diagnosis is usually obvious (Fig. 8-4). The humeral head is no longer congruous with the glenoid and is displaced lying in a subcoracoid position.

Anterior dislocations are often associated with fractures, of which there are three types:

1. A fracture of the greater tuberosity sheared off or avulsed as the humerus dislocates (15%) (Fig. 8-5).
2. Fracture of the anteroinferior corner of the glenoid (8%) known as a Bankart lesion (Fig. 8-6). These fractures may be subtle and CT can be used in such cases to clarify the site and extent of the fracture.

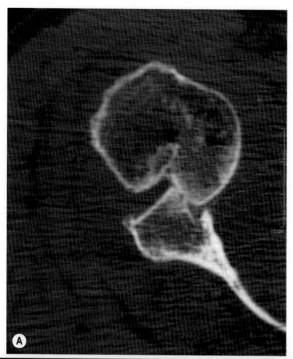

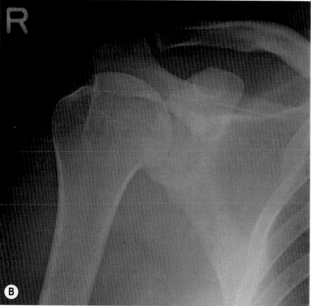

FIGURE 8-7 ■ (A) Anterior dislocation with axial oblique view on CT scan shows the effect of impaction of the glenoid on the humeral head, resulting in a V-shaped bony defect in the humeral head referred to as a Hill–Sachs lesion. (B) The humeral head is now back in joint. Note the defect in the superior contour and the vertical sclerotic line of impacted bone.

3. A V-shaped deformity of the humeral head caused by the impaction of the anterior glenoid rim on the posterosuperior humeral head. This is known as a Hill–Sachs lesion.[2] Once the humeral head is relocated, the signs of a Hill–Sachs lesion are a notch in the superolateral humeral head and a sclerotic vertical line of impacted bone (Fig. 8-7).

Careful search should be made for these fractures in all cases of anterior dislocation.

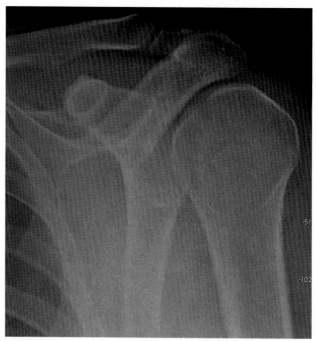

FIGURE 8-8 ■ **Posterior dislocation.** The humeral head has a round symmetrical appearance likened to a light bulb. Posterior dislocation should be suspected but can only be confirmed on the second view.

Posterior dislocation is rare[1] (<5%). The congruity of the humeral head with the glenoid often appears to be maintained on the AP view. The key observation on the AP view is that the normal asymmetrical appearance of the head is replaced by a much more spherical symmetrical appearance referred to as the 'light bulb' sign. Careful scrutiny of the second view is needed to confirm the loss of contact between the humeral head and the glenoid (Fig. 8-8). In many instances the humeral head appears symmetrical but is not dislocated. This is due to the arm being held in internal rotation such as when the arm is in a sling. Thus the second view must be used to determine whether the humeral head is in joint.

Fractures of the humeral head and proximal shaft typically occur following a fall on the outstretched arm. The humeral head is driven into the hard cortical bone of the glenoid. This results in several fracture patterns. Fractures may involve the surgical neck and the greater and lesser tuberosities. This can result in up to four major bone fragments. Comminuted fractures of the humeral head have been classified by Neer depending on the number of major fracture fragments from 1 to 4.[3] In this classification, to qualify as separate bone fragments they must be displaced by 1 cm or angled at 45° or more to the adjacent bone. Based on the above, a multiple part fracture of the humeral head which is undisplaced is classified as a Neer '1 part' fracture. This pattern accounts for the great majority (85%) of such fractures which if they are minimally displaced are not considered as separate fragments. Two-, three- and four-part fractures are seen with fractures involving, respectively, the greater and lesser tuberosities in addition to the surgical neck. Any combination of injuries may occur. Isolated fractures of greater or lesser tuberosity are most often avulsion injuries due, respectively, to the pull of supraspinatous and subscapularis muscles and are comparatively rare outside of the setting of dislocation described above.

Transverse fractures of the humerus involve either the surgical neck or the shaft inferior to this. Medial displacement of the humeral shaft occurs due to pull of pectoralis major muscle.

THE ACROMIO-CLAVICULAR JOINT

Clavicle fractures are very common; as the bone is just under the skin surface, they are easy to detect clinically. Fractures most often involve the middle third (80%). Outer-third fractures occur in 15% of cases. Medial-third fractures are uncommon, accounting for only 5% of cases.[4] The AC joint is held in place by the acromio-clavicular ligament and the two coraco-clavicular (CC) components known as conoid and trapezoid ligaments. Minor disruptions are best detected by looking at the inferior cortex of both the clavicle and the acromion. These should align. If they do not, then there is an AC joint subluxation. The normal distance between the superior surface of the coracoid and the inferior clavicle is no more than 13 mm.

Disruptions are graded from 1 to 3.[5] Grade 1 is sprain of the ligaments only. There is only minor separation, if any, at the AC joint. In grade 2 injuries the AC joint ligaments are torn but the CC ligaments are intact. In a grade 3 the CC ligaments are disrupted. As a result the coraco-clavicular distance may exceed 13 mm (Fig. 8-9). Surgical stabilisation will be required. Detecting the difference between a grade 2 and grade 3 injury may be facilitated if the affected limb is made to weight bear using weights strapped to the wrist to distract the AC joint. More recently direct visualisation of the ligaments by MRI has been suggested.[6]

THE ELBOW

There are no variations in the standard views of the elbow which are the AP and lateral.

A useful soft-tissue sign in the elbow is the fat pad sign.[7] The normal elbow has small pads of fat closely applied to the distal humerus both anteriorly and posteriorly. These are not normally visible as they lie within the bony fossae of the distal humerus. However, if there is a joint effusion such as may occur following trauma the fluid displaces the fat pads away from the humerus and out of the fossae. These fat pads can then be identified on a lateral radiograph as lucent areas. The anterior fat pad may just be visible normally but if displaced away from the humerus is abnormal. A visible posterior fat pad is always abnormal. The presence of displaced fat pads indicates an effusion[8] and if a fracture is not readily identified further careful inspection of the radiograph is needed to exclude a more subtle fracture which may have been overlooked (Fig. 8-10). In children, a supracondylar fracture is the commonest lesion to be overlooked; in adults, a radial head fracture. Note, however, that the

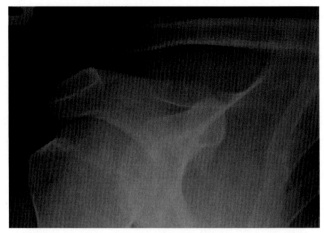

FIGURE 8-9 ■ Grade 3 injury. Distance from coracoid to clavicle is in excess of 13 mm. The coraco-clavicular ligaments will be disrupted and surgical fixation is needed.

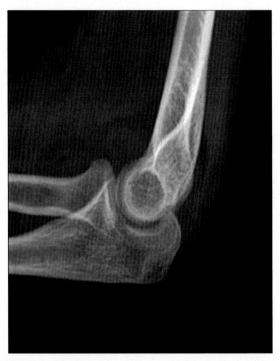

FIGURE 8-10 ■ **Displaced fat pads are visible both anterior and posterior to the humerus.** This indicates that there is a joint effusion. Careful scrutiny of the radiograph is now essential to look for a subtle injury.

absence of the fat pad sign does not exclude a fracture and effusions are not always caused by trauma.

Children

Supracondylar fractures are the commonest injury around the elbow in children.[9] Some fractures are grossly displaced with the distal bone fragment displaced posteriorly. The anteriorly displaced humeral shaft often has sharp bone edges which puts the adjacent brachial artery as well as the median and ulnar nerves in jeopardy. However, in 50% they are subtle greenstick-type injuries

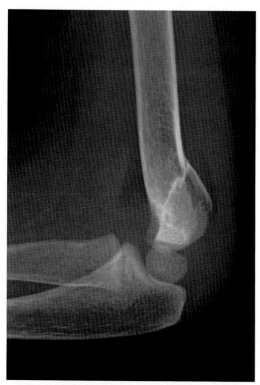

FIGURE 8-11 ■ **A subtle supracondylar fracture.** This is best identified using the anterior humeral line. A line along the anterior humeral cortex does not pass through the capitellum, which is displaced posterior to the line.

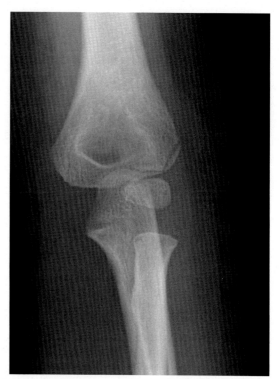

FIGURE 8-12 ■ **AP view of child's elbow.** A linear lucency is visible at the lateral epicondyle. This represents a fracture and should not be confused with a normal unfused epiphysis. The lateral epiphysis is the last to appear (CRITOL) and as only the capitellum is visible on the radiograph this cannot be the lateral epiphysis and must be a fracture.

(Fig. 8-11). Detection of subtle injuries can be facilitated by using the anterior humeral line.[10] On a lateral radiograph a line drawn down the anterior humeral cortex will pass through the capitellum such that at least one-third of the capitellum lies anterior to the line. If this rule is broken then it is very likely that there is a subtle greenstick or Salter–Harris growth plate injury of the distal humeral, allowing the distal humerus with the attached capitellum to be displaced posteriorly.[11]

The second commonest elbow injury in children is of the lateral condyle.[12] Recognition of these injuries is made difficult by the presence of developing ossification centres in the immature skeleton. There are four in the distal humerus and one each in the radius and ulna. The order of appearance with few exceptions is capitellum, radius, internal epicondyle, trochlea, olecranon, lateral epicondyle—remembered by the mnemonic CRITOL[13] from the first letter of each epiphysis. Knowedge of this order makes it possible to determine whether a bone fragment adjacent to the humerus is a normal ossification centre or represents a fracture. As the lateral epicondyle is the last ossification centre to appear, then if there is a bone fragment adjacent to the lateral aspect of the distal humerus look for the other ossification centres. If it is not possible to identify the five other centres, then the area in question must represent a fracture (Fig. 8-12). It should be noted that although there may only be a small bony component to this injury there will be a large fracture through the growing cartilaginous distal humerus.[14]

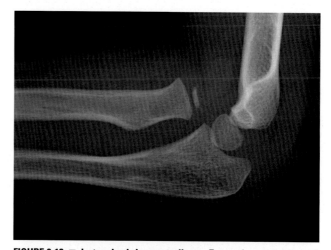

FIGURE 8-13 ■ **Lateral adolescent elbow.** Fat pads are evident. A line drawn along the proximal radius mid shaft does not pass through the capitellum. The radial head must be dislocated.

Dislocation of the radial head occurs in both children and adults. It may be difficult to appreciate on the AP radiograph but easier on the lateral. A helpful method of detecting these injuries is use of the radio-capitellar line. This line is drawn along the mid shaft of the radius proximal to the tuberosity. It should pass through the capitellum on every view; if not, the radial head is dislocated (Fig. 8-13). This rule is true also in children, although

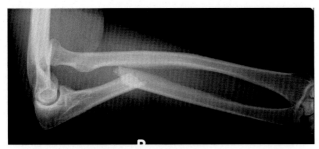

FIGURE 8-14 ■ **Radiograph of forearm.** There is an obvious fracture of the mid shaft of the ulna with angulation. When this is present there must be an abnormality of the radius. If no fracture is evident, a dislocation of the radial head is almost invariably present, as is the case here. This combination is known as a Monteggia fracture dislocation.

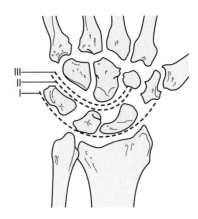

FIGURE 8-15 ■ **The carpal arcs.**

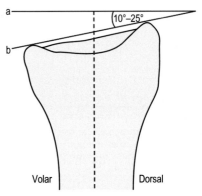

FIGURE 8-16 ■ **The normal volar angulation of the distal radius.**

care is needed in the very young when the capitellum is small.[15] There is a fracture association which must be recognised. The bones of the forearm are bound strongly at either end by strong ligaments. It is difficult to fracture one of these bones without the other, so fractures of radius and ulna occur commonly together. However, if only one bone appears fractured and, especially if the fracture is angled or overlapped, a covert injury of the other bone is very likely. This typically takes the form of a dislocation of the non-fractured bone. Thus a fracture of the ulnar shaft is often associated with a dislocation of the radial head at the elbow. This is known as a Monteggia fracture dislocation[16,17] (Fig. 8-14). Conversely a radial shaft fracture is associated with a dislocation of the ulna at the wrist. This is known as a Galeazzi fracture dislocation.

Adults

Fractures of the distal humerus in adults rarely cause diagnostic problems. Most fractures are readily apparent. Typically they involve the distal humeral condyles often with inta-articular extension into the elbow joint. Capitellar fractures are uncommon and may be difficult to see on the AP radiograph. The lateral view, however, provides the diagnosis. The displaced capitellum has an appearance like a half moon and is seen lying anterosuperior to the forearm bones. Radial head fractures[18] may involve the radial neck only or may be intra-articular, with disruption of the radial articular surface. The fat pad sign described above is useful in drawing attention to the radial head as a possible site for subtle radial head fracture. The commonest ulnar fracture is of the olecranon.[19] The fracture involves the articular surface with the proximal fracture fragment often displaced due to the unopposed pull of the triceps muscle.

THE WRIST

Standard views for evaluation of the wrist are a postero-antererior (PA) and lateral radiographs. Additional views are required when there is clinical suspicion of a scaphoid fracture.

On an AP radiograph look for the normal uniform spacing of 1–2 mm around each carpal bone and at the carpometacarpal junction. Loss of this spacing should lead to very careful inspection of the abnormal area, as often this will indicate significant carpal or carpometacarpal disruption. One should also observe the arrangement of the carpal bones into three smooth arcs. The first delineates the proximal surface of the proximal row of carpal bones (scaphoid, lunate, triquetral). The second is formed by the distal articular surface of the same bones. The third is along the proximal curvature of the capitate and hamate.[20] These arcs should normally be smooth with no steps or interruption (Fig. 8-15).

On a lateral radiograph the normal distal radius has a volar tilt of approx 10°. This represents the angle between a line drawn along the long axis of the radius and a line drawn from the dorsal to the volar rim of the radius and has a normal range of 2–20° (Fig. 8-16). Alteration of this angle occurs when there is a subtle fracture of the distal radius. Normal relationship of the distal radius and carpal bones is best assessed on the lateral view and this is discussed further in the section on carpal injuries. Displacement of the distal radial epiphysis and disruption of carpal alignment are often only evident on this view. Fractures of the triquetral will usually only be seen on the lateral radiograph. From the above it can be seen that the lateral radiograph is of critical importance in assessing wrist injuries.

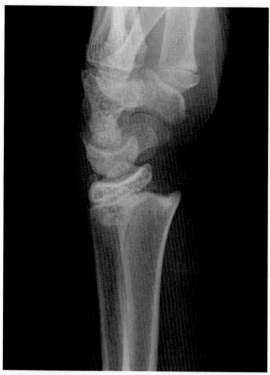

FIGURE 8-17 ■ Displacement of the distal radial epiphysis with a small fragment from the metaphysis. This is a Salter–Harris type 2 fracture.

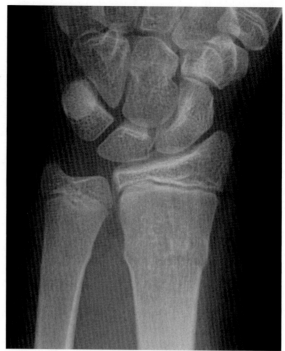

FIGURE 8-18 ■ A buckling of the radial cortex, which indicates a torus injury.

Radius and Ulna

Most commonly, injuries result from a fall on the outstretched wrist. The type of injury sustained is age related.

Children

In young children fractures of the radius proximal to the epiphyseal plate predominate in age group 6–10. These fractures often involve both radius and ulna and may be grossly displaced. After this, until epiphyseal fusion, injuries most commonly involve the epiphyseal plate and are thus Salter–Harris fractures.[9] Typically there is dorsal displacement of the epiphysis with or without an associated fracture fragment from the adjacent metaphysis, resulting in either a Salter–Harris type 1 or 2 injury (Fig. 8-17). Greenstick and buckle or torus fractures of the radius occur only in children (Fig. 8-18).

Adults

Distal radial fracture (Fig. 8-19) is the commonest wrist injury in patients over age of 40.[21] Increasing frequency with age suggests a relationship to osteoporosis. The definition of a Colles' fracture includes the following: (1) fracture of radius within 2 cm of distal radial articular surface but not involving it; (2) dorsal angulation or displacement of distal fragment; and (3) associated fracture of ulnar styloid process. Smith described a variation of the above where the distal radial fragment is displaced and angled volarly and medially. In both of these injuries the articular surface remains intact (Fig. 8-20).

Barton's fracture differs from the above due to involvement of the articular surface of the radius. It is a shearing injury through the articular surface. The term is now often incorrectly ascribed to any intra-articular fracture.

Subtle radial fractures may be detected by observing a minor disruption of the dorsal radius cortex on the lateral radiograph and alteration in the radial angle from the usual 10° volar (Fig. 8-21).

Isolated fracture of the radial styloid process, also known as Hutchinson's or chauffeur's fracture, refers to an intra-articular fracture which runs obliquely across the distal radius from the radial cortex into the joint separating the radial styloid from the parent bone.

Many fractures do not conform exactly with the original descriptions, with combination injuries common. For this reason, rather than using the eponymous names it is better to give a full description of the fracture lines, fragment displacement and angulation and extent of articular involvement.

Carpal Injuries

The scaphoid accounts for at least 60% of all carpal fractures.[21] Typically, when scaphoid injury is suspected, one or two additional radiographic projections are employed with the intention of elongating the scaphoid, projecting it clear of other carpal bones and allowing the X-ray beam to pass through the scaphoid perpendicular

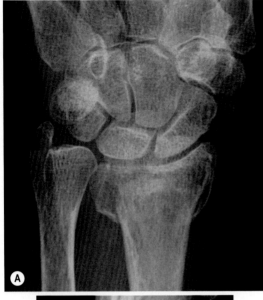

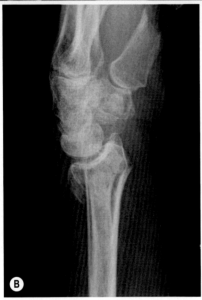

FIGURE 8-19 ■ **(A, B) A fracture of the distal radius, which on the lateral is displaced dorsally.** There is an associated fracture of the ulnar styloid. There is no intra-articular involvement. This is a Colles' fracture.

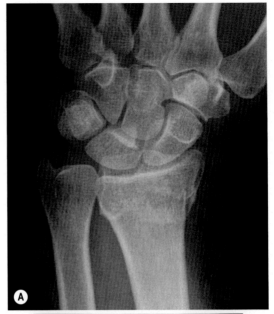

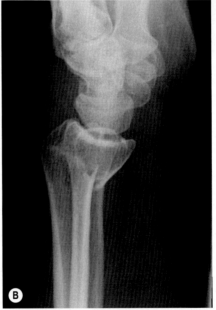

FIGURE 8-20 ■ **(A, B) Distal radial fracture with volar displacement and no intra-articular involvement.** This is a Smith's type fracture. The appearances on the AP view are virtually identical to a Colles' fracture.

to its long axis. The projections used vary but in the authors' department a second PA view with ulnar deviation plus one with the tube angled at 45° toward the elbow is obtained.

The blood supply of the scaphoid is unusual, with arteries entering distally then passing proximally to supply the rest of the scaphoid. When a fracture occurs through the waist (middle third) of the scaphoid, which is the commonest site (80% of cases), the blood supply to the proximal pole is interrupted. This results in significant risk of avascular necrosis of the proximal pole or non-union of the fracture (Fig. 8-22).

Contrary to common belief, the great majority of fractures are visible on initial radiographs.[22] Nevertheless there are a small number not identified. Accordingly, because of the risk of avascular necrosis and non-union, the patient is managed as if a fracture is present and the wrist is immobilised. The patient is then reviewed at about 10 days when further radiographs are obtained[23,24] in the belief that resorption will occur around a fracture site rendering it visible on delayed radiographs, although this is now questioned. Alternative imaging techniques are now increasingly utilised. Skeletal scintigraphy is sensitive but non-specific. MRI is now the investigation of choice and there is good evidence that this should be undertaken soon after the initial injury[25] (Fig. 8-23).

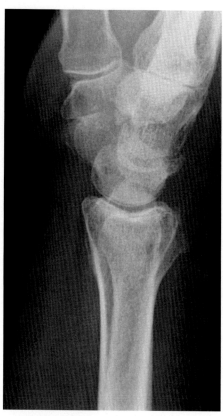

FIGURE 8-21 ■ Subtle radial fracture. There is subtle disruption of the posterior radial cortex, indicating an impacted radial fracture. The normal volar tilt of the distal radius is lost.

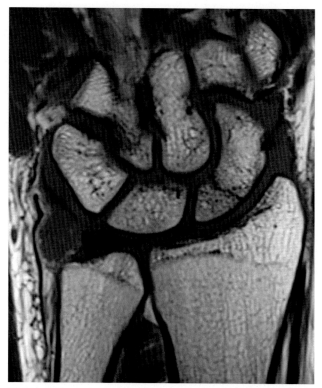

FIGURE 8-23 ■ MRI of wrist. There is a fracture through the proximal pole of the scaphoid. No fracture was visible on plain radiographs.

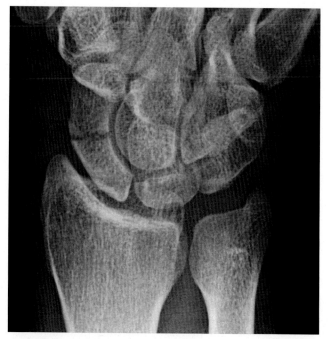

FIGURE 8-22 ■ Scaphoid fracture. There is a fracture through the waist of the scaphoid. This is highly likely to interrupt the blood supply to the proximal pole.

TABLE 8-1   Relative Incidence of Carpal Bone Fractures

Scaphoid	68.2%
Triquetrum	18.3%
Trapezium	4.3%
Lunate	3.9%
Capitate	1.9%
Hamate	1.7%
Pisiform	1.3%
Trapezoid	0.4%

After the scaphoid the triquetral is the most commonly injured carpal bone, accounting for 18–20% of injuries[26] (Table 8-1). Typically the fracture is not evident on the PA view but can be seen on the lateral as a bone fragment seen on the dorsal aspect of the wrist (Fig. 8-24). Other carpal bone injuries are all relatively rare, each of the other carpal bone accounting for only 2–3% of injuries. CT or MR has a useful role to play in these injuries, which are often difficult to detect on plain radiography.

Most carpal fractures and dislocations are caused by falling on the outstretched wrist with the wrist forced into an hyperextended position. Carpal dislocations most commonly involve the lunate.[27] On a PA radiograph the lunate normally has a trapezoid appearance. When it is dislocated, it assumes a triangular shape. There is disruption of the normal carpal arcs and the intercarpal

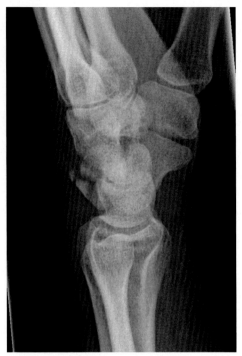

FIGURE 8-24 ■ **Small bone fragments are visible on the dorsum of the wrist.** These indicate a triquetral fracture; there was no abnormality on the AP view.

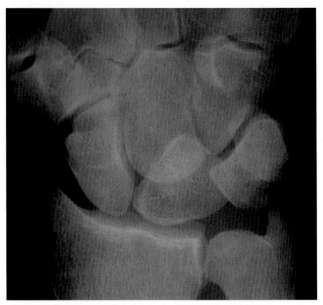

FIGURE 8-25 ■ The lunate has a triangular shape and there is disruption of the carpal arcs with loss of the normal intercarpal spaces.

spaces are lost (Fig. 8-25). It is on the lateral radiograph, however, where the diagnosis is most easily made.[28] On a normal lateral view of the wrist a vertical line drawn through the centre of the lunate should inferiorly pass through the radial articular surface and superiorly should pass through the centre of the capitate (Fig. 8-26). If this rule is broken, a carpal dislocation is certain (Fig. 8-27). Lunate dislocation is most commonly an isolated finding. The lunate will be seen displaced volar to the line. Perilunate dislocation is more common and is often associated with other carpal injuries, most commonly a fracture of the scaphoid. In this injury the lunate remains aligned with the radius but the capitate and the rest of the distal carpal row are displaced in a volar direction (Fig. 8-28).

Scapholunate disassociation is also known as rotatory subluxation of the scaphoid.[29] It is a ligamentous injury occurring with forced wrist extension. On plain radiographs the injury can be identified by noting a widening of the intercarpal distance between scaphoid and lunate; the normal gap is < 2 mm; between 2 and 4 mm suggests possible scapholunate disruption; greater than 4 mm indicates disassociation (Fig. 8-29). This is the so-called 'Terry Thomas' sign named after a 1950s comic with a gap between his front teeth.

Injuries of the Metacarpals and Phalanges

Disruption of the carpometacarpal joint may occur in isolation or may be associated with fracture of either the proximal metacarpal or the adjacent carpal bone.[30] Metacarpal fractures when present aid identification of the

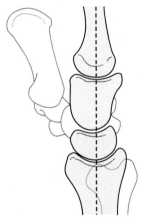

FIGURE 8-26 ■ **Normal alignment of radius, capitate and lunate as seen on a lateral radiograph.**

injury. These injuries can be detected by observation of the loss of the normal space between the distal carpal row and the base of the metacarpals (Fig. 8-30). Where there is suspicion on the standard radiograph series, a lateral of the hand may add further useful information. A common injury is that of fracture dislocation of the fifth metacarpal and this accounts for 50% of single ray dislocations in the hand.[31]

Transverse and spiral fractures of the metacarpals are common. A punch injury will typically result in a moderately angled fracture of the fifth metacarpal head. Intraarticular fractures of the base of the first metacarpal are known as a Bennett's fracture. The tendon of abductor pollicis longus attaches to the larger fragment, which will tend to displace the fracture unless it is treated with fixation (Fig. 8-31).

Most fractures of the metacarpal and phalanges are apparent on radiographs. There are three fracture types

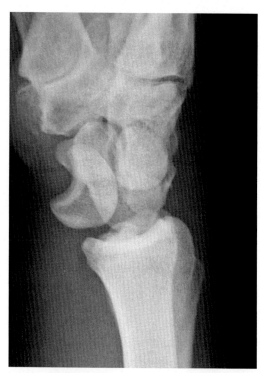

FIGURE 8-27 ■ **The lateral view of the carpal injury depicted in Fig. 8-25.** The lunate has been displaced volarly. The capitate no longer articulates with the lunate. The radius and capitate are in alignment. The lunate is rotated volarly. These are the features of a lunate dislocation.

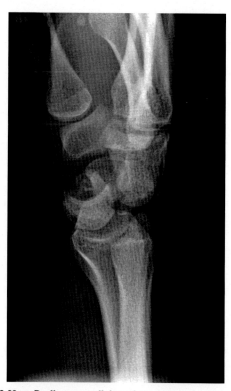

FIGURE 8-28 ■ **Perilunate dislocation.** Lateral view shows normal alignment of the radius and lunate but the capitate does not articulate with the lunate and lies dorsally. The AP view showed loss of carpal arcs and intercarpal spaces. There were also fractures of the waist of the scaphoid and triquetral. Perilunate dislocation is often associated with additional carpal fractures.

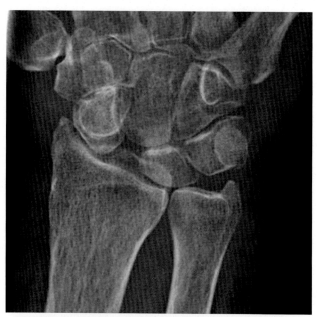

FIGURE 8-29 ■ **Widening of the gap between the lunate and the scaphoid, indicating ligament disruption.**

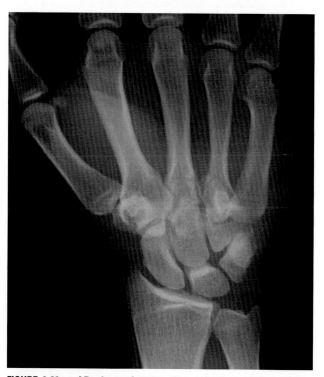

FIGURE 8-30 ■ **AP view of wrist.** There is loss of the normal spaces between the bases of the fourth and fifth metacarpals and the adjacent hamate. This indicates dislocation at the carpometacarpal junction.

worthy of particular consideration.[32] In all of these the severity and need for surgical intervention are related to the size of the fracture fragment and the extent of articular involvement.

Condylar fractures involve the articular surface of a phalanx, usually distally. These fractures will often require surgical intervention and all should be referred for specialist assessment.

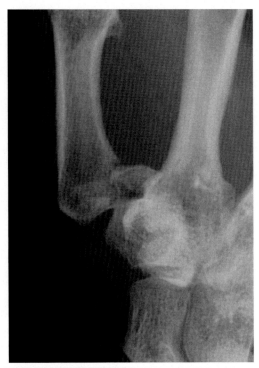

FIGURE 8-31 ■ **Bennett's fracture.** There is an intra-articular fracture of the base of the first metacarpal. The extensor pollicis longus tendon inserts onto the base of the main portion of the metacarpal and will distract and displace the fracture, rendering it unstable. Surgical fixation will be required.

Fractures at the proximal interphalageal joints on the volar aspect are due to avulsions by the volar plate, which is a fibrocartilaginous thickening of the joint capsule.

Articular fractures of the dorsal aspect of the distal phalanges involve the insertion of the extensor tendon, resulting in a mallet finger. A mallet finger deformity is very hard to produce by radiographic positioning alone and patients with a mallet deformity without a fracture frequently have extensor tendon disruption.

Many avulsion injuries of the ulnar collateral ligament of the thumb are soft-tissue ligament injuries only; however, in some cases the ligament avulses a bone fragment from the base of the proximal phalanx (Fig. 8-32). These fractures often occur in skiers, as the thumb is caught in the ski pole straps during a fall, causing hyperextension and twisting, and hence are sometimes referred to as skier's thumb.[33]

PELVIC AND ACETABULAR FRACTURES

Introduction

Fractures of the pelvic ring and acetabulum in young patients are predominantly high-energy injuries and frequently result in visceral injuries which contribute to the associated mortality and morbidity. Recognition of the patterns of pelvic ring injury informs the application of appropriate corrective forces and internal fixation in their treatment. The likelihood of life-threatening pelvic haemorrhage and bladder injury can also be surmised if the severity of the pelvic ring injury is appreciated.

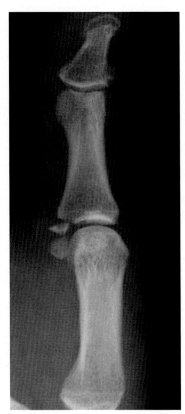

FIGURE 8-32 ■ **AP of thumb.** There is a bone fragment on the ulnar aspect of the base of the proximal phalanx. This indicates an avulsion injury at the insertion of the ulnar collateral ligament. Most of these injuries, however, are ligamentous only, with no bony involvement, and are diagnosed on clinical grounds or with MR.

Acetabular fractures have been classified by Judet and Letournel into five simple and complex types which require an awareness of acetabular anatomy and determine the surgical approach to reduction and fixation. Dependence on standard and oblique (Judet view) radiographs has recently been superseded by computed tomography (CT), with reconstructions that require a practical knowledge by the reporting radiologist. A number of CT features are important in separating fractures that require operative intervention from those that can be managed conservatively.

Avulsion injuries commonly occur in athletes, and affect the apophyseal regions in patients with an immature skeleton. Stress or repetitive injuries can also occur at the tendon insertions but are increasingly seen in the pelvic ring, acetabulum and sacrum as a result of increased sporting activity and more widespread diagnostic application of MRI. Older patients are also prone to pelvic ring injuries in the form of insufficiency fractures consequent upon underlying osteoporosis. This is particularly prevalent following pelvic irradiation.

Pelvic Ring Fractures

Anatomy

The pelvic ring constitutes the sacrum and the two innominate bones which are formed by the fusion of the ilium, ischium and pubic bones. The sacrum and innominate bones are stabilised by ligaments which are important to our understanding of pelvic injury as instability can occur in the absence of fracture as a result of ligamentous disruption. Posteriorly the sacroiliac joints are stabilised by the anterior and posterior sacroiliac ligaments, the latter being amongst the body's strongest ligaments. In the central pelvis the sacrospinous and sacroischial ligaments restrain external rotation of the innominate bones and anteriorly the superior symphyseal ligaments prevent diastasis of the symphysis. The weakest part of the pelvic ring is the anterior pelvis; hence, nearly all injuries disrupt the pubic rami or symphysis initially. Posterior pelvic disruption only occurs after the symphysis is disputed or the rami fractured.

Classification

Previous descriptions of pelvic injury have been eponymous (Malgaine fracture), encompassed presumed mechanism of injury (straddle fracture), or described the fracture appearance (open book), but these descriptions are not systematic and have been replaced with a classification borne out of the increased understanding of such injuries through the experience gained in American trauma centres.

Pennal first recognised the correlation between specific forces applied to the pelvis and patterns of fracture.[34] Subsequently, Tile in 1984 reported the increased risk of haemorrhage with the more severe injuries[35] and finally in 1986 Young and Burgess refined the classification by describing the progression of failure that occurs with particular forces.[36] They described three main patterns of fracture resulting from anterior-posterior compression (APC), lateral compression (LC) and vertical shear (VS) forces. A fourth group with hybrid appearances was described as complex (Fig. 8-33).

Anterior Compression Injuries. These injuries commonly occur during head-on collision when forces are applied in the AP plane. The least severe AP pattern of injury, the AP type 1 injury, comprises symphyseal diastasis (<2.5 cm) (Fig. 8-34) and vertical pubic rami fractures. The vertical pattern distinguishes the AP pattern from the oblique/communicated pattern in LC injuries. No significant ligament injury is encountered in AP type 1 injuries, because the pelvis is essentially stable.

AP type 2 injuries demonstrate progressive widening of the symphysis (>2.5 cm) or fracture lines consequent upon disruption of the sacroiliac, sacrotuberous and anterior sacroiliac ligaments. The posterior sacroiliac ligaments are intact. This pattern was previously referred to as the 'open-book' injury, and is unstable to external rotation forces but stable to internal rotation (Fig. 8-35).

AP type 3 injuries include additional posterior sacroiliac ligament disruption, and are unstable to forces in all directions (Fig. 8-36).

The AP type 2 injuries require a symphyseal plate to restore stability while the AP type 3 injuries require anterior and posterior stabilisation.

Lateral Compression (LC) Injury. This is the commonest pattern of injury, accounting for 57% of pelvic

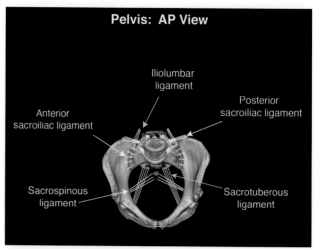

FIGURE 8-33 ■ Diagramatic representation of the pelvic ring, identifying the primary pelvic ligaments.

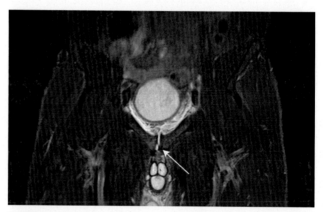

FIGURE 8-34 ■ AP type 1 pelvic ring injury, demonstrating symphyseal diastasis (arrow) and disruption of the symphyseal ligaments.

ring fractures. There are three types, LC type 1 injuries being the least severe and comprising characteristic oblique or comminuted pubic rami fractures (Fig. 8-37A) or less commonly symphyseal disruption and overlap. Such fractures are usually stable even if associated with minor compression fractures of the anterior rim of the sacroiliac joint.

LC type 2 injuries result from increased force; after the anterior pelvis fails, the innominate bone internally rotates, pivoting on the anterior margin of the sacroiliac joint, disrupting the posterior sacroiliac ligament (LC type 2a) or fracture the iliac blade (LC type 2b). These injuries are unstable to internal rotation forces.

The most severe form of lateral compression injury is the LC type 3 pattern often referred to as the 'roll-over' injury. The side of impact demonstrates the type 2 pattern but the contralateral hemipelvis is externally rotated in the pattern about to be described for AP injuries (Fig. 8-37B).

Vertical Shear. These injuries result from jumping or a fall from a height where the impact is predominantly

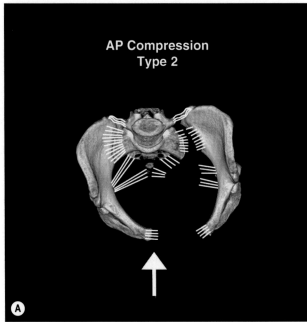

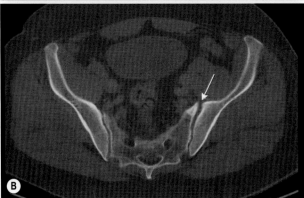

FIGURE 8-35 ■ (A) An AP type 2 pelvic ring injury. Note the disruption of the anterior sacroiliac, sacrospinous and sacrotuberous ligaments. (B) A type 2 pelvic ring injury on axial CT shows a widened anterior joint space in the left sacroiliac joint (arrow); this injury was formerly referred to as an 'open-book' injury.

unilateral. Unlike the AP and LC injuries, the vertical shear injury is of one type, consisting of complete ligamentous disruption, and is associated with multidirectional instability. The pubic rami fractures are vertical, similar to those seen in the AP injuries but the vertical shear injuries demonstrate cephalad displacement on the side of impact (Fig. 8-38).

Complex Injuries. These are uncommon and the majority demonstrate a predominant LC pattern.

Acetabular Fractures

Cross-sectional imaging of acetabular fractures with CT is now standard practice and specialised radiographic views are increasingly an investigation of the past. A good understanding of the three-dimensional anatomy is required to accurately describe and classify these injuries.

Anatomy

The acetabulum comprises a central articular portion which has a cotyloid configuration supported by the arms of an inverted 'Y' created by the anterior and posterior columns. The articular surface has anterior and posterior walls which are identifiable on AP views. The anterior column extends from the superior pubic ramus upward into the iliac blade (Fig. 8-39A), whereas the posterior column is much shorter, running upward from the ischial tuberosity (Fig. 8-39B). The iliopectineal and ilioischial lines define the anterior and posterior columns. The cotyloid articular surface and both columns are connected to the axial skeleton by the sciatic strut or buttress.

Classification

The current classification internationally adopted has an anatomical basis which influences the requirement and

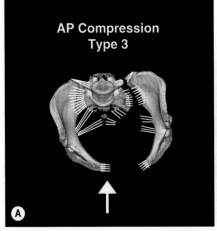

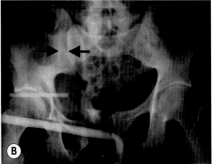

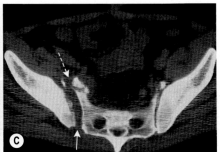

FIGURE 8-36 ■ **AP type 3 pelvic ring injury.** (A) The associated ligamentous disruption: note the disrupted posterior sacroiliac ligament. (B) A widened right sacroiliac joint (arrows): this could represent either an AP type 2 or type 3 based on radiographic appearances; however, the CT in (C) confirms a type 3 injury through the disrupted anterior aspect of the sacroiliac joint (broken arrow) and widened posterior element of the sacroiliac joint resulting from posterior ligament disruption (arrow).

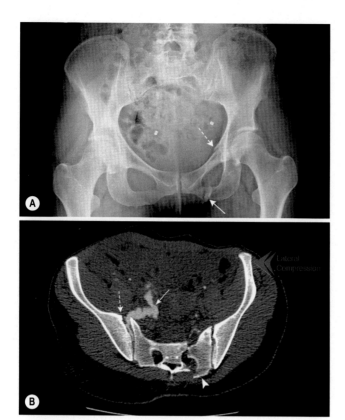

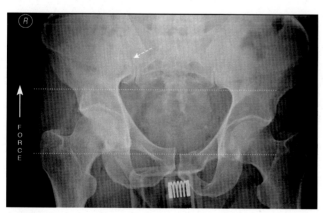

FIGURE 8-37 ■ **Lateral compression injuries.** (A) An LC type 1 injury: the superior pubic ramus fracture has an oblique orientation (broken arrow) and the inferior ramus is a segmental fracture pattern (arrow); no posterior pelvic fractures are evident. (B) A LC type 3 (rollover) injury, lateral compression and internal rotation on the left (arrowhead) and AP type 2 pattern on the right side (broken arrow). Compression fracture of the left sacral ala and active haemorrhage is also demonstrated on this enhanced CT (arrow).

FIGURE 8-38 ■ **Vertical shear injury.** Impact is sustained on the right side, the symphysis and right sacroiliac joint (broken arrow) are disrupted and the right hemipelvis is displaced cephalad.

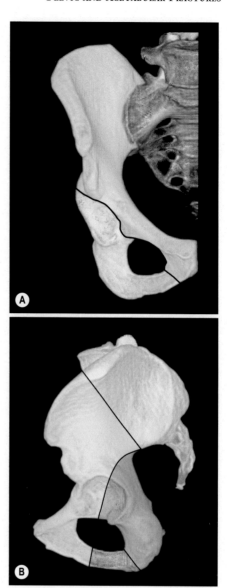

FIGURE 8-39 ■ **Acetabular anatomy.** (A) The anterior (blue) and posterior (yellow) columns coloured on a surface-rendered CT. (B) The columnar anatomy on a surface-rendered lateral projection, anterior column (blue) and posterior column (pink).

anterior column, posterior column and transverse fractures (Fig. 8-40). Complex patterns represent combinations of the elementary patterns. Common complex injuries include bicolumn, T-shaped and column injuries associated with posterior wall fractures.

Elemetary Patterns

Anterior Wall Fractures. A rare injury is often incorrectly reported when fractures involve the lateral aspect of the superior pubic ramus. These injuries in isolation are rarely displaced, do not involve a major load-bearing surface and are usually managed conservatively.

Posterior Wall Fractures. Posterior wall fractures are amongst the commonest types of acetabular injury and are commonly sustained during head-on collisions when

approach to surgical repair. The system of classification was first devised in 1964 by Judet[37] and later refined by his colleague Letournel.[38] Five basic or elementary patterns account for the majority of fractures in this classification and comprise, anterior wall, posterior wall,

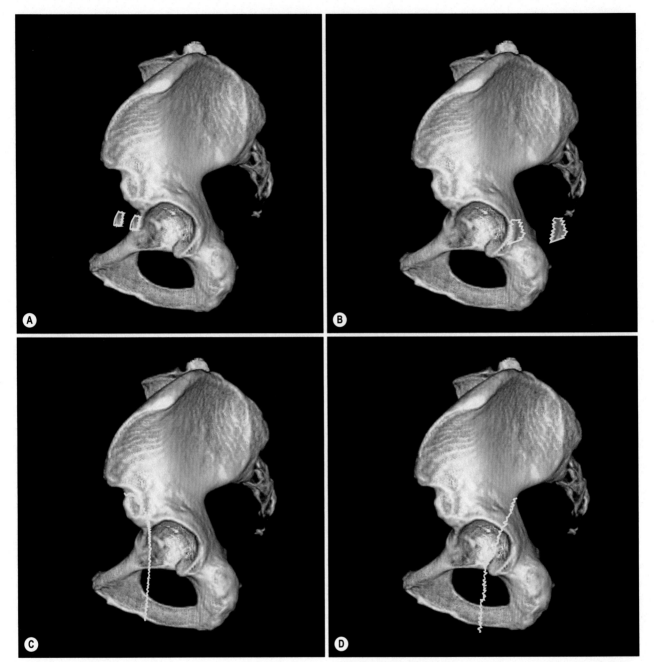

FIGURE 8-40 ■ **Elementary patterns of acetabular fractures, Judet and Letournel classification.** (A) Anterior wall fracture. (B) Posterior wall fracture. (C) Anterior column injury. (D) Posterior wall fracture.

the force along the femur in a seated individual is directed through the posterior wall, which fractures and the femoral head occasionally dislocates. The posterior wall fracture can be appreciated on the AP view but CT defines its size and displacement with or without impaction, which influences the need to reduce and fix the posterior wall (Fig. 8-41). Fractures accounting for more than 40% of the posterior wall depth will require internal fixation, as will impacted fragments.

Anterior and Posterior Column Fractures. Column fractures have a coronal fracture plane which cleaves the

acetabulum into anterior and posterior segments. Both extend through the obturator ring, a prerequisite for a column injury (Fig. 8-42). The anterior column extends anteriorly cephalad to the acetabulum, disrupting the iliopectineal line, whereas the posterior column injury extends posteriorly, disrupting the ilioischial line.

Transverse Fractures. Transverse fractures run across the acetabulum, splitting it into upper and lower halves. The ilioischial and iliopectineal lines are disrupted, but the obturator ring is intact (excluding a column injury; Fig. 8-43).

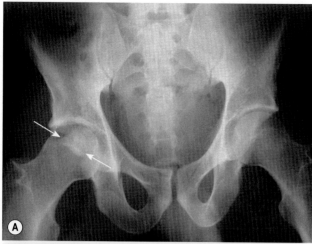

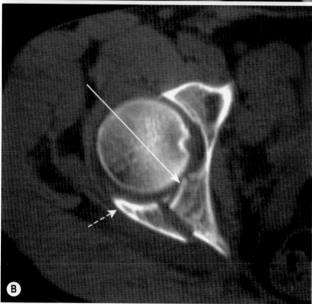

FIGURE 8-41 ■ (A) A posterior wall fracture (arrows). (B) CT of a large posterior wall fracture (broken arrow) (>40%) requiring surgical fixation with an associated impaction fracture (arrow).

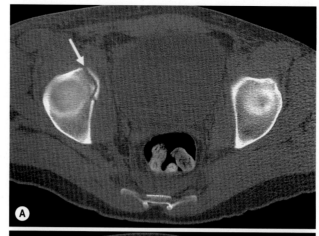

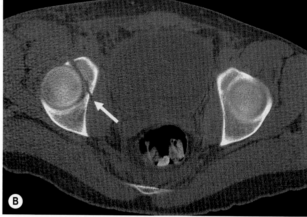

FIGURE 8-42 ■ (A, B) Sequential CT images demonstrating an anterior column fracture, extending from anterosuperior downward, splitting the acetabulum into anterior and posterior segments which then extend down through the rami and thus involve the obturator foramen.

Complex Fractures. The T-shaped and bicolumn are distinguished by the continuity between the acetabular roof and sciatic strut in T-shaped injuries, whereas the bicolumn injuries have no continuity between these structures; the spur sign refers to the disrupted sciatic strut.

Avulsion Injuries

The immature skeleton and unfused apophyses are particularly prone to injury and avulsion. The commonest sites are the anterosuperior iliac spine (sartorius origin), anteroinferior iliac spine (rectus femoris origin) and the ischial tuberosity (hamstring origin; Fig. 8-44).

These injuries may be identified on plain radiographs if a thin sliver of bone is avulsed with the apophysis through the line of provisional calcification. Alternatively, ultrasound or MRI may be requested if the plain radiographs are negative and functional disability is

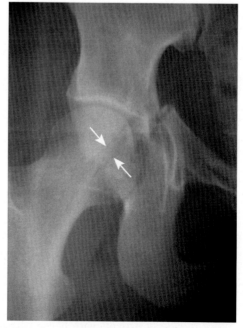

FIGURE 8-43 ■ A transverse acetabular fracture (arrows) splitting the acetabulum into upper and lower halves.

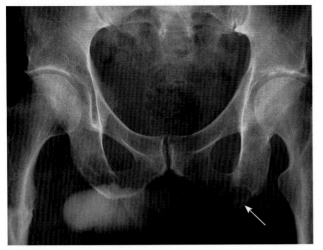

FIGURE 8-44 ■ Hamstring avulsion of the left ischial tuberosity in an adolescent sportsman (arrow).

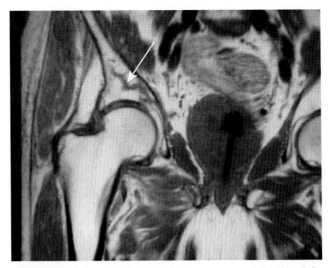

FIGURE 8-45 ■ Incomplete stress fracture (arrow) in the right acetabulum on a T1 spin-echo image, in a 20-year-old Royal Marine.

significant. Surgical repair will be considered for hamstring avulsions.

Insufficiency and Stress Fractures

Stress fractures are sustained through excessive loading, usually but not exclusively during athletic training. The vogue for distance running in particular has precipitated an increase in lower limb stress injuries, including the pelvis. Plain radiographs are usually normal and in these circumstances MRI is the preferred investigation. Stress injuries are usually associated with marrow oedema; this may have a linear orientation and occur anywhere in the pelvic ring (Fig. 8-45). The posterior column of the acetabulum and the sacrum are favoured sites due to their relatively high loading. Sacral fractures or stress reactions often parallel the sacroiliac joint. The fracture line may be identifiable but is often obscured on STIR or fat-saturated sequences and is best demonstrated on T1-SE.

CT, although good at identifying overt fractures, is less capable of identifying stress reactions without a fracture line and does not adequately assess other potential differential diagnoses relating to soft-tissue injury. Nuclear medicine is sensitive at identifying stress injuries but unless the findings are bilateral and symmetric its findings are usually non-specific.

Insufficiency fractures occur when normal loads are applied to a structurally deficient pelvic ring; these fractures are frequently multiple and characteristically are bilateral and relatively symmetric on MRI. This most commonly occurs due to osteoporosis, but other metabolic disorders predisposing to fracture include osteomalacia and parathyroid-related bone disease. Blomlie et al. have also identified insufficiency fractures as occurring in up to 79% of patients receiving radiation therapy for gynaecological malignancy, within 2 years of treatment.[39] The MRI features either resolved or improved within the duration of the study (30 months). MRI is the investigation of choice in elderly patients with pelvic pain where insufficiency fractures are suspected.

Pathological Fractures

Pathological fractures in the pelvis are not uncommon and are most frequently associated with metastatic tumour and myeloma but are also encountered with other disorders, including osteopetrosis and Paget's disease (Fig. 8-46). The diagnosis in metastatic malignancy can be supported by the confirmation of areas of other increased isotope uptake on skeletal scintigraphy. Other processes are also recognised to cause pathological fractures, including osteopetrosis and Paget's disease. Osteolysis associated with fracture can also be encountered in elderly patients following injury to the pubic rami. This process of post-traumatic osteolysis is similar to that recognised in the lateral end of the clavical following injury; it is considered that the absence of load-bearing stress at these sites is a contributory factor. The finding of fractures of the inferior and superior pubic rami is rarely caused by malignancy, helping distinguish tumour from insufficiency fractures. In post-traumatic osteolysis the margins of the fracture appear smooth and well corticated and no bony destruction is seen in the remainder of the pubic ring.

THE HIP

Fracture of the hip is one of the commonest injuries, particularly in elderly patients with osteoporosis. It is the commonest reason for admission to an orthopaedic ward.[40]

The standard view is AP of the pelvis and a lateral of the painful hip. The pelvic radiograph allows comparison of the injured hip with the uninjured side. As these patients will generally be in pain, the lateral radiograph is obtained using the so-called groin lateral projection. This is obtained with a horizontal beam with 20° cephalic angulation centred on the greater trochanter. The opposite thigh is flexed. This does not require any movement by the patient of the painful injured side.

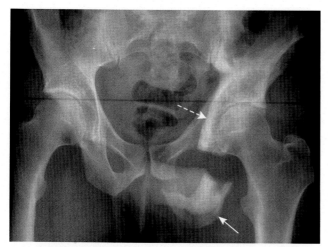

FIGURE 8-46 ■ Pathological fracture through pagetoid left ischial bone (arrow).

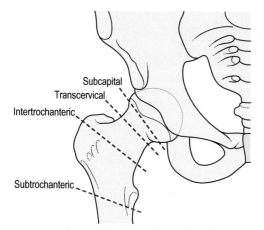

FIGURE 8-47 ■ The sites of proximal femoral fractures.

Subcapital
Transcervical
Intertrochanteric
Subtrochanteric

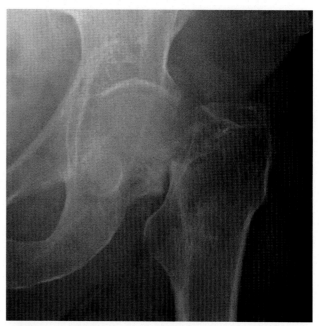

FIGURE 8-48 ■ Displaced subcapital fracture of the femoral neck. The blood supply will almost inevitably be interrupted.

Fractures are classified by location from subcapital to intertrochanteric (Fig. 8-47). Subcapital and transcervical fractures are intracapsular. The blood supply to the femoral head is derived from recurrent arteries closely applied to the femoral neck. Fractures of the neck and subcapital region interrupt this blood supply, particularly if the fracture is displaced (Fig. 8-48), resulting in avascular necrosis in 15 to 35% of patients. Such fractures are thus treated by hip replacement. Inter- and subtrochanteric fractures are extracapsular and the blood supply is not at risk. These fractures can be treated by plate and dynamic hip screw fixation.

Most fractures are readily apparent but about 15% are difficult to detect. Looking carefully at the trabecular pattern will assist in identifying these: interruption of the trabecular lines indicates a subtle fracture. Impacted undisplaced fractures may be identified by the presence of a sclerotic line and/or interruption of the normal trabecular pattern. Use of the lateral view may be extremely helpful in identifying fractures when there is uncertainty on the AP view (Fig. 8-49).

Intertrochanteric fractures, in general, are easier to identify, particularly when severely comminuted (Fig. 8-50), but some fractures may be overlooked when only minimally displaced. Care should be taken when air is trapped in an overlying skin crease. This may mimic a fracture or conversely mask an underlying fracture (Fig. 8-51).

Despite very careful observation, about 1% of fractures are initially occult and cannot be identified on radiographs. If these are not identified and the patient is encouraged to mobilise and weight-bear, then the fracture may become displaced. Because of the risk of subsequent avascular necrosis, great effort must be made to detect these fractures. In the absence of an identifiable fracture on the radiographs, the index of clinical suspicion is used to direct the use of any further investigations. Skeletal scintigraphy can identify occult fractures but may take up to 3 days before it becomes positive; MRI is specific and sensitive and is now the investigation of choice[41,42] (Fig. 8-52).

Hip fractures are often caused by underlying osteoporosis. For this reason, patients under the age of 75 who sustain a hip fracture should be assessed for underlying osteoporosis (usually by DEXA) and treated appropriately.[43]

There are two fractures which may mimic the signs and symptoms of a hip fracture. These are fractures of the pubic rami and greater trochanter. These should be looked for in every patient, but especially when no hip fracture is apparent. If found, they may well account for the patient's symptoms and preclude further investigation for occult fractures. The patient can be advised and managed appropriately.

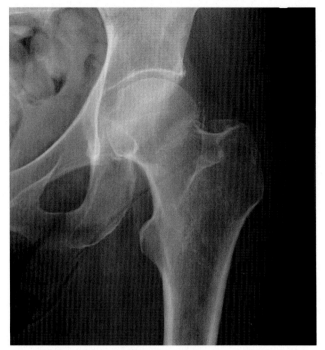

FIGURE 8-49 ■ **Subtle interruption of the trabecular lines of the femoral neck.** There is ill-defined sclerosis extending across the neck. These signs suggest an impacted fracture.

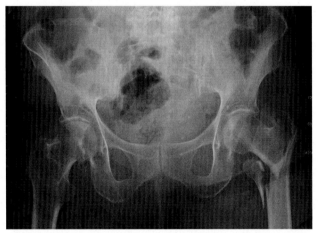

FIGURE 8-50 ■ **A comminuted intertrochanteric fracture on the left.**

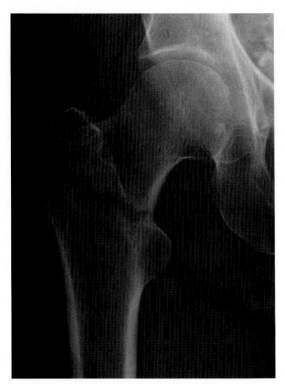

FIGURE 8-51 ■ **Air is trapped in the skin crease of the groin, producing a linear lucency traversing the underlying femur.** However, on close inspection the lucency crossing the bone is separate from the soft-tissue lucency. Thus this patient has a fracture as well as air in the groin crease.

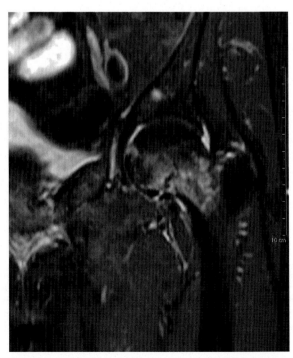

FIGURE 8-52 ■ **The AP radiograph of the hip was normal.** MRI coronal STIR shows a fracture of the inferior aspect of the femoral neck.

THE KNEE

On the AP radiograph the fibula denotes the lateral side of the knee. The medial and lateral joint spaces are normally equal. The cortices of the tibial plateau both medial and lateral are sharply defined and sclerotic. There is a useful rule of thumb aiding fracture detection. A line dropped perpendicularly from the lateral femoral condyle should meet the margin of the adjacent tibial plateau with (at most) 5 mm of bone lying lateral to the line. If this rule is broken, suspect a lateral tibial plateau fracture.

The lateral view following trauma should be obtained using a horizontal beam: that is with the patient lying flat

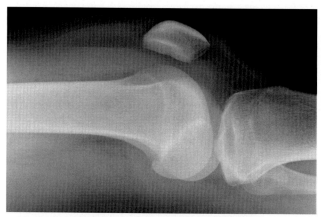

FIGURE 8-53 ■ **Horizontal beam lateral radiograph.** There is a fluid level evident within the suprapatellar pouch. The dark layer on top represents fluid fat which has layered on top of the much brighter fluid blood. The fluid fat has escaped from the bone marrow, which means there must be a fracture present.

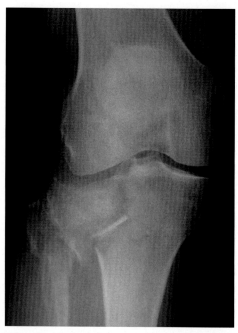

FIGURE 8-54 ■ **An obvious fracture of the lateral tibial plateau which has been depressed inferiorly.** There is an associated fracture of the fibula.

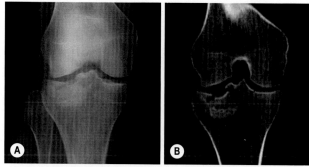

FIGURE 8-55 ■ (A) Area of sclerosis inferior to the lateral plateau indicative of trabecular condensation as a result of a plateau fracture. (B) CT demonstrates the fracture lines and also shows the degree of depression of the fracture. The sclerotic impacted trabeculae correlate with the plain radiographic findings.

and the X-ray beam parallel to the floor. This enables a useful soft-tissue sign to become evident, which is a fluid–fluid level superior to the patella lying within the suprapatellar pouch. It consists of fat layered on blood, known as a lipohaemarthrosis.[44,45] The only fat which is fluid at body temperature is marrow fat. Thus, to be evident on the radiograph there must be a break in a bony cortex, allowing fat to escape into the knee joint; this is usually accompanied by blood. If this sign is present, there must be a fracture and this is almost always visible on the radiograph with careful inspection (Fig. 8-53).

Supracondylar and condylar fractures of the femur are caused by severe trauma and usually present little diagnostic difficulty.

Fractures of the tibial plateau typically occur when the lateral side of the knee is struck, forcing the knee into valgus. The lateral femoral condyle is driven down into the lateral tibial plateau, resulting in fracturing and depression of the plateau. Medial fractures are much less common, accounting for only 10% of such injuries. Most injuries are easily detected (Fig. 8-54). Many now undergo CT, not for diagnosis but to aid surgical planning.[40] The number of fracture fragments and the degree of plateau depression will determine the need for surgery and the type. Depression of the articular surface by more than 10 mm is a key observation in this regard. Tibial plateau depression is measured as the vertical distance between the lowest point on the intact medial plateau and the lowest depressed lateral plateau fracture fragment. More subtle injuries may be detected by use of three observations:

1. Loss of clarity of the normal lateral plateau cortex.
2. Impaction of the subcortical trabeculae resulting in sclerosis (Fig. 8-55).
3. Lateral displacement of the tibial margin beyond a vertical line drawn inferiorly from the lateral femoral condyle. Normally little or no bone lies lateral to such a line (Fig. 8-56).

Small bone fragments around the knee usually signify a significant injury.[47] They should not be dismissed as flakes or chips as many are avulsion injuries by tendons or ligaments.[48] Severe force and distraction of the knee is required to avulse the bony attachments seen on the radiographs. There are two findings of particular significance.

The anterior cruciate ligament (ACL) inserts into the anterior tibial eminence. In adolescents, in particular, this bony attachment is weaker than the ligament. In some instances the ligament is avulsed from this bony attachment, resulting in a bone fragment which is seen within the joint centrally on the AP view and in the anterior half of the joint on the lateral (Fig. 8-57).

The presence of a small bone fragment adjacent to the upper lateral tibia, known as a Segond fracture,[49] is an avulsion injury by the lateral capsular ligament (Fig. 8-58). Its importance is that the mechanism of a forced varus injury that produces this finding results in a very

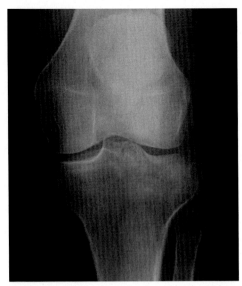

FIGURE 8-56 ■ A lateral plateau fracture with displacement of bone laterally such that a line drawn down the lateral cortex of the femur does not run smoothly onto the lateral margin of the tibia.

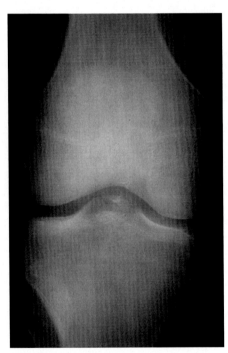

FIGURE 8-57 ■ There are small bone fragments seen centrally in the joint space projected over the tibial spines. Bone fragments in this position are due to avulsion by the anterior cruciate ligament.

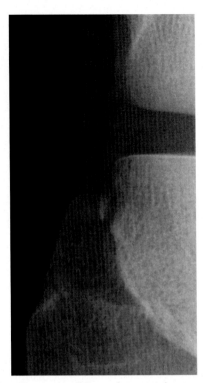

FIGURE 8-58 ■ A very small bone fragment is seen adjacent to the lateral tibia also overlapping the fibula head. This should not be misinterpreted as a minor flake injury. It indicates a high likelihood of injuries of the ACL and medial meniscus.

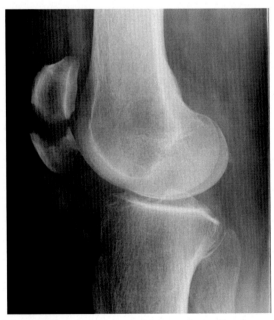

FIGURE 8-59 ■ **Lateral knee.** A horizontal patellar fracture is readily identified.

high incidence of rupture of the ACL and tears of the medial meniscus, both said to be as high as 75–100% of cases.

Patellar fracture is either transverse vertical or stellate (comminuted). Patellar injuries occur either from a direct blow or as a result of contraction of the powerful quadriceps muscles, resulting in a transverse fracture which accounts for 60% of cases. These injuries are readily visible on a lateral view (Fig. 8-59). Vertical fractures are much less common (15%) and are visible on the AP view only with difficulty because of the overlying distal femur. If a patellar injury is suspected clinically and none is seen on conventional radiographs, then an additional radiograph—the skyline (or sunrise) view—should be taken with the knee in flexion; this throws the patella off

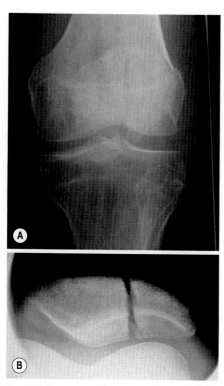

FIGURE 8-60 ■ (A) A vertical patellar fracture is seen with some difficulty. (B) If index of suspicion is high and no fracture is seen, then an additional skyline view will identify such fractures more readily.

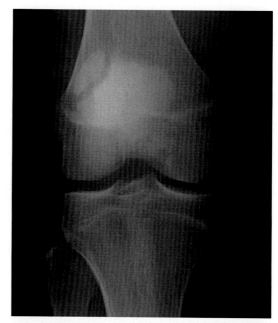

FIGURE 8-61 ■ **Bipartite patella.** The bone fragment seen arising from the superolateral quadrant of the patella is a normal variant, a bipartite patella. It should not be mistaken for a fracture.

the femur and may allow a vertical fracture to be seen (Fig. 8-60). Stellate fractures are usually caused by a direct blow to the patella. They may only be seen on the AP view with difficulty.

Bipartite patella is a normal variant. The bone fragment always occurs in the superior lateral quadrant and has well-defined sclerotic margins (Fig. 8-61). The fragment is usually larger than the defect.

Patellar dislocation is rarely evident as such on plain radiographs. Even when dislocated at the time of injury, this is usually transient and has relocated long before the patient attends the emergency department. The only occasional evidence of the dislocation is when an osteochondral fragment is displaced from the femoral condyle or avulsed from the patella by the medial patellofemoral ligament. These bone fragments may be visible on the radiograph. Again, the skyline view may be helpful in finding these small bone fragments.[50] This is another example of a small bone fragment which signifies a significant injury. It should be distinguished from an ACL avulsion injury described earlier. In the latter, the bone fragment lies centrally in the joint on both views. The former is seen often on one view only and lies away from the joint centre (Fig. 8-62).

THE ANKLE

Standard views are an AP mortice view and a lateral. The mortice view is an AP with approximately 10° of internal

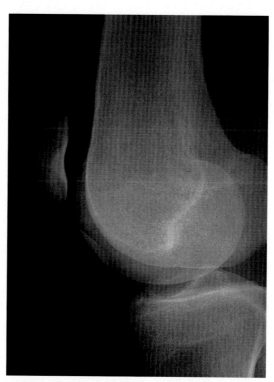

FIGURE 8-62 ■ There is a curvilinear bone fragment seen in the anterior aspect of the knee. This is not visible on an AP view. Bone fragments like this are typically found as a result of patellar dislocation, although in the majority of cases there are no radiographic abnormalities.

rotation of the foot, which projects the fibula clear of the talus, making it easier to identify fractures of these structures. The lateral radiograph of the ankle should encompass not only the distal tibia and fibula but also the calcaneus and base of the fifth metatarsal.

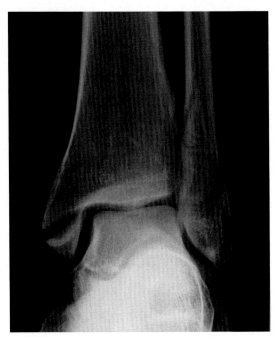

FIGURE 8-63 ■ Fractures of both medial and lateral malleolus. This represents a bimalleolar injury.

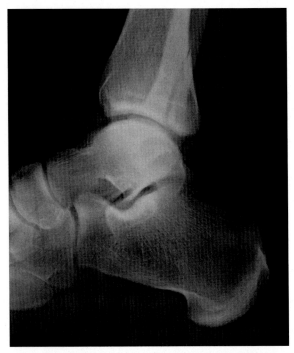

FIGURE 8-64 ■ Fracture of the posterior distal tibial tubercle often referred to (incorrectly) as the posterior malleolus. This is not visible on the AP view. These fractures are often associated with fractures of both medial and lateral malleoli and so would be termed a trimalleolar injury.

The pattern of ankle fractures depends on the position of the foot and the force applied, most often inversion, eversion and rotational injuries. Inversion injuries account for about 80% of these ankle fractures. The fractures involve the malleoli, medial and lateral either singly (unimalleolar) or in combination (bimalleolar; Fig. 8-63). There may also be an associated fracture of the posterior tubercle of the distal tibia, sometimes referred to as the posterior malleolus, resulting in a trimalleolar fracture (Fig. 8-64). Fractures of the distal fibula are often visible only on careful inspection of the lateral view.

A simple commonly used classification of malleolar fractures is the Weber classification.[51] This considers only the position of the fibular fracture in relation to the talar dome. However, the important anatomy is the syndesmosis and associated ligaments of the distal tibia and fibula. The talar dome is merely an anatomical landmark on radiographs, which can be used to try and determine whether a fracture involves the syndesmosis.

Weber A is a fracture of the distal fibula inferior to the talar dome and thus the syndesmosis will be intact (Fig. 8-65). Surgery is not usually required. Weber B fractures at the level of the talar dome may involve the syndesmosis. Surgical treatment is needed in a proportion of these injuries. Weber C fractures are proximal to the talar dome and the syndesmosis is usually disrupted in these cases (Fig. 8-66). These fractures are generally treated with internal fixation. Severity and prognosis of these injuries is also dependent on the number of malleoli involved and the degree of displacement at the fracture sites.

There are more complex comprehensive classification systems for ankle injures but these are beyond the scope of this chapter.

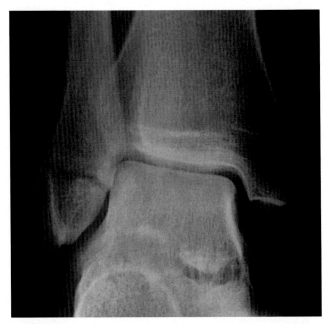

FIGURE 8-65 ■ Fracture of the distal fibula below the level of the talar dome so the syndesmosis is not disrupted. This thus represents a Weber A fracture.

With this type of ankle injury there is also the possibility of an associated high fibular fracture. This should be suspected when there is a medial malleolar fracture or widening of the medial joint space signifying ligament damage. In this circumstance there is a high likelihood

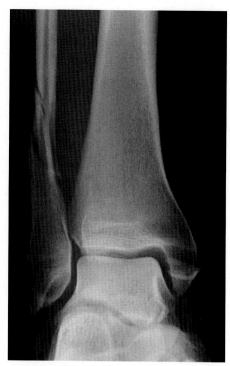

FIGURE 8-66 ■ **The fibular fracture is proximal to the talar dome.** The syndesmosis is usually disrupted in such injuries. Note there is an associated medial malleolar fracture. Therefore this is a bimalleolar Weber C injury.

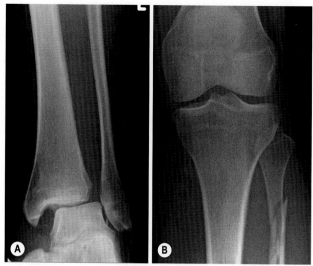

FIGURE 8-67 ■ (A) Widening of the medial joint space of the ankle or, alternatively, lateral talar shift. There must be disruption of the medial ligaments. The syndesmosis is also widened, indicating that it is also disrupted. Such injuries would normally occur in association with fracture of the distal fibula. However, none is evident here. (B) Radiograph higher up the leg, however, reveals a fibular fracture. This high fibular fracture in association with an ankle injury and is known as a Maissonneuve injury.

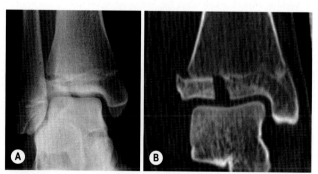

FIGURE 8-68 ■ (A) There is a fracture of the distal lateral tibia running vertically from the articular surface to the epiphyseal plate. (B) Coronal CT reconstruction shows the fracture more clearly and the degree of displacement. This is a Salter–Harris type 3 injury and is known as a Tillaux fracture.

of a lateral fibular fracture as well. If one is not visible on the ankle radiographs, it is possible that the fibula has fractured but much higher up the leg. Radiographs of this area may then reveal the fracture. This is referred to as a Maissonneuve fracture[52] (Fig. 8-67).

Tillaux fracture describes a fracture of the distal tibia resulting from external rotation. It is an avulsion injury by the anterior inferior tibiofibular ligament. The fracture involves the anterolateral aspect of the tibial articular surface. In juvenile patients with unfused skeletons this will represent a Salter–Harris type 3 injury (Fig. 8-68).

Fractures which disrupt the weight-bearing articular surface of the distal tibia result from a high-energy axial loading. These fractures are generally readily apparent and often associated with comminuted fractures of the tibia and fibula. They are referred to as pilon fractures (Fig. 8-69).

Fractures of the talar dome result from eversion/inversion injuries. The mortice view facilitates their detection when a small bone fragment is separated from the talar articular surface. The cortex of the adjacent talus is irregular, indicating the source of the bone fragment (Fig. 8-70). These fragments may need to be removed if small or fixed if large. If overlooked, continuing pain and early degenerative joint changes are likely.

Calcaneal fractures are caused by a fall from a height on to the heels. They are bilateral in 10% of cases and associated with fracture of the lumbar spine, also in 10%. However, they can also result from a simple inversion

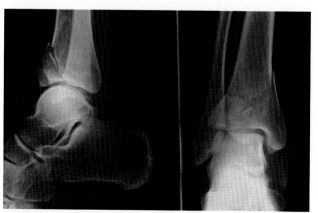

FIGURE 8-69 ■ A complex pilon fracture of the distal tibia which on the lateral view is seen to involve the articular surface with displacement of a large fragment anteriorly. This results from a high-impact injury.

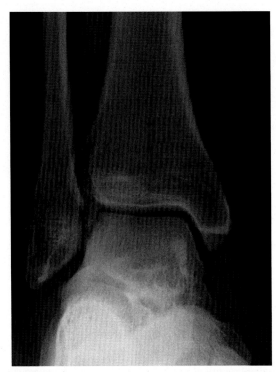

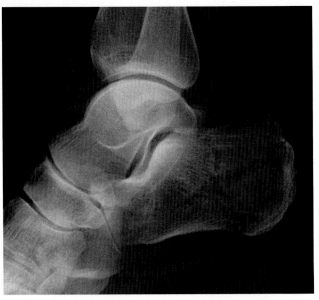

FIGURE 8-72 ■ A vertical fracture line is seen running from superior to inferior, posterior to the subarticular joint. This is therefore an extra-articular injury.

FIGURE 8-70 ■ **A fracture of the talar dome can be seen.** This injury occurs due to an inversion injury and should be carefully looked for. The mortice view facilitates its detection; a standard AP view with overlap of the fibula may make a bone fragment at this point impossible to detect.

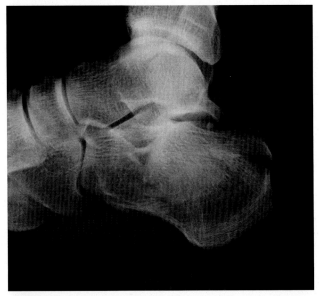

FIGURE 8-71 ■ A tongue-type fracture of the calcaneus with V-shaped fracture line extending from the posterior aspect to the body centrally. There is loss of articular congruity of the subtalar joint.

injury, especially in the osteoporotic patient. Major fractures are easily detected. There are two types of fracture. The tongue type (Fig. 8-71) involves a fracture from the posterior calcaneal cortex extending forwards to the subtalar joint. The second variety is a vertical fracture from

the superior to the inferior calcaneal margin (Fig. 8-72). Both fracture types may occur in the same patient. It is important to determine whether the fracture extends to the articular surface of the subtalar joint.[53] Articular involvement indicates a more severe injury. Whereas the lateral view of the ankle provides a satisfactory view of the calcaneus, an AP view of the ankle does not provide a second view. If calcaneal injury is suspected, a further axial projection radiograph taken at right angles to the lateral is obtained. CT is utilised to aid surgical planning, as these fractures may be very complex.[54]

Some fractures, however, are more subtle. They may be detected by using several observations:

1. Bohler's angle—this is constructed by drawing two lines through the three most superior points on the calcaneus. The first is from the superior aspect of the posterior calcaneus to the highest midpoint, which is the posterior aspect of the articular facet. The second line from this point passes anteriorly and is drawn to the superior tip of the anterior process. These two lines should normally make an angle of 30° (Fig. 8-73). In the presence of a fracture, this angle may be significantly reduced. Note, however, that a normal angle does not exclude a fracture.
2. An abnormal area of sclerosis caused by trabecular impaction signifies an impacted fracture.
3. Loss of the normal congruity of the articulation between the talus and calcaneus at the posterior subtalar joint.

Fractures of the talus most often involve the talar neck: they are uncommon and result from severe force. Fractures of the neck result from severe force driving up into the sole of the foot. It is another bone where the blood

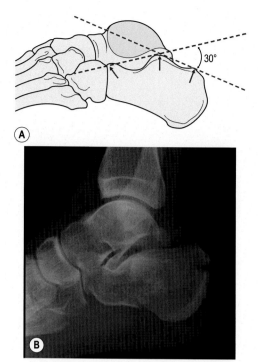

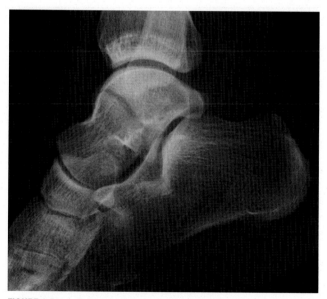

FIGURE 8-73 ■ (A) Line drawing showing how Bohler's angle is constructed and measured. (B) The calcaneus is abnormal with flattening of Bohler's angle as the highest point in the middle is depressed so that joining the three points results in an almost straight line. A posterior fracture is evident.

FIGURE 8-74 ■ A lucent line running through the talus indicates a neck fracture which is at risk of developing avascular necrosis caused by interruption of the blood supply.

supply distally may be interrupted by such a fracture with resultant avascular necrosis (Fig. 8-74).

A much more common injury is an avulsion by the joint capsule of a small flake of bone from the dorsum of the talus distally. This injury is of little clinical significance.

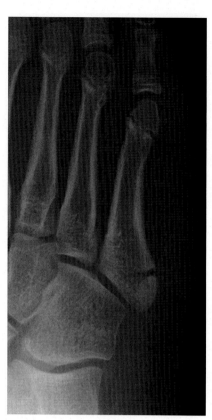

FIGURE 8-75 ■ A fracture of the base of the fifth metatarsal. At this proximal site it is an avulsion injury caused by the pull of the peroneus brevis tendon. These fractures heal well.

FOOT INJURIES

Inversion injury of the ankle may result in a fracture of the foot. It is an avulsion injury caused by the tendon of peroneus brevis muscle which inserts onto the base of the fifth metatarsal.[55] Contraction of the muscle as the ankle inverts may pull off the most proximal portion of the fifth metatarsal. The fracture is easy to see on radiographs of the foot (Fig. 8-75). However, it should also be looked for on ankle X-rays where the lateral radiograph encompasses the base of the fifth metatarsal. This injury should be distinguished from a fracture distal to the articulation between the fourth and fifth metatarsals. This is called a Jones' fracture and has a propensity to heal poorly.[56] It is also caused by inversion of the foot (Fig. 8-76).

In skeletally immature patients there is an unfused apophysis at the base of the fifth metatarsal, which should not be mistaken for a fracture. The apophysis is separated from the metatarsal by a lucency which is longitudinally orientated. Avulsion fractures lie transversely (Fig. 8-77).

Lisfranc injury refers to fractures and dislocations in and around the bases of the metatarsals.[57,58] When there is an associated fracture or the dislocation is severe, the abnormality is readily identified. Most commonly there is a fracture of the base of the second metatarsal with

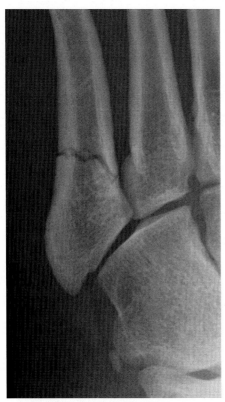

FIGURE 8-76 ■ **Fracture of the proximal shaft of the fifth metatarsal.** This is known as a Jones' fracture. Fractures at this site have a tendency to heal poorly.

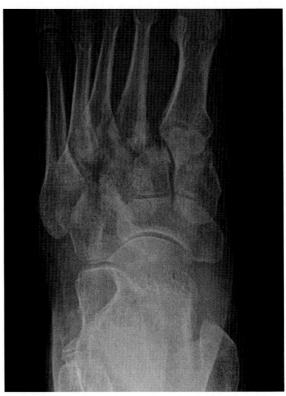

FIGURE 8-78 ■ **Lisfranc midfoot injury.** The second, third and fourth metatarsals are displaced laterally. There is a fracture at the base of the second metatarsal.

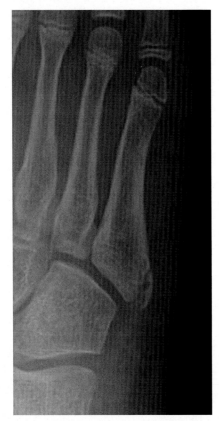

FIGURE 8-77 ■ **Immature skeleton.** The proximal apophysis of the fifth metatarsal is a normal finding and should not be mistaken for a fracture. Fractures are transverse across the bone shaft; apophyses run longitudinally. Compare with appearances of the fracture in Fig. 8-78.

displacement of the second to fifth metatarsals laterally (Fig. 8-78). More subtle injuries may be identified by observing loss of the normal alignment of the second and third metatarsal bases with their respective cuneiform bones. Normally, a line drawn down the medial cortex of the metatarsal will pass between the medial and intermediate cuneiform on the AP view. On the oblique view a line along the lateral cortex of the metatarsal should pass between middle and lateral cuneiform bones. Some injuries are not visible at all on radiographs and when there is strong index of suspicion clinically, a CT scan may reveal subtle disruptions at this joint.[59]

Stress fractures are caused by repeated low-impact trauma.[60] They are common in the foot, with a predeliction for the shaft of the second metatarsal. Stress fractures are often seen in military recruits from prolonged marching, hence the name of march fracture, but now are more common in those undertaking training for charity distance running events. They are identified radiographically not as a typical lucent line but as an area of periosteal reaction due to increased osteoclastic activity (Fig. 8-79). They are seen most commonly on those undertaking unusual increased activity such as an unaccustomed long distance walking or running.

In patients with a history of inversion injury, Table 8-2 lists injuries that can occur and should be considered when reporting.

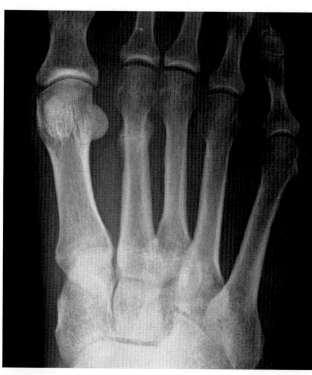

FIGURE 8-79 ■ **There is a periosteal reaction around the shaft of the distal second metatarsal.** This is the typical appearance of a stress fracture due to unaccustomed exercise. A fracture line will rarely, if ever, become visible.

TABLE 8-2 Injuries Which May Occur due to Ankle Inversion

In a patient with a history of inversion injury, consider all of the following:

Malleolar injuries	Look on lateral carefully for (a) difficult-to-see fibular fractures and (b) post-tibia fractures
High fibular fractures (Maisonneuve)	Medial fractures or talar shift and no fibular fracture visible
Talar dome fractures	
Calcaneal fractures	Look at Bohler's angle / Areas of sclerosis / Loss of articular congruity
Base of fifth metatarsal	Seen on lateral ankle X-ray

REFERENCES

1. Green A, Norris T. Gleno humeral dislocations. In: Browner B, Jupiter J, Levine A, Trafton P, editors. Skeletal Trauma, vol. 2. 3rd ed. Philadelphia: Saunders; 2003. pp. 1598–614.
2. Hill A, Sachs D. The grooved defect of the humeral head. A frequently unrecognized complication of dislocations of the shoulder joint. Radiology 1940;35:690–700.
3. Neer CS. Displaced proximal humeral fractures. 1. Classification and evaluation. J Bone Joint Surg Am 1970;52:1077–89.
4. Lazarus M, Seon C. Fractures of the clavicle. In: Buchholz RW, Heckmen JD, Court-Brown C, editors. Rockwood and Green's Fractures in Adults. 6th ed. Philadelphia: Lippincott Williams & Wilkins; 2006. pp. 1211–55.
5. Melenevsky Y, Yablon CM, Ramappa A, Hochman MG. Clavicle and acromioclavicular joint injuries: a review of imaging, treatment, and complications. Skeletal Radiol 2011;40(7):31–42.
6. Nemec U, Oberleitner G, Nemec SF, et al. MRI versus radiography of acromioclavicular joint dislocation. Am J Roentgenol 2011;197(4):968–73.
7. Goswami GK. The fat pad sign. Radiology 2002;222(2):419–20.
8. O'Dwyer H, O'Sullivan P, Fitzgerald D, et al. The fat pad sign following elbow trauma in adults: its usefulness and reliability in suspecting occult fracture. J Comput Assist Tomogr 2004;28(4):562–5.
9. Thornton A, Gyll C. Children's Fractures. New York: Saunders; 1999.
10. Rogers LF, Malave S Jr, White H, Tachdjian MO. Plastic bowing, torus and greenstick supracondylar fractures of the humerus: radiographic clues to obscure fractures of the elbow in children. Radiology 1978;128(1):145–50.
11. Shrader MW. Pediatric supracondylar fractures and pediatric physeal elbow fractures. Orthop Clin North Am 2008;39(2):163–71.
12. John SD, Wherry K, Swischuk L, Phillips WA. Improving detection of paediatric elbow fractures by understanding their mechanics. Radiographics 1996;16:1443–60.
13. Cheng JC, Wing-Man K, Shen WY, et al. A new look at the sequential development of elbow-ossification centers in children. J Pediatr Orthop 1998;18(2):161–7.
14. Sonin A. Fractures of the elbow and forearm. Semin Musculoskelet Radiol 2004;4(2):171–91.
15. Miles KA, Finlay DL. Disruption of the radiocapitellar line in the normal elbow. Injury 1989;20:365–7.
16. Eathiraju S, Mudgal CS, Jupiter JB. Monteggia fracture-dislocations. Hand Clin 2007;23(2):165–77.
17. David-West KS, Wilson NI, Sherlock DA, et al. Missed Monteggia injuries. Injury 2005;36(10):1206–9.
18. Pike JM, Athwal GS, Faber KJ, King GJ. Radial head fractures—an update. J Hand Surg Am 2009;34(3):557–65.
19. Horne JG, Tanzer TL. Olecranon fractures: a review of 100 cases. J Trauma 1981;21:469–72.
20. Gilula LA. Carpal injuries: analytic approach and case exercises. Am J Roentgenol 1979;133(3):503–17.
21. Court-Brown CM, Koval KJ. The epidemiology of fractures. In: Buchholz RW, Heckmen JD, Court-Brown C, editors. Rockwood and Green's Fractures in Adults. 6th ed. Philadelphia: Lippincott Williams & Wilkins; 2006. pp. 95–143.
22. Duncan DS, Thurston AJ. Clinical fracture of the scaphoid—an illusionary diagnosis. J Hand Surg 1985;10B(3):375–6.
23. Groves AM, Kayani I, Syed R, et al. An international survey of hospital practice in the imaging of acute scaphoid trauma. Am J Roentgenol 2006;187(6):1453–6.
24. Brookes-Fazakerley SD, Kumar AJ, Oakley J. Survey of the initial management and imaging protocols for occult scaphoid fractures in UK hospitals. Skeletal Radiol 2009;38(11):1045–8.
25. Brydie A, Raby N. Early MRI in the management of clinical scaphoid fracture. Br J Radiol 2003;76(905):296–300.
26. Gaebler C. Fractures and dislocations of the carpus. In: Buchholz RW, Heckmen JD, Court-Brown C, editors. Rockwood and Green's Fractures in Adults. 6th ed. Philadelphia: Lippincott Williams & Wilkins; 2006. pp. 857–908.
27. Kaewlai R, Avery LL, Asrani AV, et al. Multidetector CT of carpal injuries: anatomy, fractures, and fracture-dislocations. Radiographics 2008;28(6):1771–84.
28. Yeager BA, Dalinka MK. Radiology of trauma to the wrist: dislocations, fracture dislocations, and instability patterns. Skeletal Radiol 1985;13(2):120–30.
29. Nathan R, Blatt G. Rotary subluxation of the scaphoid revisited. Hand Clin 2000;16(3):417–31.
30. Fisher MR, Rogers LF, Hendrix RW. Systematic approach to identifying fourth and fifth carpometacarpal joint dislocations. Am J Roentgenol 1983;140(2):319–24.
31. Calfee RP, Sommerkamp TG. Fracture–dislocation about the finger joints. J Hand Surg 2009;34A:1140–7.
32. Yoong P, Goodwin R, Chojnowski A. Phalangeal fractures of the hand. Clin Radiol 2010;65:773–80.
33. Hintermann B, Holzach PJ, Schütz M, Matter P. Skier's thumb—the significance of bony injuries. Am J Sports Med 1993;21(6):800–4.
34. Pennal GF, Tile M, Waddell JP, Garside H. Pelvic disruption: assessment and classification. Clin Orthop 1980;151:12–21.
35. Tile M. Fractures of the Pelvis and Acetabulum. Baltimore: Williams and Wilkins; 1984. pp. 70–96.
36. Young JW, Burgess AR, Brumback RJ, Poka A. Pelvic fractures: value of plain radiography in early assessment and management. Radiology 1986;160:445–51.

37. Judet R, Judet J, Letournel E. Fractures of the acetabulum: classification and surgical approaches for open reduction. J Bone Joint Surg Am 1964;46:1615–38.

38. Letournel E. Acetabular fractures: classification and management. Clin Orthop 1980;151:12–21.

39. Blomlie V, Rofstad EK, Talle K, et al. Incidence of radiation-induced insufficiency fractures of the female pelvis: evaluation with MR imaging. Am J Roentgenol 1996;167:1205–10.

40. Parker M, Johansen A. Hip fracture. BMJ 2006;333(7557):27–30.

41. Chana R, Noorani A, Ashwood N, et al. The role of MRI in the diagnosis of proximal femoral fractures in the elderly. Injury 2006;37(2):185–9.

42. Pandey R, McNally E, Ali A, Bulstrode C. The role of MRI in the diagnosis of occult hip fractures. Injury 1998;29(1):61–3.

43. NICE Guideline CG 124. The management of hip fracture in adults. June 2011.

44. Ferguson J, Knottenbelt JD. Lipohaemarthrosis in knee trauma: an experience of 907 cases. Injury 1994;25(5):311–12.

45. Lee JH, Weissman BN, Nikpoor N, et al. Lipohemarthrosis of the knee: a review of recent experiences. Radiology 1989;173(1):189–91.

46. Markhardt BK, Gross JM, Monu JU. Schatzker classification of tibial plateau fractures: use of CT and MR imaging improves assessment. Radiographics 2009;29(2):585–97.

47. Delzell PB, Schils JP, Recht MP. Subtle fractures about the knee: innocuous-appearing yet indicative of significant internal derangement. Am J Roentgenol 1996;167(3):699–703.

48. Gottsegen C, Eyer B, White E, et al. Avulsion fractures of the knee: imaging findings and clinical significance. Radiographics 2008;28:1755–70.

49. Goldman AB, Pavlov H, Rubenstein D. The Segond fracture of the proximal tibia: a small avulsion that reflects major ligamentous damage. Am J Roentgenol 1988;151(6):1163–7.

50. Haas JP, Collins MS, Stuart MJ. The 'sliver sign': a specific radiographic sign of acute lateral patellar dislocation. Skeletal Radiol 2012;41(5):595–601.

51. Kennedy JG, Johnson SM, Collins AL, et al. An evaluation of the Weber classification of ankle fractures. Injury 1998;29(8):577–80.

52. Kalyani B, Roberts C, Giannoudis P. The Maisonneuve injury: a comprehensive review. Orthopedics 2010;33(3):190–5.

53. Matherne TH, Tivorsak T, Monu JU. Calcaneal fractures: what the surgeon needs to know. Curr Probl Diagn Radiol 2007;36(1):1–10.

54. Badillo K, Pacheco JA, Padua SO, et al. Multidetector CT evaluation of calcaneal fractures. Radiographics 2011;31(1):81–92.

55. Zwitser EW, Breederveld RS. Fractures of the fifth metatarsal; diagnosis and treatment. Injury 2010;41(6):555–62.

56. Chuckpaiwong B, Queen RM, Easley ME, Nunley JA. Distinguishing Jones and proximal diaphyseal fractures of the fifth metatarsal. Clin Orthop Relat Res 2008;466(8):1966–70.

57. Rosenbaum A, Dellenbaugh S, Dipreta J, Uhl R. Subtle injuries to the lisfranc joint. Orthopedics 2011;34(11):882–7.

58. Scolaro J, Ahn J, Mehta S. In brief: Lisfranc fracture dislocations. Clin Orthop Relat Res 2011;469(7):2078–80.

59. Kalia V, Fishman EK, Carrino JA, Fayad LM. Epidemiology, imaging, and treatment of Lisfranc fracture-dislocations revisited. Skeletal Radiol 2012;41(2):129–36.

60. Gehrmann RM, Renard RL. Current concepts review: stress fractures of the foot. Foot Ankle Int 2006;27(9):750–7.

CHAPTER 9

BONE, JOINT AND SPINAL INFECTION

Balashanmugam Rajashanker • Richard W. Whitehouse

CHAPTER OUTLINE

INTRODUCTION

EPIDEMIOLOGY

CLASSIFICATION

PAEDIATRIC MUSCULOSKELETAL INFECTIONS

ADULT MUSCULOSKELETAL INFECTIONS

DIABETIC FOOT

SEPTIC ARTHRITIS

MUSCULOSKELETAL TUBERCULOSIS

UNUSUAL MUSCULOSKELETAL INFECTIONS

DIFFERENTIAL DIAGNOSIS

MANAGEMENT

SPINAL INFECTION

INTRODUCTION

Bone and joint infections have high rates of morbidity and occasional mortality. A wide range of microbial infections can affect bones and joints, including pyogenic, mycobacterial and fungal organisms. Patients usually present with a high temperature, pain and swelling in the affected bones and/or joints. In younger patients concomitant systemic illness more often occurs. Early diagnosis at acute presentation is important to prevent chronic and recurrent infections, long-term disabilities and treatment failures. Prompt diagnosis is needed particularly in children and also after orthopaedic implant surgeries to prevent the risk of developing serious infections. A multidisciplinary team approach is necessary for effective management of these conditions. Soft-tissue and muscle infections present more acutely and may be potentially life threatening.

It can be difficult to diagnose bone infection early, especially in diabetic patients with pre-existing neuropathic bone and joint changes and in the presence of skin ulceration and cellulitis. A high degree of suspicion and use of appropriate investigations will assist diagnosis. Tuberculous infection of bones and joints pose a particular diagnostic challenge. Septic arthritis is a serious condition, which if untreated leads to destruction of cartilage and adjacent osteomyelitis, with subsequent joint ankylosis and disability. Laboratory tests including white cell count, C-reactive protein, ESR and blood culture are mandatory in the early stages to diagnose these infections. A range of radiological investigations are available currently to enable a prompt diagnosis. It is important that the radiologist is familiar with the clinical spectrum of presentations, appropriate diagnostic tests and the need to perform these without delay to enable prompt management.

EPIDEMIOLOGY

Staphylococcus aureus is the commonest organism causing bone and joint infections in any age group, accounting for up to 80% of cases of osteomyelitis. Gram-negative organisms including *Pseudomonas* and *Enterobacter* are responsible for most of the remaining 20% of cases. Acute infections of prosthetic implants are usually caused by *S. aureus*. Coagulate-negative staphylococci such as *Staphylococcus epidermidis* account for the majority of chronic osteomyelitis associated with orthopaedic implants and account for approximately 90% of pin tract infections. Bacteria adhere to bone matrix and orthopaedic implants via receptors to fibronectin and other receptor proteins. They form a slimy coat and elude the host defence mechanisms by hiding intracellularly and by developing a slow metabolic rate.[1] Osteoarticular *Listeria* infections are rare but do occur in immunocompromised patients and in prosthetic joints.[2] Polymicrobial infection occurs in the majority of osteomyelitidies occurring in the diabetic foot, comprising of mixed Gram-positive and -negative bacteria. Wound swabs are often inaccurate and dominated by contaminants. Cultures from bone biopsy or operative specimens are more reliable in planning appropriate antibiotic treatment.[3] Brodie's abscess, a true small, focal intraosseous collection of pus, is an uncommon manifestation of bone infection, except in East Africa, where reportedly it is a common occurrence.[4] *Staphylococcus aureus* is again the predominant organism cultured in these patients.

Vertebral osteomyelitis usually results from haematogenous seeding or by direct inoculation at the time of spinal surgery. *Staphylococcus aureus* is the commonest microorganism amongst others that include methicillin-resistant *S. aureus* (MRSA), streptococci and *E coli*.[5] As with other orthopaedic implants, coagulase-negative staphylococcal infections are seen after usage of fixation devices.[6]

In children, other than staphylococci, *Haemophilus influenzae* type b, *Streptococcus pneumoniae* and *Streptococcus pyogenes* also occur.[7] One of the significant changes in the epidemiology of bone and joint infections is the increasing incidence of MRSA and the emergence of multidrug resistant (MDR) organisms.[8,9]

Osteomyelitis complicating war injuries is predominantly caused by MDR organisms and include MRSA, Enterobacteriaceae and *Acinetobacter*. There is commonly a history of previous surgical procedures and these conditions usually need further more aggressive management.[10]

Fungal infections of the bone and joints are uncommon and occur predominantly in the immunosuppressed patient. Such infection may resemble tuberculous disease and present as chronic multifocal osteomyelitis or polyarthritis.[11]

CLASSIFICATION

Osteomyelitis can be classified by the type of infection or more commonly by the duration since onset of the illness. Acute osteomyelitis is defined as infection diagnosed within 2 weeks of onset of symptoms whilst subacute osteomyelitis is diagnosed if symptoms exceed 2 weeks' duration. If the infection is diagnosed months after the onset of symptoms, then it is defined as chronic osteomyelitis.[12,13] There are, however, other classifications in the literature, depending on the anatomical areas of bony involvement and on pathogenesis.[14,15]

PAEDIATRIC MUSCULOSKELETAL INFECTIONS

Paediatric, unlike adult, bone infections more commonly occur in healthy bones, without pre-existing trauma, etc. The usual mode of infection is haematogenous, via the arterial blood supply. Acute haematogenous osteomyelitis (AHO) is the most common form of bone infection in children. About 50% of cases occur in children less than 5 years of age and it is twice as common in boys than in girls. Immunocompromised children and children with underlying haematological disorders such as sickle cell disease are more prone to these infections.[16] Infections are commonest in long bones such as the femur, tibia or humerus, with most cases limited to single bone involvement. Less than 10% of cases involve two or more locations,[17] the corollary of which is that multifocal involvement does not exclude acute osteomyelitis (the same is true for septic arthritis).

Pathophysiology

Haematogenous spread is the most common route to bones and joints, though implantation at trauma or surgery and spread from contiguous infection may also occur. Infection usually starts in the metaphysis due to its rich blood supply. From here the infection may spread to the bone cortex and penetrate the loosely attached periosteum, eliciting a periosteal reaction. It may perforate the periosteum and spread to adjacent muscles and soft tissues, forming abscesses. Less commonly, the infection may spread to the epiphyseal plates and joints, causing septic arthritis. In neonates, the metaphyseal capillaries form a connection with the epiphyseal plate, thus increasing the chance of joint infection. In later infancy, these vessels atrophy and there is thickening of the cortex, thus reducing the risk of growth plate involvement and septic arthritis.

Staphylococcus aureus accounts for approximately 60–90% of childhood AHO, followed by group A β-haemolytic streptococci (10%). Other causes include *H. influenzae* and *S. pneumoniae*. *Salmonella* infections were historically common in patients with sickle cell disease but this seemed to reflect the organism prevalence in the population. *Pseudomonas* infections can be seen after puncture wounds of the feet. In neonates, again, *S. aureus* infections predominate, but group B streptococcus and *E. coli* infections are also common.[16,18]

Clinical Features

A few well-recognised clinical presentations of bone and joint infections are seen in children.

Acute osteomyelitis, more common in boys, usually occurs between ages 1 and 10 years. The lower limbs are usually involved. Children usually present with pain and reluctance to use the affected limb. The cardinal signs of acute inflammation, including pain, redness and swelling, may not be present initially, may develop later and may be associated with systemic illness. Often pain is localised and prompt diagnosis and treatment offers a good prognosis.

Chronic osteomyelitis has a more insidious onset over a few weeks and is more difficult to diagnose. There is usually minimal loss of function. Systemic signs are usually absent, but local tenderness may be present. Radiographs are usually helpful as bone changes are usually present by the time medical attention is sought. Chronic osteomyelitis is further discussed under adult infections.

Septic arthritis is also twice as common in boys, with a peak incidence below 3 years of age. Symptoms include pain and swelling around the joint with reluctance to move the limb. Pseudo-paralysis and painful passive movements may be present. There are systemic symptoms and there is rapid progression of symptoms. Diagnosis is more difficult in neonates. The joint is warm and ultrasound can demonstrate a joint effusion. The lower limbs are usually involved, particularly the hip or knee.

Neonatal osteomyelitis and septic arthritis are probably different manifestations of the same condition: 75% of the children are not severely ill and present as failure to thrive. Prognosis is not as good as there is usually a delay in diagnosis.

Disseminated staphylococcal disease presents as a rapidly progressive severe life-threatening illness with virulent bacteraemia and multiorgan involvement, but fortunately is rare.

Investigations and Management

Thorough clinical examination and laboratory investigations are extremely important in diagnosis, before imaging evaluation is performed. Conventional radiography is still one of the most important investigations for diagnosis. The other imaging investigations, ultrasound, CT, MRI and scintigraphic studies are also used. The risk/benefits and costs of these tests, their radiation exposure, requirements for sedation or anaesthesia need to be assessed carefully as investigations are planned.

Plain Radiographs

In acute osteomyelitis, plain radiographs are extremely useful to exclude other lesions such as fractures, Perthes' disease and slipped femoral epiphysis. In septic arthritis the joint space is initially expanded with fluid and may give rise to some asymmetry in the position of the epiphysis, but ultrasound is more reliable to demonstrate fluid in the joint. In subacute osteomyelitis, periosteal reaction, new bone formation and occasionally lucent lesions (Brodie's abscess) in the metaphysical region may be seen. Chronic osteomyelitis shows bone sclerosis, destruction, and periosteal new bone formation.

Ultrasound

Ultrasound has an important role in demonstrating increased joint fluid early in acute septic arthritis and is also used to guide aspiration of the joint effusion for diagnostic and therapeutic purposes (Fig. 9-1). In septic arthritis the cellular debris-laden effusion may be echoic, rendering it less conspicuous. Demonstrating movement of this debris by varying the US probe pressure during the examination may reduce false-negative interpretation. Subperiosteal abscess can be demonstrated as hypoechoic fluid along the bone surface in acute and subacute disease. Soft-tissue abscesses can also be seen as hypoechoic fluid with thick walls that may show increased colour Doppler flow. Direct aspiration under ultrasound guidance and culture and sensitivity of the aspirate is extremely helpful to confirm diagnosis and for further treatment with the appropriate antibiotics. Soft-tissue abnormalities can also be demonstrated with ultrasound, though MRI is more reliable.

Computed Tomography

This investigation is less useful in a paediatric population due to its radiation dose and lack of specific advantages, and MRI is preferred.

Magnetic Resonance Imaging

MRI is the investigation of choice for the diagnosis of acute, subacute and chronic osteomyelitis with high sensitivity and specificity. The characteristic signs of acute osteomyelitis in children include bone marrow oedema, which is seen as low T1 signal in the bone marrow, along with high signal on T2 and STIR images.[19] Abscesses are seen both early and late in disease, as well-defined

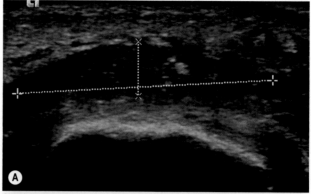

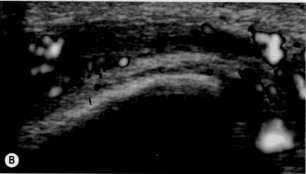

FIGURE 9-1 ■ **Septic arthritis in a child.** (A) Ultrasound of the right knee in a limping 3-year-old child demonstrates the presence of echogenic fluid in the prepatellar bursa. (B) There is increased colour Doppler flow in the surrounding soft tissues and wall of the bursa. The finding of an infected bursa should arouse the possibility of adjacent septic arthritis.

low-signal collections on T1, high signal similar to fluid on T2 images, with enhancing walls on post contrast sequences (Fig. 9-2). This may be seen in the bone, adjacent soft tissues or subperiosteal location due to the loose attachment of the periosteum to the underlying bone in children. Septic arthritis is diagnosed by the presence of a joint effusion, abnormal bone marrow signal localised to either side of the joint or synovial thickening which also shows post contrast enhancement. Physeal involvement is characterised by low T1 and hyperintense T2 signal along the growth plate associated with widening of the growth plate and enhancement on post contrast imaging (Fig. 9-3). Later in the course of the infection, chondrolysis occurs.

Fat-saturated T1-weighted (T1W) images with intravenous contrast medium can increase confidence in the diagnosis of osteomyelitis and also help diagnose complications such as septic arthritis, physeal involvement, intra-osseous, subperiosteal and soft-tissue abscesses. Intravenous gadolinium is most useful to identify non-enhancing abscess collections within a background of soft-tissue and bone marrow oedema and to aid differentiation between granulation tissue and true abscess. It is generally not useful if unenhanced images show no evidence of soft-tissue or bone marrow oedema. The merits of administering intravenous contrast agents should be weighed against its injudicious use in children.[20]

The rim sign is seen in chronic osteomyelitis as a low-signal area of fibrosis surrounding an area of active

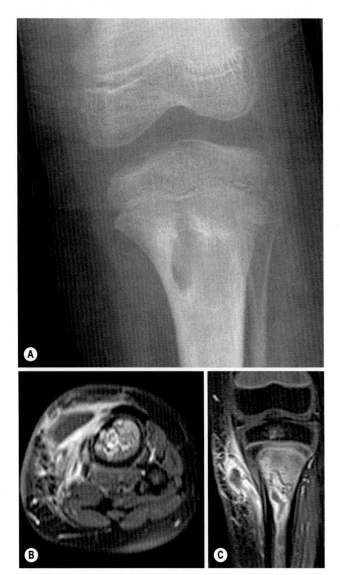

FIGURE 9-2 ■ Osteomyelitis with abscesses in a child. (A) AP radiograph of the left knee showing a lucent metaphyseal lesion of the tibia with surrounding sclerosis. (B) Axial and (C) coronal post-contrast T1-weighted fat-saturated images confirm the presence of a bone abscess, with surrounding oedema of the metaphysis. There is also focal epiphyseal involvement and an abscess in the medial soft tissues.

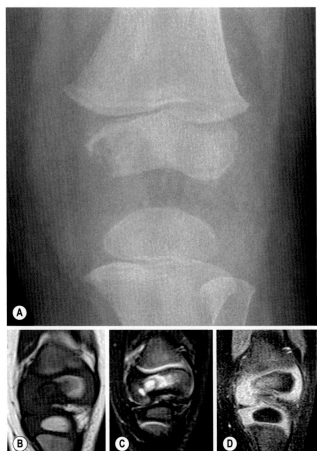

FIGURE 9-3 ■ Osteomyelitis in an 18-month-old child. (A) AP radiograph shows irregularity, erosion and rarefaction of the femoral epiphysis. (B) Coronal T1W image showing low T1 signal at the site of epiphyseal destruction, loss of normal fat signal and destruction of medial aspect of left femoral epiphysis. (C) Coronal STIR image demonstrates high signal in the affected epiphysis. (D) Coronal T1 fat-saturated enhanced image demonstrates abnormal enhancement in the affected medial epiphysis due to active infection.

infection. Active infection has high signal on T2, whereas the rim has low signal on all sequences. There may also be thickening and remodelling of cortex due to chronic infection. Periosteal reaction may not be present at this stage. Bone abscess is seen as fluid signal surrounded by a thick wall that has low signal on T1 and significant enhancement. Abscesses may extend through the cortex into the surrounding soft tissues with the formation of sinuses. There is high T2 signal return from surrounding soft tissues, with loss of normal fat signal on T1 and T2 images (Fig. 9-4).

Post-surgical or interventional procedures cause bone signal changes that can persist for up to 12 months. Hence, whenever possible, MRI should be obtained before any interventions are performed, to avoid the need

for additional procedures.[21] Whole-body MRI may be useful to demonstrate multiple sites of involvement.

Nuclear Medicine

In early stages, three-phase ^{99m}Tc-MDP skeletal scintigraphy may be useful for demonstrating increased radioactivity in the affected bone and also for demonstrating multifocal disease. Increased activity may be seen in dynamic perfusion, early blood pool and delayed images. However, such uptake is non-specific and may be seen in other conditions including trauma and tumours. Use of Ga-67 citrate and [111]indium-labelled leucocytes will increase the specificity for infection up to 80%.[13]

Chronic Recurrent Multifocal Osteomyelitis (CRMO)

This uncommon form of non-bacterial inflammatory osteomyelitis occurs in children, usually less than 18

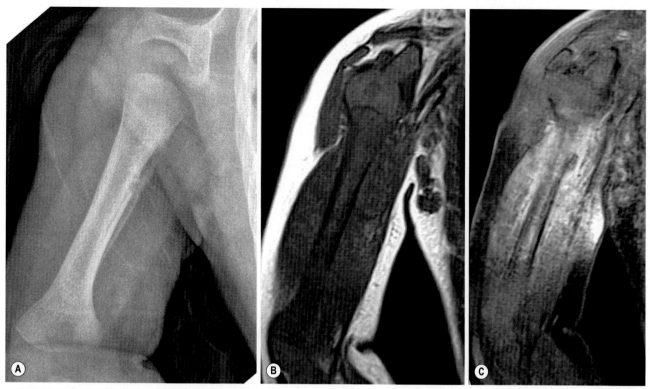

FIGURE 9-4 ■ **Osteomyelitis of the humerus in a child.** (A) Plain radiograph of a child with humeral osteomyelitis showing abnormal texture of medullary bone, with cortical destruction and periosteal reaction. (B) Coronal T1 and (C) fat-suppressed PD-weighted images show low T1 signal in bone marrow, which is hyperintense on the fat-suppressed PD image. Periosteal reaction, cortical destruction and adjacent soft-tissue oedema (seen as low T1 and high T2 signal abnormality) is also evident.

years of age. The aetiology is not known, but may be related to autoimmune disorders due to its association with inflammatory bowel disease and psoriasis-like skin conditions. A genetic aetiology is also postulated due to an association with mutation of the *LPIN2* gene. It is characterised by recurrent bouts of inflammatory arthritis and features of osteomyelitis which undergo spontaneous remission. It is more common in the lower limbs and may be symmetrical. Metaphyseal lesions occur in approximately 75% of cases. Symptoms are vague and it may present as monoarthritis or polyarthrits. When a single site of disease is present, the term chronic non-bacterial osteomyelitis is used.[22] There may be mild elevation of inflammatory markers but lab diagnosis is generally not helpful. Cultures do not reveal any organisms. Plain radiographs may reveal osteolytic lesions with surrounding sclerosis. Whole-body MRI can be helpful by identifying multiple sites of the disease, some of which may be asymptomatic. Typically MRI reveals periostitis, bone marrow oedema and signs of transphysitis.[23] Many lesions may heal spontaneously, though symptoms may persist for several years. Diagnosis is made by exclusion and from clinical history and typical radiological findings affecting multiple sites and recurrent negative cultures and bone biopsy. Majeed syndrome is an autosomal recessive disorder comprising a triad of CRMO, congenital dyserythropoietic anaemia and inflammatory dermatosis.

SAPHO Syndrome

This is considered as a form of CRMO and occurs in children and young adults, commonest between the second and third decades of life.[23] It is characterised by the presence of synovitis, acne, pustulosis, hyperostosis and osteitis (SAPHO). Skin manifestations and osteoarticular involvement commonly occur. Skin manifestation includes palmoplantar pustulosis and acne. There is bilateral symmetric pain and swelling of the bones and joints. The metaphyses of the tubular bones are commonly affected, though flat bones and axial skeletal sites may also be affected. Biopsy demonstrates acute and chronic inflammatory cells. Relationship to *Propionibacterium acnes* has been postulated but is debatable.[24] Treatment is by non-steroidal anti-inflammatory drugs (NSAIDs) in the first instance but severe cases may need immunosuppressive treatment.

Sclerosing Osteomyelitis of Garré

This is a chronic form of osteomyelitis, usually occurring in children, and commonly affects the mandible. This is considered as a form of CRMO affecting the mandible. Patients present with pain and hard swelling of the mandible. Initial findings include lytic lesions of the mandible associated with sclerosis. With disease progression there is non-suppurative ossifying periostitis with subperiosteal new bone formation and sclerosis.[25] The diagnosis can be made presumptively by radiology, and biopsy reveals features of chronic osteomyelitis, with cultures usually negative.[23]

Necrotising Fasciitis

This is a rapidly progressive life-threatening infection occurring in young children and more common in males. This condition also occurs in adults. Risk factors include immunocompromise, diabetes, intravenous drugs or alcohol abuse and patients with peripheral vascular disease. The condition is polymicrobial in origin, and includes Gram-positive aerobes like group A β-haemolytic streptococcus, *S. aureus*, Gram-negative organisms like *E. coli*, *Pseudomonas aeruginosa* and anaerobes like *Bacteroides*. *Clostridium* infection leads to a gas-producing necrotic infection, gas gangrene, which is rapidly progressive and leads to systemic toxicity and shock. Characteristically, the gas is intramuscular in gas gangrene, giving rise to gas loculi that are elongated and aligned with the muscle fascicles, whilst more globular gas loculi are seen in fasciitis, when a gas-forming organism is present.

The infection involves deep subcutaneous tissues and is associated with a high mortality. Infection causes thrombosis of small blood vessels, leading to necrosis and rapidly involving several facial planes. The condition has been associated with trauma, burns, eczema and varicella infections. The extensive soft-tissue damage leads to multi-organ failure and shock.[26]

Ultrasound can be useful in diagnosing the abnormal muscle echo texture, but MRI is more reliable and is needed to assess the extent of tissue damage and demonstrate the spread of infection along the facial planes. CT may also be useful, but MRI is preferred due to better soft-tissue contrast and lack of radiation. Emergency surgical debridement is needed to stop the progress of this fulminating condition; relevant imaging must therefore be performed immediately.

ADULT MUSCULOSKELETAL INFECTIONS

Spontaneous musculoskeletal infections in adults are less common than in children and are usually due to trauma, previous surgery or underlying immunodeficiency disorders. Trauma and open wounds can result in seeding of bone with microorganisms and to development of osteomyelitis. Whilst haematogenous infection is common in childhood osteomyelitis, in adults, it is mostly responsible for vertebral osteomyelitis. Apart from trauma, infection can also develop in prosthetic implants after surgery. Underlying conditions like diabetes, vascular insufficiency, decubitus ulcers and sinuses can predispose to development of osteomyelitis in adults. Osteomyelitis is classified by the time since onset, as described earlier.[27,28]

Pathogenesis

Healthy adult bone is usually resistant to infection, but when affected can be difficult to treat. The presence of dead bone and implants make it difficult to treat by antimicrobial agents and removal of the debris and the prosthetic implants is necessary to eradicate the infection. The bacteria attach to the bone matrix and orthopaedic implant devices by developing receptors to fibronectin and other structural proteins. They develop a slimy coat and a very slow metabolic rate, hide in intracellular locations and are thus able to elude host defences and antibiotics. The presence of implants also causes cell dysfunction which decreases the ability of polymorphonuclear cells to phagocytise bacteria. Reactions between the bacteria and the host defences cause release of cytokines and consequent osteolysis.[29]

Patients with sickle cell disease are prone to developing enteric bacterial osteomyelitis. In sickle cell disease, there is impaired gut defence due to sickling in the vasculature of gut. This enables the entry of organisms into the bloodstream, and haematogenous spread of infection into the bones. Typically this is *Salmonella* infection but this probably reflects the prevalence of *Salmonella* in countries where sickle cell disease is common.[30]

Clinical Features

Clinical features are variable, but acute infections generally present with pain, swelling and redness of the affected area associated with systemic illness. Joint swelling, reduced mobility and features of overlying cellulitis may be present. In chronic infections, discharging sinuses may be present. Treatment may render chronic osteomyelitis inactive, but reactivation may occur, with recurrence of symptoms (pain, swelling, erythema, fever) and new radiographic features (bone destruction, periosteal reaction). Characteristic radiographic features of chronic osteomyelitis include intraosseous cavities which may contain separated fragments of necrotic bone (a sequestrum) with the surrounding bone becoming thickened and sclerotic (involucrum). The cavity may communicate with the surrounding soft tissue through cloacae in the involucrum, with sinus tracks to soft-tissue abscesses or cutaneous ulcers. Extrusion of sequestra may occur through these sinuses.

Investigations and Management

Laboratory investigations may demonstrate an increased white cell count, elevated C-reactive protein and ESR. In acute infections blood cultures may be positive. Culture of the pus from discharging sinuses is also useful, but generally has a low yield rate for microorganisms. Table 9-1 summarises the main imaging findings in acute, subacute and chronic osteomyelitis.

Plain Radiographs

In acute infections, plain radiographs are useful to exclude other lesions such as fractures or malignancy. Focal abnormalities occur in acute osteomyelitis, usually in the metaphyseal region. These are commonly lytic lesions with a narrow zone of transition but bone sclerosis can also occur. There may be associated soft-tissue abnormalities. In subacute osteomyelitis, periosteal reaction

TABLE 9-1   Imaging Findings in Osteomyelitis

	Plain Radiograph	CT	MRI	NM
Acute	Minimal findings Soft-tissue swelling may be seen	Not useful	Bone marrow oedema can occur as early as 24–48 h, seen as low T1, and high T2 signal	May show increased uptake, but takes a few days
Subacute	Lucent or sclerotic lesion, periosteal reaction, soft-tissue swelling	Cortical and marrow abnormalities, including abscess, periosteal reaction, soft-tissue oedema and abscess	Bone marrow changes, cortical abnormalities seen as thickening, bone abscess, periosteal reaction, increased T2 signal in soft tissues, abscess formation. Post-gadolinium T1W sequences outline abscess cavities clearly	Three-phase bone scintigram, [111]indium WBC scan and combined studies are useful, especially to assess multifocal involvement. PET-CT generally not used in this context, but may be useful in exceptional circumstances
Chronic	Bone sclerosis, cortical thickening, sequestrum and cloaca, bone destruction, resorption and deformities	Much better than plain radiographs to demonstrate cloaca and sequestrum, periosteal new bone formation and abscess	Better soft-tissue and bone marrow resolution to demonstrate medullary and cortical changes, sequestra and cloaca well demonstrated, useful to outline soft-tissue abscess and sinus tracts	Generally useful if there is a problem with diagnosis. Combined WBC and bone marrow scintigram is useful. May highlight multiple sites of involvement

and cortical thickening also occur. As the disease progresses, bone sclerosis, thickening, resorption and destruction resulting in deformities may occur (Fig. 9-5). Septic arthritis can destroy the joint, resulting in joint fusion and deformities.

Ultrasound

Ultrasound is a simple, non-expensive bedside investigation that can be extremely useful in the acute setting with ease of performing interventions in the same setting. Cellulitis is easily demonstrated as oedema and thickening of the subcutaneous tissues.[31] This creates a cobblestone pattern due to anechoic strands randomly traversing the subcutaneous tissues.

Infective bursitis is demonstrated by the presence of excess fluid in the bursa, wall thickening with increased colour Doppler flow due to inflammatory changes in the affected bursa. Prepatellar and olecranon bursae are the most commonly affected. Fluid aspiration for diagnosis by microscopy and culture under ultrasound guidance also offers therapeutic benefit.

Tenosynovitis shows thickening of the tendon sheath associated with fluid surrounding the tendon itself. There may be non-compressible thickening of the tendon sheath which also demonstrates increased colour Doppler flow due to hyperaemia.[32] It is difficult to differentiate inflammatory tenosynovitis from infection, and aspiration and cytology will confirm the diagnosis (Fig. 9-6).

In the appropriate clinical setting, septic arthritis is confirmed by the presence of fluid in the affected joint and can usually be readily demonstrated by ultrasound, though turbid fluid may be echogenic and more difficult to see. Ultrasound is particularly useful in the hip, where guided diagnostic aspiration can be performed. Early diagnosis can avoid serious consequences, especially in children, where an effusion can be the only sign localising infection to that joint. In the hands, wrists and feet joints,

diagnostic aspiration under ultrasound reduces the risk of contamination of other compartments.[26] Thickening of the synovium is seen in septic arthritis associated with lack of compressibility and increased colour Doppler flow due to the presence of inflammation, but can also be seen in other inflammatory and non-inflammatory arthritis.

Abscesses are usually well defined and show hypoechoic or anechoic fluid within, usually with a thick capsule which shows increased Doppler flow. Subperiosteal abscesses can also be demonstrated by ultrasound before a periosteal reaction is evident radiographically, but osteomyelitis generally needs further cross-sectional imaging. Pyomyositis shows abnormal echogenicity in early stages, but in later stages abscess formation is seen (Fig. 9-7). With prosthesis-related infection, ultrasound can be extremely useful to demonstrate fluid collections and diagnostic aspiration can be performed at the same time.

Computed Tomography

High-resolution, multiplanar reconstruction and wide availability result in CT being commonly used in the diagnosis and assessment of osteomyelitis. The main disadvantages of CT are exposure to ionising radiation and limited soft-tissue contrast.

The advantages of CT are that it can demonstrate periosteal reaction, subtle bone erosion, cortical destruction, abscess formation and soft-tissue swelling. CT may also demonstrate thickening of trabeculae and medullary abnormalities. In chronic osteomyelitis CT is better than MRI for the demonstration of cortical destruction and demonstrating the presence of gas (Fig. 9-8). CT is also superior to MRI in the demonstration of sequestra (Fig. 9-9), involucra and cloacae and can guide therapeutic options.[33] Soft-tissue abnormalities can be seen with CT, but MRI is superior for demonstrating these (Fig. 9-10).[34]

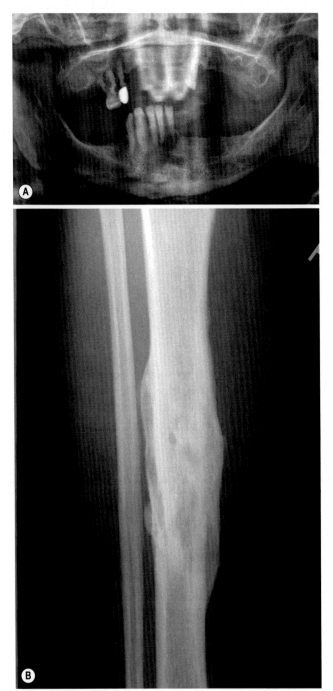

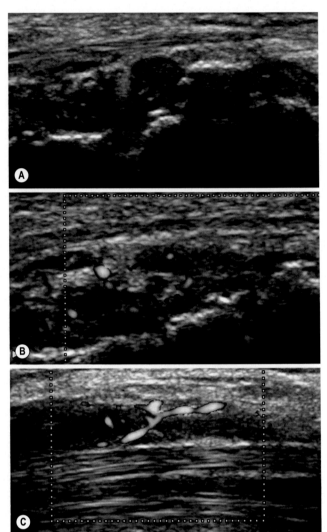

FIGURE 9-6 ■ **Ultrasound extremities.** (A) Ultrasound of the foot shows non-compressible synovial thickening with (B) increased colour Doppler flow over the dorsum of the foot. (C) Tenosynovitis of extensor tendons with synovial thickening and fluid around the extensor tendons of the hand. There is also increased colour Doppler flow suggesting active inflammation. These signs are rather non-specific and are associated with inflammatory conditions, but are also an important early findings in septic arthritis. If clinical symptoms are suspicious, diagnostic aspiration should be performed.

FIGURE 9-5 ■ **Chronic osteomyelitis.** (A) Plain radiograph of the mandible in an elderly patient shows increased bone density and cortical thickening on the left side due to chronic osteomyelitis. There is bone destruction from an associated dental abscess around the roots of the remaining incisors and caries in the remaining right upper molar tooth. (B) Chronic osteomyelitis of the tibia. There is cortical thickening and chronic periosteal new bone formation, forming an involucrum around an indistinct medullary cavity. There is a cloaca.

In the spine, CT is much more sensitive in demonstrating trabecular destruction and end-plate erosions than conventional radiography. Paravertebral abscesses may be demonstrated clearly with CT. Vertebral disc space narrowing is not reliably detected on axial images and requires sagittal reconstructions. Spinal canal stenosis and associated fractures of bones can also be clearly demonstrated.[35] In the absence of trauma, the presence of fat/fluid levels in the soft tissues around the bone, especially when associated with spongy bone destruction is an important and specific sign of underlying osteomyelitis.[29]

Periprosthetic infection may be demonstrated by CT. Artefacts due to beam hardening, from high density metallic prosthetic components can be minimised by using an extended CT number scale, a high kVp, acquiring data in thin sections then generating thicker section maximum intensity projection reformations and the use of iterative image reconstruction software designed to suppress metal artefacts.

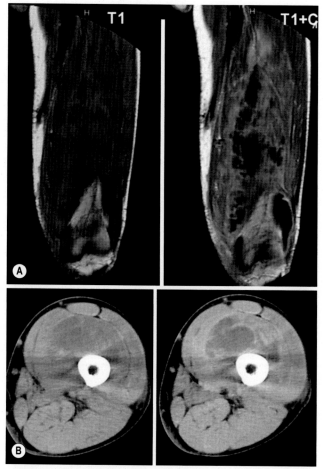

FIGURE 9-7 ■ **Pyomyositis.** (A) Coronal T1 pre- and post-contrast show an extensive intramuscular collection in the vastus inter-medius with irregular enhancing walls and septae. (B) Axial CT images before and after intravenous enhancement also demonstrate these features.

Magnetic Resonance Imaging

MRI has high accuracy and can be positive as early as 3–5 days after the onset of infection. The good soft-tissue contrast, high diagnostic accuracy and wide availability of MR imaging makes this the investigation of choice in suspected osteomyelitis.

T1- and T2-weighted (T2W) spin-echo (SE) sequences should be obtained in at least two planes: axial and coronal or sagittal. A short tau inversion recovery (STIR) sequence or fat-suppressed T2 sequence is useful to identify the bone marrow oedema and soft-tissue oedema easily. Usual slice thickness is 3–4 mm (Fig. 9-11).[36] Fat-suppressed images can identify ulceration, abscess formation and sinus tracts due to the accentuated fluid signal against a background of suppressed soft-tissue and marrow signals. Gadolinium-enhanced T1-weighted SE images with fat saturation help improve diagnostic confidence, although the overall sensitivity and specificity do not change significantly (Fig. 9-12).[33]

Bone marrow oedema is one of the earliest signs of osteomyelitis. In acute osteomyelitis there is increase in intramedullary water due to oedema, inflammation and ischaemia, resulting in areas returning low T1 signal and

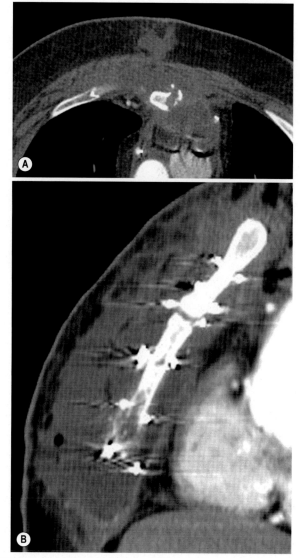

FIGURE 9-8 ■ **Subacute osteomyelitis of the sternum.** (A) Axial CT and (B) sagittal reconstruction through the sternum showing features of osteomyelitis following sternotomy. There is bone destruction and sclerosis along the margins of the sternotomy and a large abscess around the sternum extending to the mediastinum and subcutaneous tissues and containing a gas loculus. Osteomyelitis of the sternum also occurs in intravenous drug abusers.

increased T2 signal; this is even better appreciated on fat-saturated or STIR images. The marrow oedema is usually ill defined in its early stages. Later on with more localised bone destruction the oedema and signal changes appear well defined.[36]

Bone marrow oedema is more extensive in osteomyelitis than in degenerative or infective arthritis. Cortical disruption may lead to the development of periosteal reaction. Cortical disruption is seen as a break in the normal low signal of the cortical bone. Periostitis shows as thin linear pattern of oedema with enhancement, surrounding the outer cortical margin. Chronic periostitis and periosteal reaction are seen as thickening of low signal of cortical bone in both T1- and T2-weighted images.

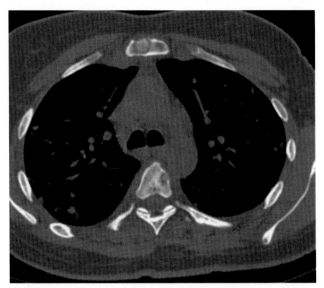

FIGURE 9-9 ■ **Chronic osteomyelitis with sequestra.** Axial CT thorax demonstrates lytic destructive bone lesions containing central sequestra in the sternum and spine. Pulmonary nodules are also present, due to disseminated TB.

In subacute osteomyelitis, an intramedullary abscess (Brodie's abscess) may be seen. The central fluid component has low-to-intermediate T1 signal and hyperintense T2 signal, surrounded by a sclerotic rim which has low T1 and T2 signal (Fig. 9-13).

The MR characteristics of a sequestrum are similar to the bone it is derived from. If it is from cortical bone, it has low signal, with a higher signal if derived from cancellous bone. The exudate in the presence of active infection tends to show a low T1 signal and high T2 signal, which may show enhancement, which is seen to surround the central sequestrum. The involucrum has the signal of normal living bone, but is commonly thickened and sclerotic and may show oedema. A cloaca is seen as a high signal defect in cortical bone at the edge of a cavity. Collections of pus may be seen extending from the cloaca to the subcutaneous tissue (Fig. 9-14).[36]

Soft-tissue oedema is demonstrated as low T1 signal on the background of high signal of the subcutaneous fat and has hyperintense signal compared to normal fat on T2 images. Fat-saturated proton density-weighted images and STIR images can demonstrate the soft-tissue changes more clearly.[37]

MR imaging can be useful in differentiating between acute osteomyelitis and acute bone infarction, especially after intravenous gadolinium contrast agents. Those with osteomyelitis showed a thick, irregular peripheral enhancement around a non-enhancing centre. Medullary infarctions show thin, linear rim enhancement or a long segment of serpiginous central medullary enhancement.[38]

Metal artefact suppression MRI techniques are useful for imaging close to prostheses. These include avoidance of gradient-echo sequences, use of STIR rather than fat suppression, acquiring the images on a high image matrix with a wide bandwidth and repeating sequences with swapped phase and frequency.

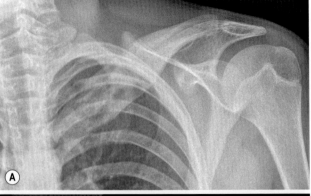

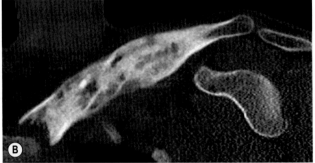

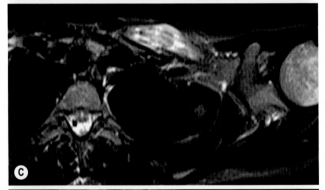

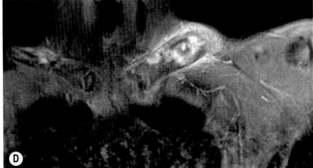

FIGURE 9-10 ■ **Chronic osteomyelitis clavicle.** (A) Plain radiograph of the left clavicle show features of chronic osteomyelitis. There is sclerosis and diffuse periosteal new bone formation. (B) CT of the clavicle shows diffuse bone sclerosis with multiple cavities and cloaca (arrow). (C, D) MR axial T2W and coronal PD fat-saturated images confirm the above findings. The cloaca is clearly seen in coronal images as a focus of hyperintense signal surrounded by a low signal area (arrow).

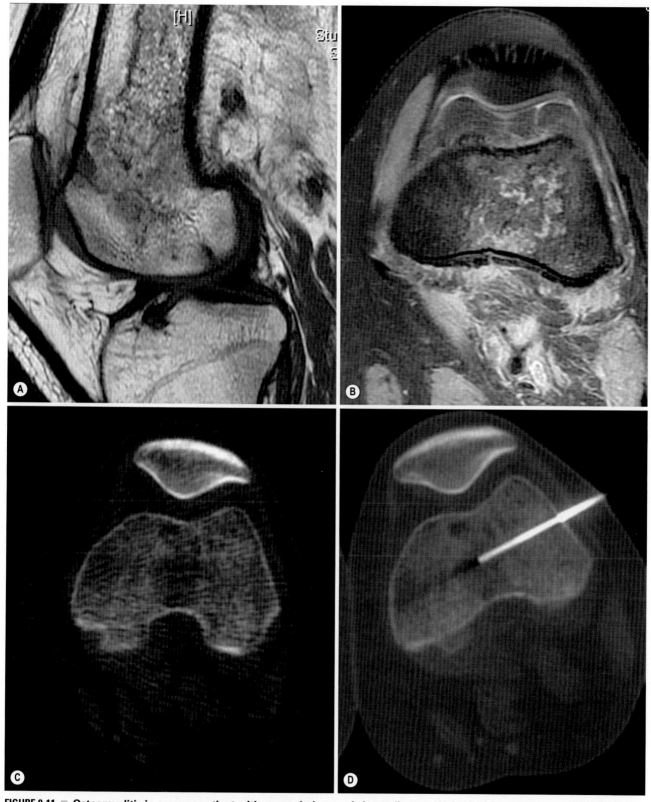

FIGURE 9-11 ■ **Osteomyelitis in a young patient with congenital cyanotic heart disease.** (A) Sagittal T2 and (B) axial PD STIR images demonstrate abnormal area of the medullary bone in the metaphysis extending into the epiphysis. There is associated soft-tissue oedema seen clearly on the PD images. (C) Axial CT through the epiphyseal region shows patchy trabecular bone lysis. (D) Subsequent biopsy confirmed the diagnosis of osteomyelitis.

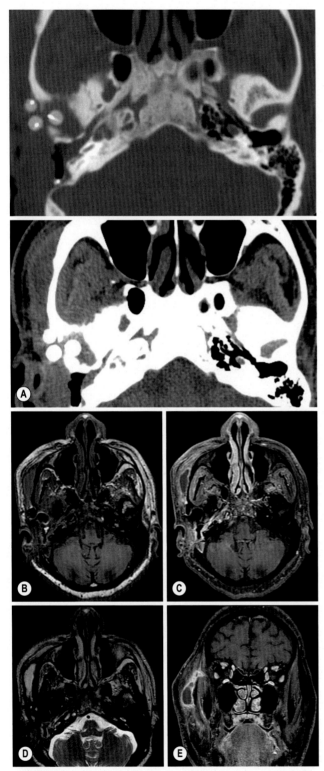

FIGURE 9-12 ■ Osteomyelitis of the zygoma as a complication of middle ear infection. (A) Axial CT image on bone and soft-tissue windows shows soft-tissue filling the right middle ear associated with bone destruction around the temporomandibular joint, antibiotic-impregnated beads within the bone cavity and an abscess around the arch of the zygoma. (B) Axial T1-weighted image, (C) axial fat-suppressed post-enhanced T1-weighted image, (D) axial T2-weighted image and (E) coronal fat-suppressed enhanced T1-weighted image all demonstrate the perizygomatic abscess, evidence of infection in the right middle ear and artefact from the metal wire in the antibiotic beads.

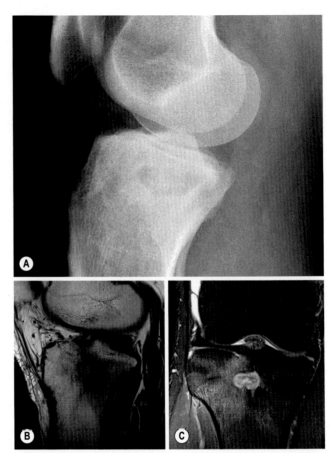

FIGURE 9-13 ■ Brodie's abscess of the tibia. (A) Lateral plain radiograph of the right tibia shows a well-defined lucent lesion with surrounding sclerosis, features of Brodie's intramedullary bone abscess. (B) Sagittal T1-weighted and (C) coronal PD-weighted with fat suppression show the well-defined Brodie's abscess with surrounding bone oedema.

Nuclear Medicine

Three-phase skeletal scintigraphy is generally useful in the diagnosis of osteomyelitis. However, in the presence of previous trauma, metal devices, neuropathic joints and pre-existing bone conditions, this becomes less reliable and indium and gallium studies play a role. The limiting factor in these investigations is the need for a second investigation such as MRI to confirm the diagnosis due to poor specificity and spatial resolution (Fig. 9-15).

PET-CT has some clear advantages over the conventional. Normal bone cortex has only low FDG uptake and the normal medulla shows slightly increased uptake compared to cortical bone. Hence, in osteomyelitis, increased uptake is a sensitive sign, but it is also positive in trauma, inflammatory diseases, and normal healing processes up to four months after surgery.

Prosthetic joint infection: differentiation between infection and loosening is paramount in the management of these cases, as infection may need removal of the metal prosthesis. FDG may not be accurate here, as hypercellular marrow around a prosthesis secondary to inflammation may show increased uptake both in loosening and infection. Combined [111]indium-labelled leucocytes and

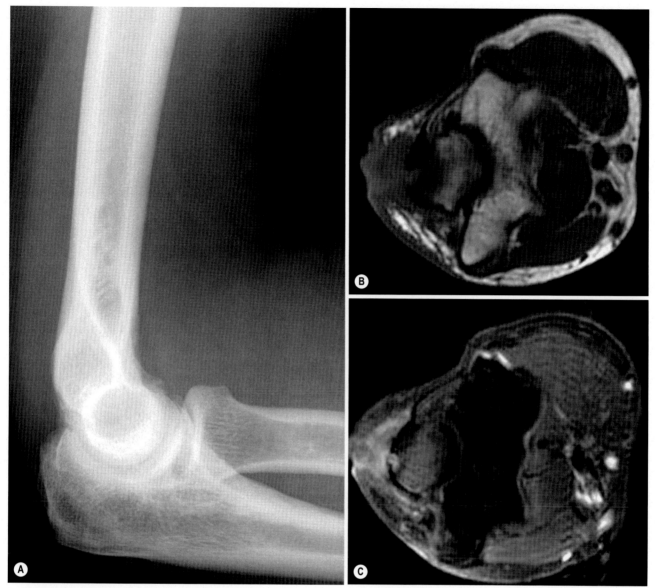

FIGURE 9-14 ■ **Osteomyelitis of the olecranon with a cloaca.** (A) Lateral radiograph of the right elbow shows abnormal bone texture of the olecranon with thinning of the cortex and a focal lytic area due to chronic osteomyelitis. (B) Axial T1-weighted and (C) T1 fat-saturated enhanced images showing abnormal bone marrow signal with low T1 signal which shows enhancement after intravenous contrast medium. There is a well-defined defect in the cortex which represents the cloaca (arrow), with formation of an abscess in the overlying subcutaneous tissue.

^{99m}Tc-sulphur colloids have an accuracy of more than 90% in diagnosing prosthetic infection and are the agents of choice (Figs. 9-16 and 9-17).[39]

Combined skeletal and gallium scintigraphy is the nuclear medicine investigation of choice in diagnosing spinal osteomyelitis and is valuable when there are contraindications for MRI. Gallium SPECT can also be equally useful. However, the procedure requires several patient visits to the department. PET-CT certainly has advantages in this respect and can be useful to diagnose vertebral osteomyelitis and also in localisation of abscesses (Fig. 9-18).

The investigation of choice for diagnosing diabetic foot infections is a labelled leucocyte study with an accuracy of 80%. Combined bone–leucocyte scintigraphy is the investigation of choice in detecting osteomyelitis on the background of neuropathic joints. PET-CT does not appear to have a definitive role in this setting.[40]

Osteomyelitis Secondary to Prosthetic Devices

Infections seen within 3 months of implant surgery are called 'early' and occur due to contamination during surgery or in the early postoperative days. The usual causative organism is *S. aureus*. Subacute infections occur between 3 and 24 months after the implant surgery and are usually caused by virulent coagulase-negative

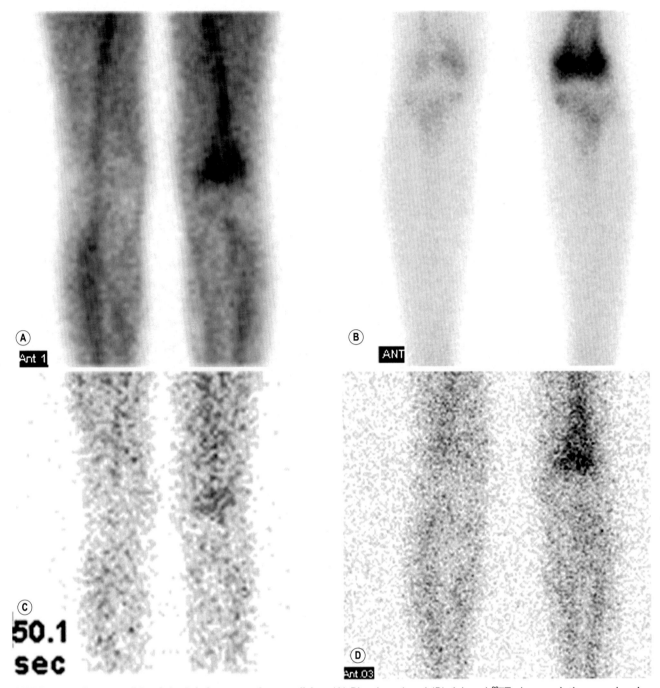

FIGURE 9-15 ■ **Osteomyelitis of the left femur: nuclear medicine.** (A) Blood pool and (B) delayed 99mTc bone scintigrams showing increased uptake in the left femoral condyle. (C) First circulation (selected image at 50 s) and (D) 3 days delayed 111In-labelled white cell scintigram showing increased uptake in the same area confirming the presence of osteomyelitis.

staphylococci or *S. epidermidis*. Chronic infections occur after 24 months and are usually due to haematogenous spread of infections from other sources.[8]

Diagnosis of prosthetic infections can be a clinical challenge and may warrant removal of the prosthetic device. Because of the similarities in the imaging appearances of aseptic loosening and prosthetic infection, no single investigation is conclusive. Plain radiography may not be useful in diagnosis but may demonstrate soft-tissue swelling or evidence of loosening. MRI has its

limitations due to the presence of artefacts from the metalwork, but sometimes is useful especially after intravenous gadolinium administration to demonstrate bone marrow oedema and fluid collections. Ultrasound is generally the investigation of choice to diagnose fluid collections around the prosthetic device and also to perform diagnostic aspirations for culture and sensitivity. CT with contrast also can demonstrate the presence of deeper collection that is not clearly seen on ultrasound. CT-guided aspirations can also be performed in deeper

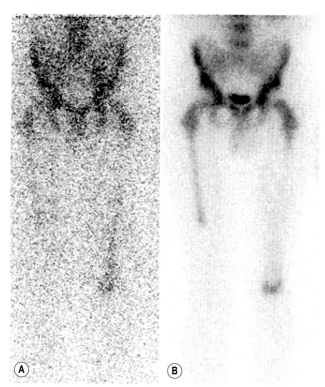

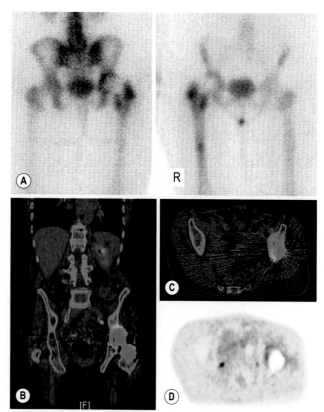

FIGURE 9-16 ■ **Osteomyelitis of left femur.** Combined ^{111}In and ^{99m}Tc-sulphur colloid bone scintigram. This is currently the gold standard for prosthesis-related bone infection. (A) Sulphur colloid is taken by normal bone marrow of left femur. (B) ^{111}In-labelled white cells accumulate around the site of infection only.

FIGURE 9-17 ■ **Prosthesis infection.** (A) Anterior and posterior views of a ^{99m}Tc-MDP bone scintigram showing increased uptake around a hip prosthesis. This was proved to be due to infection, though loosening or any other problem around the hip can produce increased uptake. Confirmation with MRI or ultrasound would be necessary. (B) Coronal reformatted fused PET-CT, (C) axial fused PET-CT and (D) axial PET images showing increased uptake around the prosthesis. Again this is non-specific and further evaluation would be warranted to confirm the diagnosis.

collections that cannot be clearly visualised on ultrasound (Fig. 9-19).

Skeletal scintigraphy is widely available and shows increased uptake of tracer around prostheses in the presence of infection. The appearance is generally due to osteolysis and thus can be similar in aseptic loosening. Gallium imaging, the uptake of which is related to inflammation in general, increases the overall accuracy to about 70–80%, but this is still less than satisfactory to separate infection from aseptic loosening.[41,42]

Combined labelled leucocyte and ^{99m}Tc-sulphur colloid imaging is currently the gold standard for imaging of prosthetic infections.[42] Sulphur colloid is taken up in normal marrow whilst labelled leucocytes accumulate at sites of infection as well as bone marrow. Hence if there is activity in the labelled leucocyte images in the suspected area without corresponding activity on sulphur colloid images, then prosthetic infection is confirmed with an accuracy of 95%. There are, however, several limitations including costs, the labour intensive in vitro labelling process, availability, and inconvenience for elderly and unwell patients. ^{111}In-labelled polyclonal immunoglobulin lacks specificity. ^{99m}Tc-sulphur colloid does not consistently differentiate infection from aseptic inflammation.[43]

Anti-granulocyte scintigraphy (AGS) with monoclonal antibodies or antibody fragments labelled with ^{99m}Tc has a reasonably high discriminating ability to identify prosthetic infection with a sensitivity of 83% and specificity of 80%.[44] PET-CT may also play a role in diagnosis of prosthetic infection, but is not widely used for this purpose at the current time and its role is still debatable.[43]

DIABETIC FOOT

Radiology plays an important role in the multidisciplinary approach to management of diabetic foot infections and osteomyelitis. The high risk of amputation in these patients if diagnosis is delayed necessitates the need for prompt and accurate investigation and treatment. The lifetime risk of foot ulceration in diabetic patients is as high as 25% and more than 50% of these become infected, which may need hospitalisation. Osseous involvement occurs in 20–50% of cases.[45,46]

Microangiopathy is the major initiating event in the cascade of foot infection and ulceration in these patients. Microangiopathy reduces the end-organ perfusion reserve despite revascularisation, contributing to development of bone and soft-tissue infections.

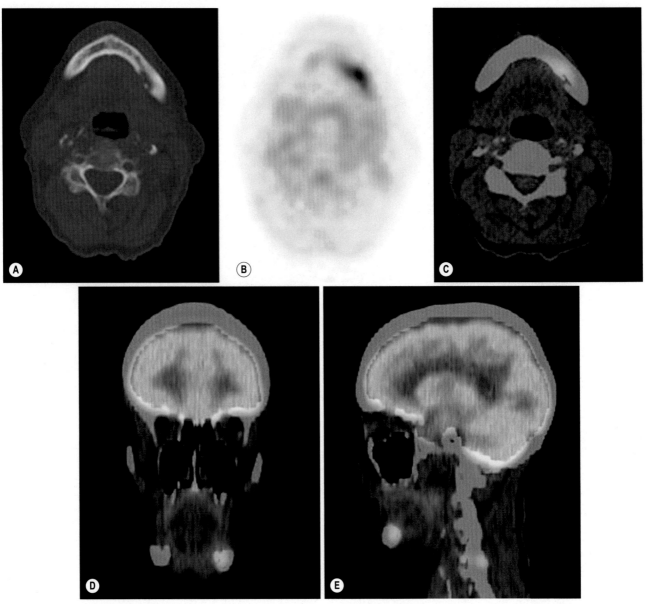

FIGURE 9-18 ■ **PET-CT in osteomyelitis.** (A) Axial CT through the mandible shows a lytic area with thickening of the adjacent mandible. (B) Axial PET image, and (C) axial, (D) coronal and (E) sagittal PET-CT fusion images show abnormal uptake of tracer in the left mandible, suggesting active infection.

A combination of motor, sensory and autonomic neuropathy contributes to development of foot ulcers, impaired healing and superadded infections.

The cause of foot infection is usually polymicrobial, commonly *S. aureus*, followed by *S. epidermidis*. Extension of soft-tissue infection into the bone causes osteomyelitis.

The clinical presentation of patients with diabetes and a foot complication is extremely important in the diagnostic algorithm. A warm, swollen foot with intact skin is probably an acute Charcot neuroarthropathy, whilst the presence of a cutaneous ulcer that can be probed down to the underlying bone surface is almost 100% diagnostic of underlying osteomyelitis. Imaging tests need to be over 95% sensitive and specific to alter these pre-test likelihoods.

The American College of Radiology introduced appropriateness criteria to select the appropriate imaging investigation(s) which will provide the most help in the management of diabetic osteomyelitis.[47]

Plain Radiography

Plain radiography of the toes, forefoot, foot, ankle or heel (tailored to the suspected site of infection) have Appropriateness Criteria score of 9 (9, most appropriate, to 1, least appropriate) in the diagnosis of osteomyelitis in diabetic foot infections in all forms of clinical presentations (Figs. 9-20 to 9-22). Radiographs have a sensitivity of 60% and specificity of 80% in the diagnosis of acute osteomyelitis in diabetic foot infections.[46]

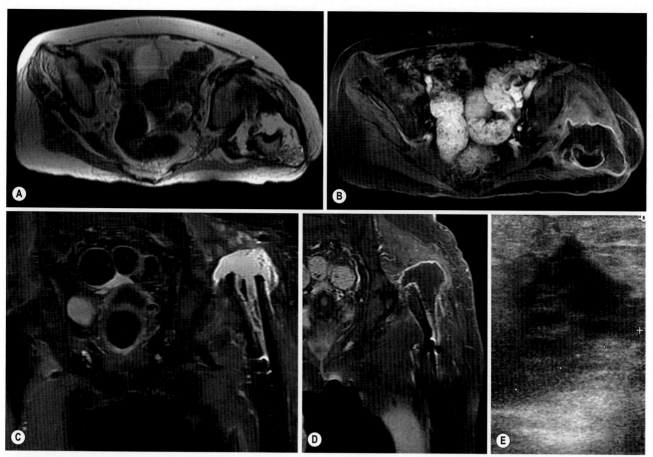

FIGURE 9-19 ■ **Girdlestone procedure infection.** (A) Axial T2W, (B) axial fat-suppressed post-contrast T1W, (C) coronal STIR and (D) coronal fat-suppressed post-enhanced T1W images through the left hip demonstrate a large abscess in the left hip after removal of a prosthesis. (E) The abscess was localised with ultrasound and aspiration of fluid under ultrasound guidance was performed. Culture of the fluid grew *Listeria monocytogenes.*

The earliest changes include soft-tissue swelling with loss of fat planes, though this is a rather non-specific finding.[48] The classic findings include the triad of *osteolysis, periosteal reaction and bone destruction.* These changes, however, take 10–20 days to be apparent on radiography. The changes may progress to destruction of the cortex, increased bone sclerosis due to sequestrum formation or loss of blood supply with bone necrosis. Bone resorption and auto-amputation occurs in chronic cases. The appearances are often difficult to assess in the presence of associated neuropathic arthropathy. Serial radiography is usually necessary to assess progressive changes. When the diagnosis of osteomyelitis is uncertain, use of MRI with or without contrast or three-phase skeletal scintigram is suggested.

Magnetic Resonance Imaging

After initial radiography, MRI is the investigation of choice in the evaluation of pedal osteomyelitis.[47] Bone marrow and soft-tissue abnormalities are usually demonstrated much earlier compared to plain radiographs. MRI has a sensitivity of 90% and specificity of 82.5% in the diagnosis of osteomyelitis[49] and is superior to ^{99m}Tc bone scanning, plain radiography and white blood cell studies.

High-resolution MRI examines the affected digit or foot with an extremity coil using thin slices (3–4 mm) and a small field of view (8–10 cm). Markers may be helpful for localisation of skin ulceration and clinical sites of swelling, giving increased accuracy of reporting. The patient is usually supine, or the forefoot may be imaged in the prone position with toes in an extremity coil. Imaging in at least two planes is needed for diagnosis and cross-referencing. Axial views are good for the anatomy of tendons and compartments. Sagittal and coronal views help to demonstrate ulcers and sinus tracts, especially when used with fat saturation. A combination of T1 SE, T2 SE or PD Fat Sat and STIR images may be used in different planes. Intravenous contrast medium is often useful. T1 is good for demonstrating the anatomy of bones and tendons. T2/STIR sequences are good for the demonstration of fluid and oedema. Intravenous contrast medium may help to define abscesses and sinuses clearly, but does not have proven value.[50-52]

MR may demonstrate bone marrow oedema, periosteal reaction, cellulitis, joint effusion, sinus tracts, foot ulcerations and callus formation and evidence of gangrene (Fig. 9-22).

Bone marrow oedema is seen as hyperintense signal on T2 imaging, accompanied by corresponding low signal intensity on T1 images. Absence of corresponding

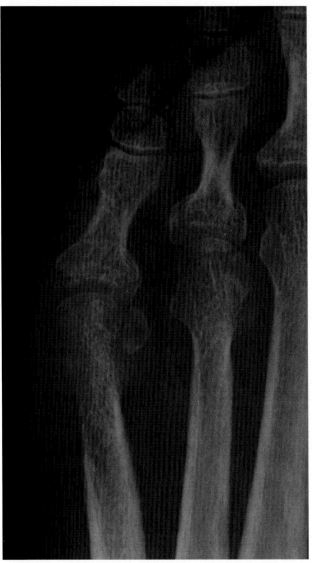

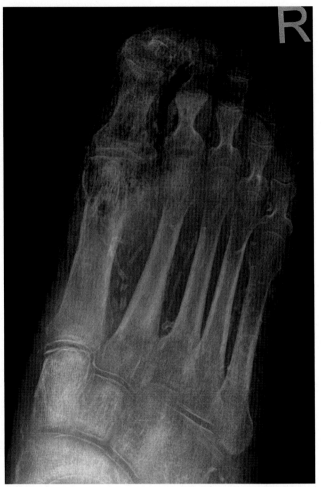

FIGURE 9-21 ■ Diabetic foot complication. Oblique radiograph of the foot shows extensive vascular calcification. There is gas in the soft tissues of the great toe; this more commonly occurs due to air forced in through an open ulcer than a gas-forming organism infection. The loss of soft tissue around the great toe indicates ischaemic mummification of the toe.

FIGURE 9-20 ■ Diabetic foot osteomyelitis. Cortical bone destruction is evident along the lateral edges of the fifth metatarsal head and base of the adjacent proximal phalanx, with overlying soft-tissue abnormality due to cutaneous ulceration.

low signal changes on T1 images is more likely to represent osteitis than osteomyelitis, even if bone marrow enhancement is present.[53,54] STIR sequences are useful to assess bone marrow oedema, but may overestimate disease by exaggerating high signal against the suppressed signal from normal soft tissues. Periosteal reaction is seen as low signal separated from the cortical bone by high signal fluid collection or oedema; it is usually seen in the metatarsals.[55] Periosteal reaction other than in metatarsals should raise the possibility of infection.

An intraosseous fluid collection is highly indicative of abscess formation. The penumbra sign is also a sign indicative of osteomyelitis; this is an area of intermediate signal on T1 image, surrounding a central low signal area representing the fluid collection. Joint effusion is evidenced by presence of fluid signal in the joint space associated with thickened (and enhancing) synovium.

Skin ulcers are represented as breaches in the skin signal intensity, usually low on T1 and T2 images, and have T2 a hyperintense signal around them caused by oedema. There may be hypertrophy of the edge of the ulcer, which is indurated and has low T2 signal. Sinus tracts are demonstrated as linear fluid containing tracts, hyperintense on T2 images, better seen on fat-saturated T2 or STIR sequences. If the tract is healing or healed, fluid may not be seen and the tract may yield low T2 signal; tract walls will enhance, producing a tramline appearance. Cellulitis is seen as soft-tissue oedema caused by infection and inflammation of the subcutaneous tissue. The normal subcutaneous fat yields high T1 and T2 signal; in cellulitis, low T1 signal and hyperintense T2 signal on fat-saturated sequences are present.[56]

In the diabetic foot it is often difficult to diagnose infections on the background of changes associated with neuropathic joints. This remains the prime diagnostic challenge in imaging of the diabetic foot. Both osteomyelitis and neuropathic osteoarthropathy can demonstrate bone marrow oedema, soft-tissue oedema, joint effusion and enhancement; the conditions often coexist and

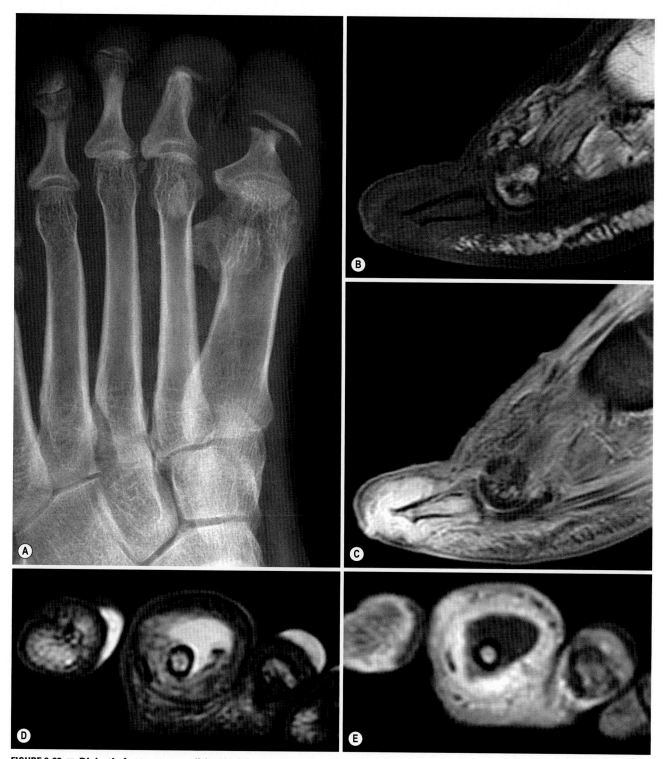

FIGURE 9-22 ■ **Diabetic foot osteomyelitis.** (A) DP radiograph in a diabetic patient showing complete destruction of distal phalanges and most of the middle phalanges of the 2nd–4th toes and the terminal phalanx and bone around the interphalangeal joint of the great toe. This 'sucked candy' appearance can be due to chronic neuropathy, however. (B) Sagittal T1W and (C) sagittal PDW fat-saturated images show the presence of bone marrow oedema, which has low T1 and high T2 signal. There is bone destruction and abscess formation around distal phalanx of the second toe. (D) Coronal PDW fat-saturated and (E) coronal T1 fat-saturated images following intravenous contrast medium demonstrate the extent of abscess formation, confirming active osteomyelitis.

correlation with clinical features is always recommended. There are, however, some features which may help to differentiate between the two and enable one to come to a conclusion of osteomyelitis, in the background of neuropathic joints. Some of these features will be briefly discussed below.

Neuropathic changes include multiple bone involvement, joint deformity, subluxation or dislocation, cortical fragmentation, low signal changes in subchondral bone on both T1 and T2 images, correlating with osteosclerosis on plain radiography. Periosteal new bone is seen exclusively in the metatarsals and phalanges. Neuropathic disease tends to affect intertarsal and tarsometatarsal joints in 60% cases followed by MTP joints in 30%.[57]

Single bone involvement usually favours osteomyelitis. Neuropathy is primarily an articular disease; thus bone marrow oedema may be juxta-articular, centred on subchondral bone, whereas oedema from osteomyelitis may be more diffuse and generally on one side of the joint. However, inflammatory or infective arthritis also tends to produce subchondral distribution of bone oedema. Associated soft-tissue changes, cellulitis, abscess formation and sinus tract suggest infection.

Joint effusion may be present in neuropathic joints with or without infection. However, superadded infection tends to produce thick rim enhancement, whereas neuropathic joint effusion without infection has thin rim enhancement.[56] Bone fragmentation and proliferation, subluxation and dislocations can occur in neuropathic joints with or without infection. Increased erosion occurs after infections, though it is also seen in neuropathic joints without infection.

Intra-articular bodies are more common in neuropathic joints with or without infection. Soft-tissue-related fluid collections are seen more often and are larger near infected joints. Soft-tissue signal abnormalities due to oedema are seen in both entities, but loss of subcutaneous fat signal is seen more with infection. Though ulceration is seen near both infected and non-infected joints, sinus formation is seen only in the presence of underlying osteomyelitis or septic arthritis.

Bone marrow signal abnormalities are seen in both, but intensity and extent of signal abnormalities are greater in the presence of infection. Bone marrow oedema associated with osteomyelitis has low T1, high T2 or STIR signal and shows post-contrast enhancement. Subchondral bone cysts are seen more in neuropathic joints without infection.[56]

Imaging of post-amputation diabetic patients for infection at the amputation margin is also a clinical challenge. The criteria for diagnosis of infection are the same as above after surgery, though it should be borne in mind that signal changes secondary to oedema from surgery should not be mistaken for osteomyelitis. Surprisingly little postoperative oedema is seen after amputation in these patients.[53]

SEPTIC ARTHRITIS

Most septic arthritis results from haematogenous seeding of the synovial membrane.[58] Because synovium lacks a basement membrane infection easily spreads into the joint. Infection can also spread from other source of infections, including endocarditis, sepsis, intravenous drug abuse and inoculation of foreign bodies.

Patients usually present with sudden onset of monoarticular arthritis, associated with systemic symptoms and clinical signs of a joint effusion. Joint effusion may be difficult to detect in shoulders, hips and sacroiliac joints. The knee joint is most commonly affected. Hips, shoulders or ankles are also commonly affected. Sternoclavicular joint infections occur in intravenous drug abusers.[59] In one study, the metatarsophalangeal joint was most commonly affected, followed by small joints of the foot, knee, sacroiliac joints and joints of upper limbs.[60]

Early diagnosis is critical in septic arthritis to avoid disabling outcomes. Delay in diagnosis may lead to development of cartilage and bone destruction due to the release of enzymes by the action of neutrophils, synovial cells and bacteria leading to permanent disability.[61] Before the era of MRI, early imaging findings in septic arthritis were considered non-specific and it was essentially a clinical diagnosis.[62] MRI has improved the diagnostic confidence of septic arthritis and clinical outcome.

Plain radiographs are not diagnostic in early septic arthritis but may reveal signs suggestive of a joint effusion. Subsequent cartilage destruction will result in joint space narrowing, provided the joint is not held open by an effusion. Lysis of the subchondral bone plate, erosions and adjacent bone destruction then occurs (Fig. 9-23). When these latter features are evident the prognosis is poor and diagnosis and urgent management should be achieved before these features have developed. Joint effusion, synovial thickening and increased vascularity can be demonstrated with ultrasound and this is more useful in small and superficial joints. CT may be useful if MRI is contraindicated. CT will reveal joint effusions, and may show bone erosions, bone destruction and synovial enhancement. CT or fluoroscopy may be used for guiding diagnostic aspiration, if ultrasound is difficult.

MRI findings in septic arthritis have now been well established and can occur as early as 24 hours after the onset of infection. MRI is especially useful in deep joints like shoulders and hips where clinical examination is difficult. Gadolinium-enhanced MRI with fat suppression has a sensitivity of 100% and specificity of 77% (Fig. 9-24).[63] There is usually a joint effusion, particularly in the larger joints, which may also be seen in other forms of arthritis. The degree of effusion is not reliable in differentiating between infective and non-infective arthritis. Enhancement of the joint effusion may be present.[60] There may be decrease in the perfusion of the bones. Synovial thickening may be present which is seen as intermediate signal on T2 images. Thickened synovium usually shows significantly more enhancement, compared to normal synovium. Synovial enhancement and joint effusion have the highest correlation with clinical diagnosis of septic arthritis.[60] High-resolution ultrasound may be more useful to demonstrate synovial thickening, especially in smaller joints. Synovial thickening is due to inflammation and vascular proliferation. Synovial outpouring may be present due to increased fluid pressure within the joint.

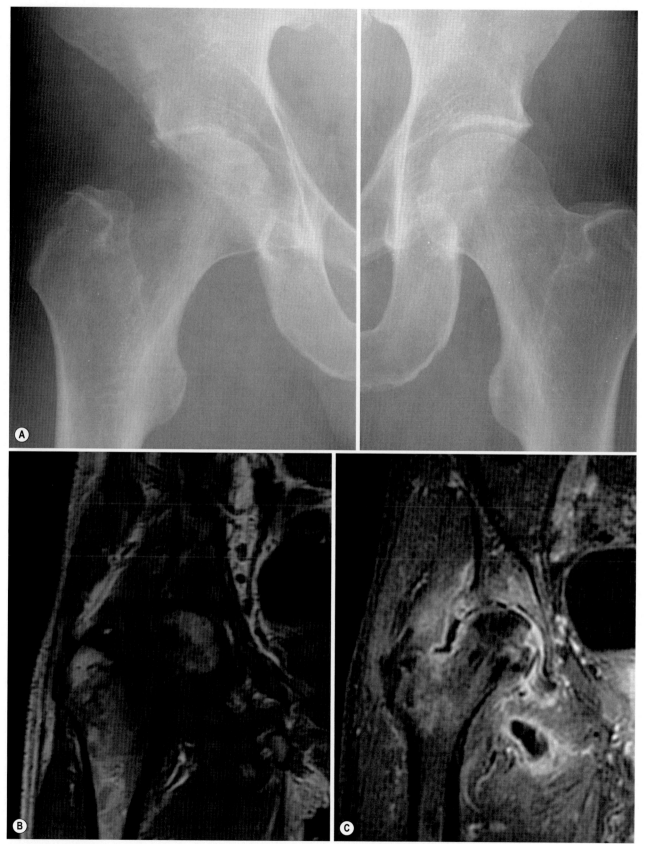

FIGURE 9-23 ■ **Septic arthritis.** Late presentation, three weeks after onset of symptoms in an intravenous drug user. (A) Plain radiograph demonstrates loss of joint space, marked reduction in bone density of the femoral head and partial destruction of the subchondral bone plate in the lateral part of the femoral head. (B) Coronal T1W and (C) enhanced fat-suppressed T1W images show a joint effusion with surrounding enhancement, enhancing bone marrow oedema and an abscess in the adjacent medial soft tissues. Despite immediate surgical arthrotomy and joint washout, the prognosis for this articulation is poor.

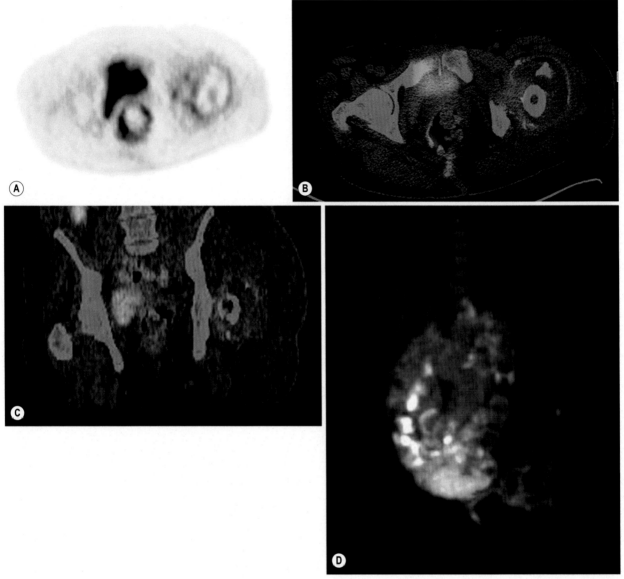

FIGURE 9-24 ■ **Septic arthritis.** (A) Axial PET and (B) axial and (C) coronal fused PET-CT images showing uptake of ^{18}F-FDG along the wall of an abscess cavity surrounding the dislocated proximal left femur after removal of an infected prosthesis. (D) PET MIP image outlines the abscess cavity and sinus tracks.

Septic arthritis progresses to destruction of articular cartilage and then the subchondral bone plate, which can be seen as irregularity of articular cartilage with high signal changes on T2 images with associated bony irregularities and erosions. Bone marrow signal abnormalities may occur due to oedema, and is usually not very extensive. The presence of extensive bone marrow changes, especially low signal on T1 images, should alert one to the possibility of underlying osteomyelitis.[62] Soft-tissue signal abnormalities may also be seen around the affected joints due to inflammation. Cellulitis may develop in muscles, leading to abscess formation in extreme cases.

The diagnosis of septic arthritis is made on the basis of a combination of clinical symptoms and radiology findings. The final diagnosis is made on the presence of positive culture on arthrocentesis, which can be performed under ultrasound, CT or fluoroscopy. Ultrasound is useful for small joints, hips, knees, ankles, paediatric patients and pregnant women. The shoulder, sternoclavicular and sacroiliac joints are more difficult with ultrasound and may require fluoroscopic or CT guidance. If pus is aspirated, as much fluid as possible should be aspirated to achieve decompression.[64] If there is only minimal fluid, saline irrigation of the joint may be performed and the aspirate sent for culture.[65] If culture is negative, a WBC count of more than 50,000/mL is useful to make a diagnosis of septic arthritis.[66] Material for culture should be obtained urgently and antibiotic therapy instigated as soon as possible. Relevant imaging should be performed as soon as possible and should not delay treatment.

MUSCULOSKELETAL TUBERCULOSIS

Tuberculous infections of the bones and joints are common in the developing countries, but are being seen with increasing frequency in developed countries due to increases in immigrant populations and the incidence of HIV, AIDS and other immunosuppressive conditions.

The causative organism is *Mycobacterium tuberculosis*. Haematogenous spread of the bacillus from a primary or reactivated focus in the body, to the bones or vertebrae (see below), is the most common mechanism of bone infection.[67]

Several forms of musculoskeletal tuberculosis are seen, which include tuberculous spondylitis, osteomyelitis, septic arthritis (Fig. 9-25), dactylitis, multifocal bone tuberculosis and soft-tissue infections.[68] Spinal TB is the most common form of tuberculous bone infection and accounts for about 50% of all musculoskeletal infections.[68,69] It is discussed separately in the section on spinal infection.

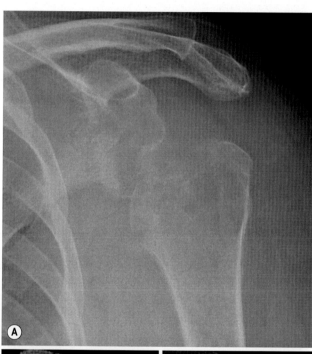

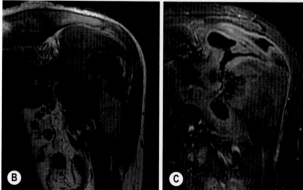

FIGURE 9-25 ■ Tuberculous arthritis. (A) Plain radiograph demonstrates extensive bone destruction in the glenoid and humeral head. This appearance in the humeral head has been termed 'caries sicca' (dry rot). (B) MR coronal T1W and (C) coronal enhanced fat-suppressed T1W sequences demonstrate a large joint effusion, extending into the adjacent soft tissues with surrounding enhancing walls and the bone destruction also evident on plain radiograph.

Pathogenesis

Pathologically chronic granulomas develop and are characterised by multinucleated giant cells, lymphocytes and macrophages, with central caeseating necrosis. In the spine this causes rarefaction and destruction of the vertebral end-plates and infection then spreads to adjacent discs.[68] There is late preservation of the intervertebral disc due to a lack of proteolytic enzymes which is somewhat dissimilar to pyogenic spinal infections where disc destruction is an early feature. In long bones, tuberculous arthritis usually starts as a bone infection in the metaphysis, which spreads to the epiphysis and then to the joint. Haematogenous spread is a less common mode of spread in tuberculous arthritis.

In the bones there is rarefaction, trabecular destruction, progressive demineralisation and bone and cartilage destruction. The consequent lytic lesions are well defined, with little surrounding bone regeneration and periosteal reaction. Para osseous abscess formation, called cold abscesses (as they are not warm or tender), may occur. Further extension into the soft tissues leads to sinus formation and skin ulceration.

Investigations (Table 9-2)

Plain Radiography

Plain radiographs are useful in established infection, but in acute infections abnormality is absent or subtle. Small bones may ultimately demonstrate abnormal marrow changes which include lytic lesions with rather thick and well-defined borders. Bony destruction may also be seen in established cases with joint deformities.

Computed Tomography

CT is more sensitive than plain radiographs to demonstrate cortical and trabecular bone destruction, and

TABLE 9-2 Features Which Aid in Distinguishing Pyogenic from Tuberculous Infection

Pyogenic Infection	Tuberculous Infection
Clinical symptoms are more acute and severe, with systemic toxicity and raised acute inflammatory markers	Insidious onset, less toxic, present as chronic infections
Subchondral bone marrow oedema prominent	Less prominent
Bone erosions less common	More common
Destruction of articular cartilage more common	Cartilage destruction occurs, but less common
Irregular synovial thickening, that shows avid post-contrast enhancement	Synovial thickening is smooth, and shows enhancement
Surrounding soft-tissue changes are prominent, ill-defined and more extensive	Well-defined inflammation and abscess with little surrounding signal changes, cold abscess
Usually a single site	Multiple sites of involvement common

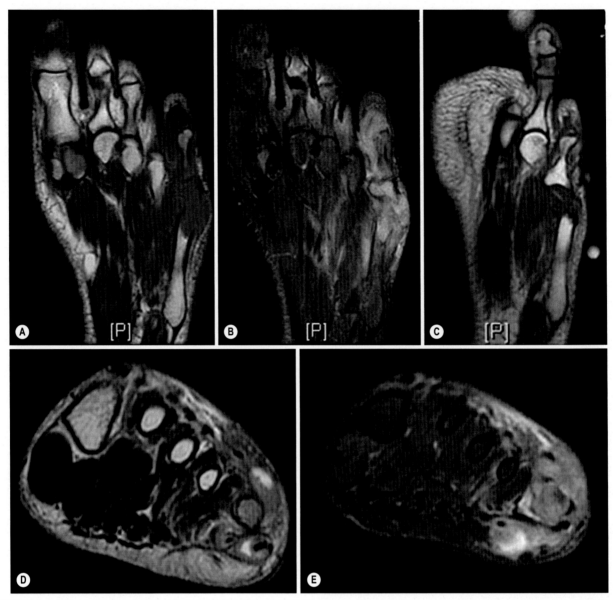

FIGURE 9-26 ■ **Tuberculous arthritis.** (A) Axial T1W, (B) axial PDW with fat suppression, (C) coronal T2 and (D) coronal PDW with fat-suppression images showing tuberculous septic arthritis with destruction of the head of the fifth metacarpal, associated with abscess formation. There is extension of the abscess into the subcutaneous tissues with sinus formation. (E) Axial T1W image, after chemotherapy for TB, showing significant improvement.

periosteal reaction. CT is generally useful for planning guided interventions—drainage of abscesses or planning/ guiding bone biopsies.

Magnetic Resonance Imaging

MRI can be useful in distinguishing between tuberculous and pyogenic arthritis, but the features show considerable overlap (Fig. 9-26). Bony erosions are more commonly seen in tuberculous arthritis compared to pyogenic arthritis. Subchondral bone marrow oedema is more prominent in pyogenic arthritis, best seen on T2 images with fat suppression. This may be better seen after gadolinium enhancement. Articular cartilage destruction may

be seen in both, but is earlier and more prominent in pyogenic arthritis.[70] Synovial thickening demonstrated as intermediate T2 signal is seen in both conditions. After gadolinium enhancement, synovial changes are more easily analysed and show smooth thickening in tuberculous arthritis compared to irregular thickening in pyogenic arthritis (Fig. 9-27). Surrounding soft-tissue changes are irregular and ill-defined in pyogenic arthritis, while in tuberculous infection tend to be better defined. Abscess cavities in tuberculous infection tend to have smooth and thin walls, with less prominent surrounding inflammation as these are cold abscesses (Fig. 9-28), whereas pyogenic abscesses tend to be more thick walled with pronounced surrounding inflammation.[70,71]

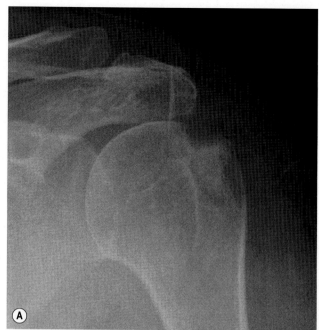

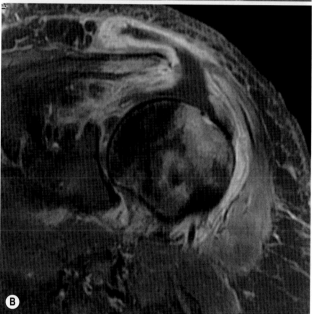

FIGURE 9-27 ■ Pyogenic septic arthritis. (A) Plain radiograph demonstrates a large acute bone erosion at the superior margin of the humeral head articular surface, in a patient with acute sepsis after shoulder arthroscopy. (B) MR coronal-enhanced fat-suppressed T1W image demonstrates marked thickening and enhancement of the synovium, marrow oedema and surrounding soft-tissue enhancement.

UNUSUAL MUSCULOSKELETAL INFECTIONS

Atypical Mycobacterial Musculoskeletal Infections

Atypical mycobacterial infections are also on the rise and are more resistant to treatment than tuberculosis.[72]

Musculoskeletal infections occur in approximately 5–10% of atypical mycobacterial infections. Most osseous infections are caused by *Mycobacterium kansasii* and *M. scrofulaceum*, followed by *M. avium-intercellulare* and *M. fortuitum*. The mode of infection may be haematogenous or by direct inoculation from surgical implants or trauma. Patients present with similar symptoms as mycobacterial infections but may be milder and more protracted. Fevers, chills, malaise and weight loss may occur. Early radiographic manifestation includes soft-tissue swelling due to inflammatory changes and regional hyperaemia. General radiographic observations include a tendency for metaphyseal or diaphyseal involvement. Bone resorption, osteolysis with periosteal reaction and bone marrow oedema occur, but take several weeks to be evident radiographically. Multiple sites of involvement, well-defined lytic lesions with marginal sclerosis and osteopenia are less striking than that seen in tuberculosis. In subacute and chronic forms bone abscess, sequestrum, involucrum and cloaca formation occur with the formation of sinus tracts. Spinal involvement, monoarticular arthritis and soft-tissue infections of tenosynovitis, septic bursitis or carpal tunnel syndrome occur and have radiographic changes similar to tuberculous disease.

Hydatid Disease

Infection of bone by the parasitic tapeworm *Echinococcus* is rare, accounting for less than 5% of cases of hydatidosis. Spinal and pelvic sites are commonest. Uni- or multiloculate intraosseous cysts which may expand the bone and extend into adjacent soft tissues are seen but are not specific. Serological tests are positive.

Bone Infections in Sickle Cell Disease

Sickle cell disease is an autosomal recessive condition that occurs as a result of a defect in haemoglobin S, affecting the β-chain. The mild, heterozygous form of the disease is called sickle cell trait, which results in a carrier status, without symptomatic disease. The effect of sickle cell disease is abnormal sickling of red blood cells within the capillaries and blood vessels, which result in vascular occlusion and infarction affecting various organs, called a 'sickling crisis'. Bone infarction can occur, resulting in severe pain. The effect of autosplenectomy due to recurrent splenic infarcts and the presence of bone infarcts predispose these patients to bone infections. Infection is usually caused by *Salmonella* organisms, the source of infection being the gut, followed by staphylococci infections.[73] Long bones and small bones are commonly affected. Radiographic appearances are similar to other forms of osteomyelitis, but a diagnostic challenge can occur due to pre-existing replacement of fatty marrow by red marrow secondary to intramedullary marrow hyperplasia causing abnormal bone marrow signal in the absence of infection. Also aseptic infarction can cause severe bone pain and can cause abnormal signal changes on MRI imaging and be confused with infection. Familiarity with the patterns of MRI appearances of bone infarcts and normal red bone changes is necessary to avoid overdiagnosis of osteomyelitis.

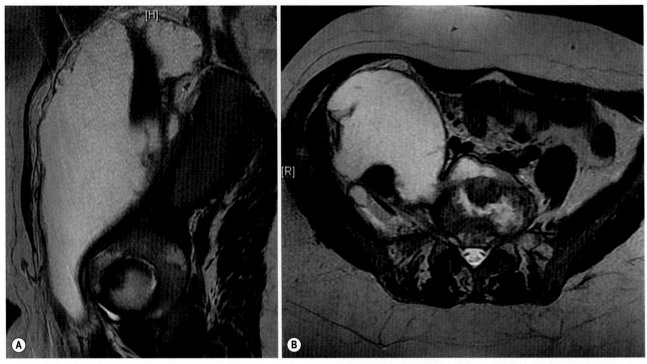

FIGURE 9-28 ■ Tuberculous 'cold' abscess. (A) MR sagittal and (B) axial T2W sequences demonstrate a large abscess extending over the surface of the psoas muscle in the pelvis, arising from tuberculous discitis at L4/5.

Bone infarcts typically affect small tubular bones of the hands and feet in children and long bone in adults. Lucency and periosteal reaction occurs in the early stages, which may proceed to sclerosis and bone infarcts and destruction. Avascular necrosis of the epiphyses of the femoral and humeral head is common and can be bilateral.

Blood cultures can be positive in up to 50% of cases and are essential for diagnosing osteomyelitis. Radiographic changes of bone infection are usually subtle in the early stages and may not be evident for up to 10 days after the onset of infection. Osteolysis and periosteal reaction are the initial findings. MRI is the optimal investigation for diagnosing bone infection as it can demonstrate bone marrow changes, abscesses, and periosteal reaction and helps to differentiate from bone infarction and avascular necrosis.[74] Bone infarcts tend to have a serpiginous appearance on MRI and avascular necrosis affects typical sites. Septic arthritis is less common than osteomyelitis. Combined leucocyte-labelled and Tc-sulphur colloid imaging may also help to differentiate between infection and infarction. Early diagnosis and treatment is important in preventing long-term complications in these patients.

Musculoskeletal Fungal Infections

High-risk patients for fungal infections include immunosuppressed HIV-positive patients, organ transplant recipients and patients on chemotherapy and long-term corticosteroids. Travel to endemic areas also increases the risk of infection. Infection occurs through skin inoculation or by the haematogenous route, usually via the lungs.

They cause granuloma formation and may show soft-tissue nodules, discharging sinuses, chronic multifocal osteomyelitis and joint infection.[75] Mixed sclerotic and lytic lesions can occur. Synovial thickening and features of chronic granulomatous arthritis are present and resemble osteoarticular tuberculosis.

Aspergillus fumigatus infection occurs via haematogenous spread from invasive pulmonary aspergillosis. The spine is most commonly affected, but infection can occur in other joints. Multifocal osteomyelitis, septic arthritis and discitis can occur. Diagnosis is made by synovial or bone biopsy.

Blastomycosis is endemic in the western United States, and bone infection affects the spine and lower limbs. Radiological features include those of chronic arthritis. Osteolytic lesions resembling bone tumours may occur and need bone biopsy for diagnosis.

Candida osteomyelitis presents as a lytic lesion without significant periosteal reaction, in immunosuppressed patients. Arthritis affects the larger joints.

Cryptococcosis occurs in immunosuppressed patients and may proceed to disseminated infection affecting larger joints, osteolytic lesions in flat bones and avascular necrosis.

Mycetoma tends to cause granulomatous infection of plantar subcutaneous tissue and proceed to cause chronic osteomyelitis, with multiple discharging sinuses. Mixed sclerotic and lytic lesions of bone are seen on radiographs. Chronic infection of the bones and soft tissues of the foot due to fungae or actinomycetes implanted by penetrating injury from thorns was described as 'Madura foot'. The soft-tissue abscesses in this condition characteristically contain multiple small cavities, each with a low

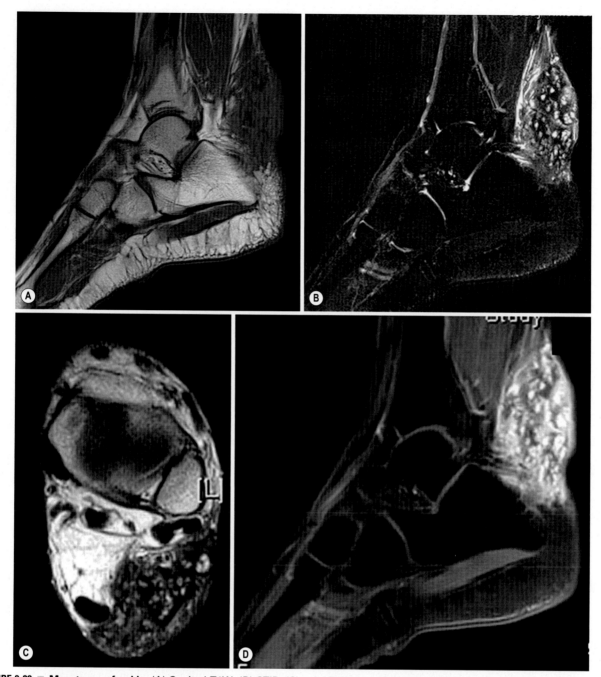

FIGURE 9-29 ■ **Mycetoma of ankle.** (A) Sagittal T1W, (B) STIR, (C) axial T2W and (D) sagittal fat-saturated enhanced T1W images of the ankle. A subcutaneous lesion demonstrating multiple low signal rings with central low signal dots on the T2W image and multiple avid ring enhancements with contrast is seen. The appearances on imaging mimicked a haemangioma, but the 'dot in a ring' appearance is typical of a mycetoma, which was confirmed on biopsy. (Courtesy of Dr R Mehan, Bolton Royal Hospital.)

signal centre on T2W MR imaging (the dot in a ring sign) (Fig. 9-29).

Musculoskeletal Infections in HIV Patients

Bone and joint infections were originally considered relatively rare in patients with HIV infections.[76,77] Infection is usually caused by opportunistic organisms like *Candida*, *Clostridium* and *Mycobacterium avium* complex. However, more recent studies show musculoskeletal infections as a relatively common manifestation in HIV patients.[78] The incidence also increases in IV drug-using HIV-infected patients. Apart from musculoskeletal manifestations of painful articular syndrome and non-infectious arthritis, musculoskeletal infections also occur in HIV patients. These include infectious myositis, septic arthritis, osteomyelitis and tuberculous arthritis.[78] Patients present with fever and arthritic symptoms, commonly affecting knees or ankles. *Staphylococcus aureus*, *Salmonella* and *Penicillium* infections were the commonest seen in these groups.

Radiographic findings include periarticular osteopenia, osteolysis and soft-tissue swellings and share similarities to other forms of osteomyelitis. Outcomes were generally poor in patients with bone infections.

DIFFERENTIAL DIAGNOSIS

Several other disorders may mimic osteomyelitis. *Inflammatory arthritis* may mimic septic arthritis in its early stages and a good clinical history is often the clue to diagnosis. As discussed earlier, both conditions may give rise to joint effusion, synovial thickening and post-contrast enhancement, though symptoms are usually severe with septic arthritis. *Bone infarcts* may mimic osteomyelitis in the acute stages and clinical features and laboratory tests often help in diagnosis. Bone infarcts have serpiginous appearances on MRI imaging, whilst osteomyelitis demonstrates more significant bone marrow oedema and post-contrast enhancement. *Tumours* are an important differential diagnosis in osteomyelitis and share several imaging features, including bone marrow oedema and contrast enhancement. Both lytic and sclerotic lesions with wide zones of transition and cortical destruction can occur with tumours and infection. Biopsy is sometimes needed to confirm the diagnosis and needs liaison with referring clinicians and pathologists. It is axiomatic that biopsy material should always be sent for both histological and microbiological assessment. Acute *diabetic neuropathic joints* are also difficult to differentiate from infection, as discussed earlier in detail. *Degenerative arthritis* can also cause diagnostic difficulties on imaging and clinical symptoms and history is important in management. *Granulomatous diseases* like giant cell tumour or Langerhans cell histiocytosis can also mimic infections of bone. Deposition diseases such as amyloidosis may also cause focal erosive bone lesions similar to infection.

MANAGEMENT

Good clinical history and thorough clinical examination is the most important step in early diagnosis of these infections. Laboratory tests are extremely useful in many instances to highlight the presence of acute infections. Blood cultures should be obtained whenever possible, before the start of treatment with antibiotics, as it helps in choosing the appropriate antibiotics. Culture of pus from sinus tracts, abscess cavities and effusions should also be performed whenever possible to obtain a microbiological diagnosis. It is important to have a multidisciplinary approach to choose appropriate investigations.

Percutaneous biopsy is an alternative to surgery in appropriate circumstances, being cost-effective and less invasive. Percutaneous bone or soft-tissue biopsy may be performed under ultrasonic, fluoroscopic or CT guidance to obtain a definitive diagnosis. This is a relatively safe procedure and extremely useful to confirm the diagnosis as the histological yield from the procedure is high. Abscess cavities and soft-tissue aspirates also require culture and sensitivity, along with cytology and histology, to analyse typical features of certain infections, like

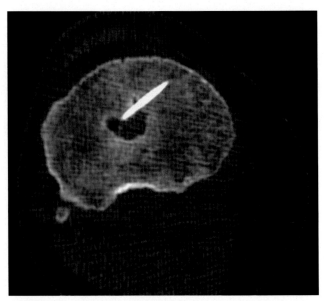

FIGURE 9-30 ■ **CT-guided bone biopsy.** Diagnosis of bone infection is confirmed by bone biopsy. CT remains the most useful tool for planning and guiding biopsy.

caseating necrosis in tuberculosis. Discussion with the referring team is necessary to plan the appropriate route for biopsy, in case the lesion in question turns out to be a malignancy. Departmental protocols should be present to ensure rapid transfer of specimens to the microbiology department in the appropriate transport medium.

Histological examination may reveal changes that are compatible with acute or chronic osteomyelitis. In acute osteomyelitis, there are acute inflammatory cells, neutrophils, congestion and thrombosis of medullary and periosteal blood vessels and necrotic bone. Chronic osteomyelitis shows lack of neutrophils, areas of fibrosis in bones, macrophages, lymphocytes and histiocytes.

Bone biopsy can be usually performed as an outpatient procedure under CT or fluoroscopic guidance (Figs. 9-8 and 9-30). The procedure is performed under local anaesthesia, augmented with nitrous oxide analgesia or conscious sedation if required. The coaxial bone biopsy technique is the one that is commonly used. Once the penetrating cannula is placed on the surface of the lesion, a biopsy needle is inserted and specimen is aspirated.[79] Positive culture rates are usually low and are about 35% for long bones. Cultures from the spine may reveal a higher yield rate, perhaps by sampling the infected disc. Surgical biopsies produce similar yields and thus carry no advantage over percutaneous biopsy. Positive culture rates are very low once antibiotic therapy has been instigated.

Treatment of osteomyelitis and soft-tissue infections needs aggressive antibiotic therapy, surgical debridement and removal of prostheses, depending on the severity of infection. Follow-up is necessary to assess response to treatment and modify treatment accordingly. Septic arthritis requires immediate arthrotomy and joint lavage and optimal antibiotic therapy, adjusted as required by discussion with the microbiologist.

SPINAL INFECTION

Vertebral Osteomyelitis

The incidence of vertebral osteomyelitis is 2.4/100,000 population per annum and tends to increase with increase in age.[80] Vertebral osteomyelitis may be acute, subacute or chronic.

Vertebral osteomyelitis may be pyogenic, tuberculous or rarely fungal, such as *Candida*. Several studies have shown pyogenic infections to be the most common cause, followed by tuberculosis even in TB endemic areas.[81] In some areas brucellosis appears to be the most common.[82]

Pyogenic Vertebral Osteomyelitis

Acute pyogenic vertebral osteomyelitis is usually from haematogenous seeding. Direct extension from adjacent soft-tissue infections and direct inoculation of infection during surgery are also common. The usual causative pathogen is *S. aureus*, but in the presence of spinal implants, coagulase-negative staphylococcal infection also occurs. Low-virulence coagulase-negative staphylococcal infection occurs in prolonged bacteraemia after pacemaker infections.[80] The primary site of infection in acute vertebral osteomyelitis may be urinary tract infections, skin or soft-tissue infections, vascular access sites, septic arthritis or bursitis and endocarditis. There may be underlying disease, including diabetes, coronary artery disease, immunosuppression, cancer or renal failure on dialysis (Fig. 9-31).[80,83]

Pyogenic infection almost always begins in the intervertebral disc. From here, infection spreads into the end-plate and along the longitudinal ligaments. There is ischaemia and necrosis of the disc associated with abscess formation. Contiguous end-plate destruction occurs with extension of the abscess into the paravertebral soft tissues.

Symptoms

Back pain is the commonest clinical presentation and is present in 86% of patients. The lumbar spine is most commonly affected (58%), followed by thoracic (30%) and cervical spine (11%).[83] Vertebral osteomyelitis is complicated by direct seeding in different compartments, including epidural, paravertebral and disc space abscess, with the paravertebral location being the commonest.[84] Systemic signs such as fever may not always be present. Severe sharp pain should alert one to the possibility of epidural abscess. Motor and sensory involvement may occur depending on the degree of spinal cord compression. Neurological complications are particularly common in cervical vertebral infections.

Investigations

Usual inflammatory markers: raised white cell count with neutrophilia. Elevation of the CRP and ESR is invariably present. Blood cultures may be positive in up to 58% of patients. Higher yield rates up to 77% can be obtained from bone biopsy cultures.

Plain Radiographs. Plain radiographs are not very sensitive in acute vertebral osteomyelitis, but are useful in subacute or chronic conditions. Early changes may be seen as minor end-plate irregularities but MRI is much more sensitive. End-plate destruction, paravertebral soft-tissue swelling and kyphoscoliosis are present in established osteomyelitis. In the acute setting, plain radiographs are mandatory to exclude other lesions, such as metastases or fractures.

Computed Tomography. CT is generally only used when there are contraindications to MRI. Enhanced images with multiplanar reformats help to delineate the lesion and demonstrate the extent of any abscess. The main role for CT in vertebral osteomyelitis is to plan and direct the biopsy, thereby confirming the diagnosis and obtaining material for culture (Fig. 9-32).

Magnetic Resonance Imaging. MRI is the investigation of choice for vertebral osteomyelitis and should be promptly arranged, especially in the presence of neurological symptoms and signs, as it also excludes other causes such as intervertebral disc prolapse and malignancy. Motor and sensory symptoms depend on the degree and level of spinal cord or cauda equina involvement.

MRI is extremely sensitive and has 90% accuracy in the diagnosis of acute vertebral osteomyelitis.[85–87] The imaging features are typical for infective discitis and osteomyelitis, and in many instances these entities can be differentiated from tuberculous osteomyelitis. Typically, one disc space and the two adjacent vertebral bodies are involved. The disc usually yields low signal on T1- and increased signal on T2-weighted images associated with loss of the intranuclear cleft. There is destruction of the end-plates of the adjacent vertebrae above and below the disc space. There is adjacent bone marrow oedema and inflammatory tissue. The bone marrow oedema shows as low signal on T1 and high signal on T2 and STIR images, involving the vertebral bodies and end-plates. As the infection proceeds untreated, this may lead to vertebral destruction and collapse. Epidural and/or paraspinal abscess may be noted as high signal fluid collections on T2 images. Intraspinal collections or granulation tissue may cause cord compression. Gadolinium-enhanced T1 images with fat saturation are useful to define the extent and effects of epidural or paravertebral abscess collections (Fig. 9-33). STIR images of the whole spine may be useful to assess multilevel involvement.

In pyogenic osteomyelitis there is usually homogeneous and diffuse enhancement of the vertebral bodies as opposed to the heterogeneous and localised enhancement seen in tuberculous vertebral osteomyelitis. Disc abscess with rim enhancement is more common in pyogenic infections, whilst vertebral intraosseous abscess with rim enhancement occurs more commonly in TB. Paraspinal abscesses are more commonly associated with TB than with pyogenic infections.[87]

Several recent studies have demonstrated the usefulness of diffusion-weighted imaging and apparent diffusion coefficient (ADC) values to differentiate between

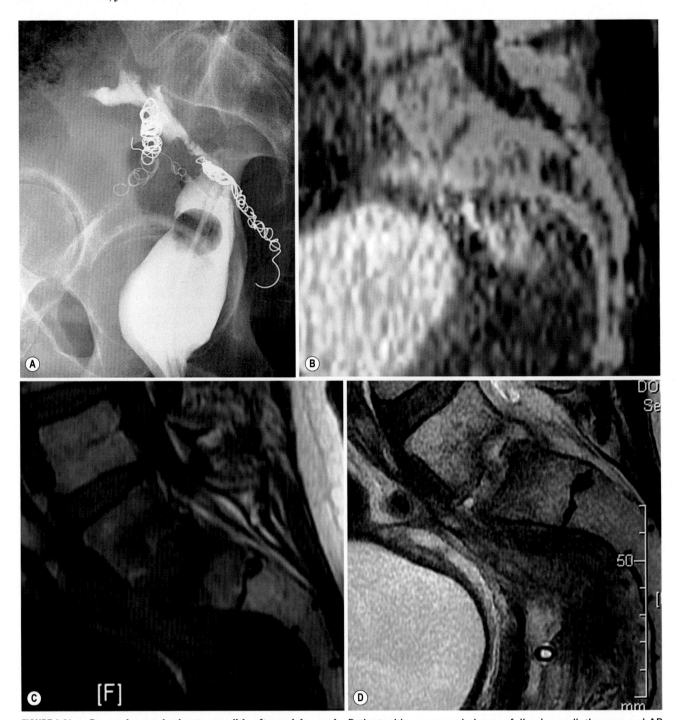

FIGURE 9-31 ■ **Pyogenic vertebral osteomyelitis after pelvic sepsis.** Patient with a presacral abscess following radiotherapy and AP resection for rectal cancer. (A) Contrast enema showing a sinus track to the prevertebral region at L5/S1. (B) Sagittal fused PET-CT image shows increased uptake of FDG tracer in the presacral region, but not the disc. (C, D) Sagittal T1 and T2 images show the presacral abnormality consistent with granulation tissue extending to the L5/S1 disc, with typical appearances of infective discitis.

infectious and malignant causes of spinal involvement, although results are still somewhat inconsistent.[88,89]

Nuclear Medicine. Skeletal scintigraphy is less important than it was, as most centres rely on MRI. Three-phase [99mTc] bone scintigraphy has about 67% accuracy, but positive results are seen only after a few days. It is also less sensitive to the detection of epidural abscess.

[111Indium] leucocyte scintigraphy and antileucocyte scintigraphy are more specific, but have sensitivity of around 20%, and hence are not generally useful. Gallium imaging is also a useful adjunct to MRI in the evaluation of spinal infections (Fig. 9-34). Because of limited availability, PET-CT is generally not used in the diagnosis of vertebral osteomyelitis but has been found to be useful in some studies.[90]

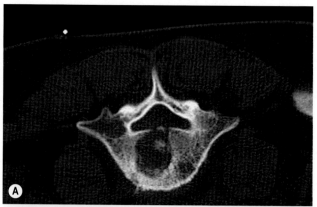

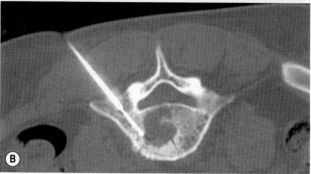

FIGURE 9-32 ■ **CT-guided vertebral body biopsy.** (A) Preliminary CT with a wire marker on the skin, from which the skin entry site can be measured and marked. (B) CT-guided bone biopsy of the intramedulllary abscess showing needle positioned at the margin of the abscess. Biopsy of the wall for histology, aspiration of the abscess and (if the latter is unsuccessful) gentle instillation and reaspiration of sterile saline for culture is performed.

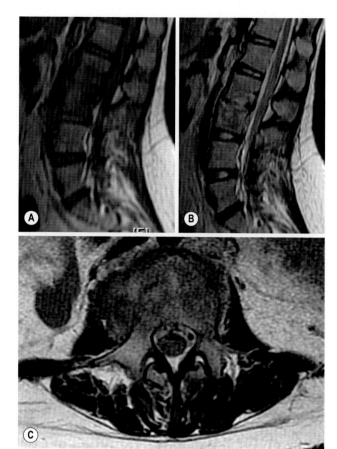

FIGURE 9-33 ■ **Bacterial infective discitis.** (A, B) Sagittal T1W and T2W images through the spine show involvement of the L2/3 disc with destruction of adjacent end-plates and oedema in the vertebral bodies of L2 and L3. (C) Axial T2W image at the same level shows a paravertebral abscess extending on the right from the involved disc (arrow).

Treatment

Acute vertebral osteomyelitis is usually treated with intravenous antibiotics. Image-guided intervention under CT may be necessary for diagnostic purposes and CT or ultrasound is used for guiding the drainage of abscesses. Surgery is usually required in the presence of implants; in chronic infections due to treatment failure, removal of the implant is generally recommended.

Tuberculous Vertebral Osteomyelitis

Tuberculosis of the spine is still prevalent in developing countries and in TB endemic areas. Poverty, malnutrition and overcrowding predispose to the development of primary tuberculous infection. It is increasingly seen in developed countries in the immigrant population and also increases with the increase in incidence of pulmonary tuberculosis due to immunosuppressive conditions, including HIV infection and AIDS. Tuberculosis of the spine is usually a secondary infection, with spread to the spine occurring by the haematogenous route, usually from primary lung or genital tract infection. Spinal tuberculosis accounts for approximately 50% of all musculoskeletal tuberculous infections.[91,92]

Spinal tuberculosis is most common around the thoracolumbar junction. The incidence decreases on either side of this level but may occur at any level.[92] Infection usually occurs at the anterior ends of vertebral bodies and spreads under the longitudinal ligament to involve contiguous vertebrae. Skip lesions may also occur due to haematogenous spread.

The vertebral body is commonly affected; posterior element involvement is rare but is seen particularly in Asian patients. Three patterns of vertebral body involvement are seen.[92,93]

A paradiscal lesion is the most common form of involvement of spinal tuberculosis. There is involvement of subchondral bone adjacent to an intervertebral disc, with reduction in disc height.

Anterior lesions occur due to spread of infection under the periosteum and anterior longitudinal ligament resulting in loss of blood supply to the vertebral body with development of necrosis and infection. Abscess formation may occur with resultant stripping of the periosteum from the vertebral body, causing scalloping and multiple-level involvements.

Central lesions involve the centre of the vertebral body with loss of height resulting in vertebra plana.

'Gibbus' deformities occur due vertebral body collapse manifesting as acute angulation in the spine. Paraspinal

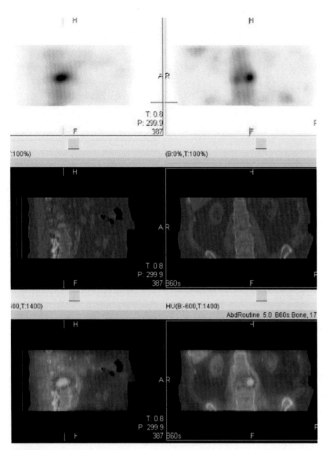

FIGURE 9-34 ■ **Vertebral osteomyelitis: gallium SPECT CT showing vertebral osteomyelitis as hot spots involving the vertebral bodies.** (Courtesy of Dr Ewa Novosinska, Royal Free Hospital, London, UK.)

TABLE 9-3	Differentiation between Pyogenic and Tuberculous Vertebral Osteomyelitis on Imaging	
Pyogenic Spinal Infection		**Tuberculosis of Spine**
1. Lumbar spine involvement common		More common in thoracic spine
2. Commonly single site with disc space infection and involvement of two adjacent vertebra		Multilevel involvement and skip lesions are common. Spread may occur along anterior longitudinal ligament
3. Disc abscess with end-plate destruction occurs		Intraosseous and paraspinal abscess occurs more frequently
4. Significant surrounding inflammation with diffuse oedema of vertebral bodies		Inflammation is more localised and formation of cold abscess
5. Enhanced images show diffuse vertebral body enhancement, irregular enhancement of thick-walled abscesses		Enhancement of vertebral bodies more localised and show rim enhancement of thin-walled abscess cavities

abscess formation also occurs and typically shows no significant signs of inflammation; hence such abscesses are called cold abscesses (9, 14, and 15).

Table 9-3 summarises features that may help to distinguish pyogenic from tuberculous spinal infection.

Plain Radiographs

In acute infections, plain radiographs may be normal. In subacute infection, bone lucency may be seen in vertebral bodies. End-plate changes and destruction occur with reduction in the intervertebral disc space. Cold abscess formation may cause paraspinal soft-tissue density on AP films. Chronic infection can cause sclerosis of the bone and end-plates, bone destruction with compression fractures and deformities. Gibbus is an acute angulation seen in the spine on lateral views, due to vertebral compression fractures. Other deformities such as kyphosis and scoliosis also occur.

Computed Tomography

The role of CT is usually limited to guiding biopsy but is also useful if there are contraindications, poor patient tolerance or lack of availability of MRI.

Early infection tends to show bone rarefaction and destruction. End-plate changes are more accurately evaluated than on plain radiographs. Sclerosis is seen in advanced disease.

Sagittal reconstructions of thin-section acquisition shows vertebral body and end-plate changes clearly. Vertebral body collapse and posterior wall retropulsion can be clearly identified even in its early stages. Spinal canal stenosis and cord compression due the bone destruction or soft-tissue inflammatory component can be clearly identified. Intravenous enhancement increases the diagnostic accuracy, outlining the inflammatory granulation tissue and also the thick irregular wall of abscess cavities. Paraspinal cold abscesses are also better seen on CT after intravenous contrast medium. Spinal canal encroachment secondary to vertebral body destruction can be assessed. Multilevel involvement and end-plate changes are also well shown on CT, which is particularly used for planned intervention of spinal tuberculosis. Common indications include drainage of cold abscesses, vertebral body or intervertebral disc biopsy.

Magnetic Resonance Imaging

MRI is the investigation of choice for assessment of tuberculous vertebral osteomyelitis. Usually the affected area of the spine is imaged, but in tuberculous osteomyelitis, it may be be useful to perform imaging of the whole spine to exclude skip lesions. Sagittal T1, T2 and STIR images are obtained with axial T2 images through the involved vertebral bodies (Fig. 9-35).

MRI can also be reliably used to differentiate between tuberculous and pyogenic vertebral osteomyelitis. Patients with tuberculous vertebral osteomyelitis have a significantly higher incidence of a well-defined paraspinal abnormal signal, thin- and smooth-walled abscess cavities, particularly at paraspinal or intraosseous locations, sub-ligamentous spread to three or more vertebral levels and involvement of multiple vertebral bodies. In

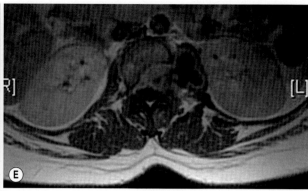

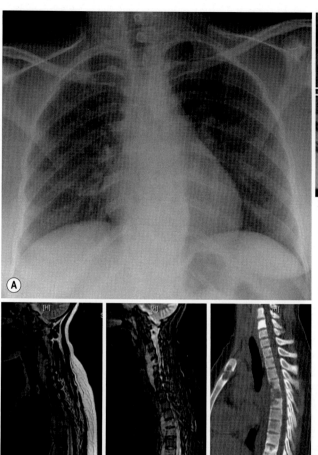

FIGURE 9-35 ■ **Multilevel involvement in tuberculous spondylitis.** Multilevel involvement is a common presentation in tuberculous vertebral osteomyelitis. This may be caused by spread along the anterior longitudinal ligament. Multilevel haematogenous borne skip lesions also occur. (A) Chest radiograph shows no evidence of underlying pulmonary TB, but there is a mild scoliosis and widened paravertebral soft-tissue planes around the lower thoracic spine. (B, C) Sagittal T2W and STIR images demonstrate multilevel involvement with subligamentous extension at multiple sites. Note the preservation of the intervertebral discs. (D) Sagittal reformatted CT demonstrates lytic lesions at the sites of bone involvement, with surrounding sclerosis. (E) Axial enhanced MRI of lumbar vertebrae shows chronic bone destruction and a large left paraspinal collection which extends laterally to abut the left kidney.

tuberculous spondylitis, there is also an increased incidence of thoracic spine involvement.[94]

Involvement of vertebral bodies and extension to the epidural and paravertebral spaces are commoner than disc space involvement. Bone marrow oedema is seen as low signal on T1 images, but the presence of corresponding high T2 signal may be variable.[95]

In paradiscal lesions, T1 images show low signal with loss of height of disc spaces, with high T2 signal, endplate destruction and paraspinal abscess formation (Fig. 9-36). With anterior lesions there is low T1 and high T2 signals involving the vertebral body, with preservation of disc signal and height. Central lesions involve the centre of the vertebral body and MRI shows abnormal signal of the vertebral body associated with collapse and vertebra plana, classically with preservation of adjacent discs.[96]

Whole-spine fat-suppressed STIR or T2 images are extremely useful to identify high signal bone marrow oedema in vertebral bodies and also high signal in the affected discs, which should be conspicuous against the background of very low signal from adjacent normal vertebrae. Gadolinium-enhanced images are useful for confirmation, revealing enhancement of the bone marrow oedema in affected vertebral bodies. T1 fat-saturated images before and after enhancement are useful to identify abscesses within the vertebral bodies or paravertebral soft tissues. These are typically cold abscesses and hence do not show significant surrounding inflammatory reaction, but there is uniform enhancement of the thin walls (Fig. 9-37). Enhanced images allow accurate assessment of extension and also evaluate the extent of spinal cord compression.[87,92,93]

Though posterior element involvement is not common in tuberculosis of the spine, studies have been published involving only the posterior elements. Posterior element involvement is most common in the thoracic spine, and tends to affect the lamina most commonly, followed by pedicles and articular processes. Spinal cord involvement was seen in many of these patients.[96]

Unusual Spine Infections

Candida albicans is rare but can cause spinal infections.[97] *Aspergillus fumigatus* infections of the spine are extremely rare but occur in immunocompromised people and chronic granulomatous disease. Diagnosis is difficult without microbiology and imaging features are similar to tuberculous disease.[98,99] Treatment is with antifungal

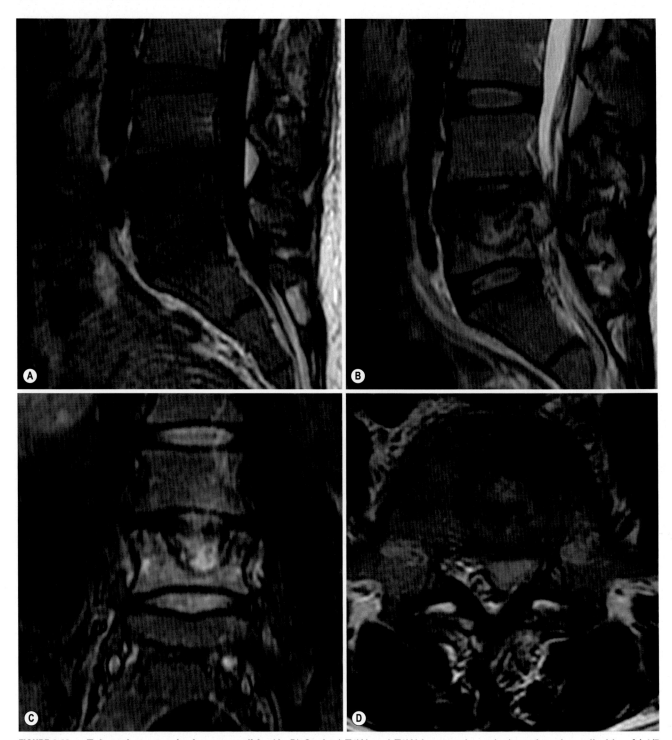

FIGURE 9-36 ■ Tuberculous vertebral osteomyelitis. (A, B) Sagittal T1W and T2W images through the spine show discitis of L4/5 vertebra extending to superior end-plate of L5 vertebra, extending to the vertebral body. There is also extension of the abscess into the spinal canal. (C) Axial T2 image at the same level shows the well-defined vertebral body abscess. The abscess component extends into the thecal sac and causes compression of nerve roots on the left. (D) Coronal PD SPIR image shows the well-defined abscess, with relatively little inflammation of surrounding soft tissue, the so-called 'cold abscess'.

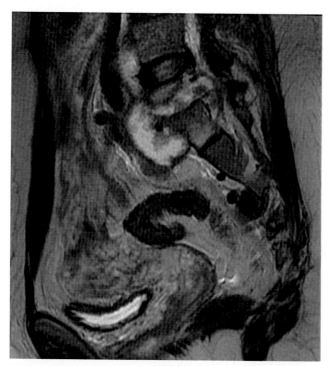

FIGURE 9-37 ■ **Tuberculous vertebral abscess presenting as psoas abscess.** This young lady was referred for pelvic MRI with a diagnosis of complex ovarian cyst. Pelvic MRI showed this to be psoas abscess extending from spinal TB (see Fig. 9-28). Sagittal T2W image shows the vertebral origin of the psoas abscess. Note the thick, irregular wall to the abscess and the subligamentous spread superiorly, both characteristic of TB.

agents. Atypical *Mycobacterium* infections with *M. intercellulare* and pneumococcal infections have also been reported but are rare.

REFERENCES

1. Ciampolini J, Harding KG. Pathophysiology of chronic bacterial osteomyelitis. Why do antibiotics fail so often? Postgrad Med J 2000;76:479–83.
2. Charlier C, Leclerq A, Cazenave B, et al. *Listeria monocytogenes*-associated joint and bone infections: a study of 43 consecutive cases. Clin Infect Dis 2012;54:240–8.
3. Mackowiak PA, Jones SR, Smith JW. Diagnostic value of sinus-tract cultures in chronic osteomyelitis. JAMA 1978;239:2772–5.
4. Olasinde AA, Oluwadiya KS, Adegbehingbe OO. Treatment of Brodie's abscess: excellent results from curettage, bone grafting and antibiotics. Singapore Med J 2011;52:436–9.
5. Yoon SH, Chung SK, Kim KJ, et al. Pyogenic vertebral osteomyelitis: identification of microorganism and laboratory markers used to predict clinical outcome. Eur Spine J 2010;19:575–82.
6. McHenry MC, Easley KA, Locker GA. Vertebral osteomyelitis: long-term outcome for 253 patients from 7 Cleveland-area hospitals. Clin Infect Dis 2002;34:1342–50.
7. Pääkkönen M, Kallio PE, Kallio MJ, Peltola H. Management of osteoarticular infections caused by *Staphylococcus aureus* is similar to that of other etiologies. Analysis of 199 staphylococcal bone and joint infections. Pediatr Infect Dis J 2012;31:436–8.
8. Montanaro L, Testoni F, Poggi A, et al. Emerging pathogenetic mechanisms of the implant-related osteomyelitis by *Staphylococcus aureus*. Int J Artif Organs 2011;34:781–8.
9. Calhoun J, Manring M, Shirtliff M. Osteomyelitis of the long bones. Semin Plast Surgery 2009;23:59–72.
10. Murphy RA, Ronat JB, Fakhri RM, et al. Multidrug-resistant chronic osteomyelitis complicating war injury in Iraqi civilians. J Trauma 2011;71:252–4.
11. Corr PD. Musculoskeletal fungal infections. Semin Musculoskelet Radiol 2011;15:506–10.
12. Harik N, Smeltzer M. Management of acute hematogenous osteomyelitis in children. Expert Rev Anti Infect Ther 2010;8: 175–81.
13. Krogstad P. Osteomyelitis. In: Feigin RD, Cherry JD, Feigin, Demmler-Harrison GJ, Kaplan SL, editors. Cherry's Textbook of Pediatric Infectious Diseases. 6th ed. Philadelphia: Saunders, Elsevier; 2009. pp. 725–42.
14. Waldvogel FA, Medoff G, Swartz MN. Osteomyelitis: a review of clinical features, therapeutic considerations, and unusual aspects (second of three parts). N Engl J Med 1970;282:260–6.
15. Cierny G III, Mader JT, Pennick J. A clinical staging system for adult osteomyelitis. Clin Orthop Relat Res 2003;414:7–24.
16. Frank G. Musculoskeletal infections in children. Paediatric Clin N Am 2005;52:1083–106.
17. Nelson JD. Acute osteomyelitis in children. Inf Disease Clin North Am 1990;4:513–22.
18. Blickman JG, van Die CE, de Rooy JW. Current imaging concepts in pediatric osteomyelitis. Eur Radiol 2004;14(Suppl 4):L55–64.
19. Erdman WA, Tamburro F, Jayson HT, et al. Osteomyelitis: characteristics and pitfalls of diagnosis with MR imaging. Radiology 1991;180(2):533–9.
20. Averill LW, Hernandez A, Gonzalez L, et al. Diagnosis of osteomyelitis in children: utility of fat-suppressed contrast-enhanced MRI. Am J Roentgenol 2009;192:1232–8.
21. Kan JH, Hilmes MA, Martus JE, et al. Value of MRI after recent diagnostic or surgical intervention in children with suspected osteomyelitis. Am J Roentgenol 2008;191:1595–600.
22. Girschick HJ, Raab P, Surbaum S, et al. Chronic non-bacterial osteomyelitis in children. Ann Rheum Dis 2005;64:279–85.
23. Khanna G, Sato TS, Ferguson P. Imaging of chronic recurrent multifocal osteomyelitis. Radiographics 2009;29:1159–77.
24. De Souza A, Solomon GE, Strober BE. SAPHO syndrome associated with hidradenitis suppurativa successfully treated with infliximab and methotrexate. Bull NYU Hosp Jt Dis 2011;69:185–7.
25. Belli E, Matteini C, Andreano T. Sclerosing osteomyelitis of Garré periostitis ossificans. J Craniofac Surg 2002;13:765–8.
26. McHenry CR. Determinants of mortality for necrotising soft tissue infections. Am Surg 1993;59:304–8.
27. Howell WR, Goulston C. Osteomyelitis: an update for hospitalists. Hosp Pract (1995) 2011;39(1):153–60.
28. Carek PJ, Dickerson LM, Sack JL. Diagnosis and management of osteomyelitis. Am Fam Physician 2001;63:2413–20.
29. Ciampolini J, Harding K. Pathophysiology of chronic bacterial osteomyelitis. Why do antibiotics fail so often? Postgrad Med J 2000;76:479–83.
30. Burnett MW, Bass JW, Cook BA. Etiology of osteomyelitis complicating sickle cell disease. Pediatrics 1998;101:296–7.
31. Loyer EM, DuBrow RA, David CL, et al. Imaging of superficial soft-tissue infections: sonographic findings in cases of cellulitis and abscess. Am J Roentgenol 1996;166:149–52.
32. Bureau NJ, Chhem RK, Cardinal E. Musculoskeletal infections: US manifestations. Radiographics 1999;19:1585–92.
33. Pineda C, Espinosa R, Pena A. Radiographic imaging in osteomyelitis: the role of plain radiography, computed tomography, ultrasonography, magnetic resonance imaging, and scintigraphy. Semin Plast Surg 2009;23:80–9.
34. Fayad LM, Carrino JA, Fishman EK. Musculoskeletal infection: role of CT in the emergency department. Radiographics 2007; 27:1723–36.
35. Golimbu C, Firooznia H, Rafii M. CT of osteomyelitis of the spine. Am J Roentgenol 1984;142:159–63.
36. Tang JSH, Gold RH, Bassett LW, Seeger L. Musculoskeletal infection of the extremities: evaluation with MR imaging. Radiology 1988;166:205–9.
37. Erdman WA, Tamburro F, Jayson HT, et al. Osteomyelitis: characteristics and pitfalls of diagnosis with MR imaging. Radiology 1991;180:533–9.
38. Umans H, Haramati N, Flusser G. The diagnostic role of gadolinium enhanced MRI in distinguishing between acute medullary bone infarct and osteomyelitis. Magn Reson Imaging 2000;18: 255–62.
39. Palestro CJ, Love C, Tronco GG, et al. Combined labeled leukocyte and technetium 99m sulfur colloid bone marrow imaging

for diagnosing musculoskeletal infection. Radiographics 2006;26: 859–70.

40. Love C, Tomas MB, Tronco GG, Palestro CJ. FDG PET of infection and inflammation. Radiographics 2005;25:1357–68.

41. Palestro CJ, Torres MA. Radionuclide imaging in orthopedic infections. Semin Nucl Med 1997;27:334–45.

42. Palestro CJ. Nuclear medicine, the painful prosthetic joint, and orthopedic infection. J Nucl Med 2003;44:927–9.

43. Love C, Marwin SE, Palestro CJ. Nuclear medicine and the infected joint replacement. Semin Nucl Med 2009;39:66–78.

44. Pakos EE, Trikalinos TA, Fotopoulos AD, Ioannidis JP. Prosthesis infection: diagnosis after total joint arthroplasty with antigranulocyte scintigraphy with ^{99m}Tc-labeled monoclonal antibodies—a meta-analysis. Radiology 2007;242:101–8.

45. Singh N, Armstrong DG, Lipsky BA. Preventing foot ulcers in patients with diabetes. JAMA 2005;293:217–28.

46. Donovan A. Current concepts in imaging diabetic pedal osteomyelitis. Radiol Clin North Am 2008;46:1105–24.

47. Schweitzer ME, Daffner RH, Weissman BN, et al. ACR Appropriateness Criteria on suspected osteomyelitis in patients with diabetes mellitus. J Am Coll Radiol 2008;5:881–6.

48. Capitol GM. Assessment and management of foot disease in patients with diabetes. N Engl J Med 1994;331(13):854–60.

49. Kapoor A, Page S, Lavalley M, et al. Magnetic resonance imaging for diagnosing foot osteomyelitis: a meta-analysis. Arch Intern Med 2007;167:125–32.

50. Craig JG, Amin MB, Wu K, et al. Osteomyelitis of the diabetic foot: MR imaging-pathologic correlation. Radiology 1997;203: 849–55.

51. Marcus CD, Ladam-Marcus VJ, Leone J, et al. MR imaging of osteomyelitis and neuropathic osteoarthropathy in the feet of diabetics. Radiographics 1996;16:1337–48.

52. Miller TT, Randolph DA Jr, Staron RB, et al. Fat-suppressed MRI of musculoskeletal infection: fast T2-weighted techniques versus gadolinium-enhanced T1-weighted images. Skeletal Radiol 1997; 26:654–8.

53. Donovan A, Schweitzer ME. Use of MR imaging in diagnosing diabetes-related pedal osteomyelitis. Radiographics 2010;3: 723–36.

54. Johnson PW, Collins MS, Wenger DE. Diagnostic utility of T1-weighted MRI characteristics in evaluation of osteomyelitis of the foot. Am J Roentgenol 2009;192:96–100.

55. Ledermann HP, Morrison WB, Schweitzer ME. MR image analysis of pedal osteomyelitis: distribution, patterns of spread, and frequency of associated ulceration and septic arthritis. Radiology 2002;223:747–55.

56. Ahmadi ME, Morrison WB, Carrino JA, et al. Neuropathic arthropathy of the foot with and without superimposed osteomyelitis: MR imaging characteristics. Radiology 2006;238:622–31.

57. Tan PL, Teh J. MRI of the diabetic foot: differentiation of infection from neuropathic change. Br J Radiol 2007;80(959):939–48.

58. Goldenberg DL. Septic arthritis. Lancet 1998;351:197–202.

59. Dubost JJ, Fis I, Denis P, et al. Polyarticular septic arthritis. Medicine 1993;72:296–310.

60. Karchevsky M, Schweitzer ME, Morrison WB, Parellada JA. MRI findings of septic arthritis and associated osteomyelitis in adults. Am J Roentgenol 2004;182:119–22.

61. Tehranzadeh J, Wang F, Mesgarzadeh M. Magnetic resonance imaging of osteomyelitis. Crit Rev Diagn Imaging 1992;33: 495–534.

62. Weishaupt D, Schweitzer ME, Alam F, et al. MR imaging of inflammatory joint diseases of the foot and ankle. Skeletal Radiol 1999;28:663–9.

63. Hopkins KL, Li KC, Bergman G. Gadolinium-DTPA-enhanced magnetic resonance imaging of musculoskeletal infectious processes. Skeletal Radiol 1995;24:325–30.

64. Lin HM, Learch TJ, White EA, Gottsegen CJ. Emergency joint aspiration: a guide for radiologists on call. Radiographics 2009;4: 1139–58.

65. Resnick D. Diagnosis of Bone and Joint Disorders. 4th ed. Philadelphia: Saunders; 2002.

66. Kwack KS, Cho JH, Lee JH, et al. Septic arthritis versus transient synovitis of the hip: gadolinium-enhanced MRI finding of decreased perfusion at the femoral epiphysis. Am J Roentgenol 2007;189: 437–45.

67. Moore SL, Rafii M. Imaging of musculoskeletal and spinal tuberculosis. Radiol Clin North Am 2001;2:329–42.

68. De Vuyst D, Vanhoenacker F, Gielen J, et al. Imaging features of musculoskeletal tuberculosis. Eur Radiol 2003;13:1809–19.

69. Harisinghani MG, McLoud TC, Shepard JA. Tuberculosis from head to toe. Radiographics 2000;20:449–70.

70. Hong SH, Kim SM, Ahn JM, et al. Tuberculous versus pyogenic arthritis: MR imaging evaluation. Radiology 2001;218:848–53.

71. Suh JS, Lee JD, Cho JH, et al. MR imaging of tuberculous arthritis: clinical and experimental studies. J Magn Reson Imaging 1996;6: 185–9.

72. Theodorou DJ, Theodorou SJ, Kakitsubata Y, et al. Imaging characteristics and epidemiologic features of atypical mycobacterial infections involving the musculoskeletal system. Am J Roentgenol 2001;176:341–9.

73. Piehl FC, Davis RJ, Prugh SI. Osteomyelitis in sickle cell disease. J Pediatr Orthop 1993;13:225–7.

74. Ejindu VC, Hine AL, Mashayekhi M, et al. Musculoskeletal manifestations of sickle cell disease. Radiographics 2007;27: 1005–21.

75. Corr PD. Musculoskeletal fungal infections. Semin Musculoskelet Radiol 2011;15:506–10.

76. Berman A, Espinoza LR, Diaz JD, et al. Rheumatic manifestations of human immunodeficiency virus infection. Am J Med 1988;85: 59–64.

77. Calabrese LH. The rheumatic manifestations of infection with the human immunodeficiency virus. Semin Arthritis Rheum 1989;18: 225–39.

78. Olivé A, Pérez-Andrés R, Tena X, Louthrenoo W. Musculoskeletal manifestation of HIV. J Clin Rheumatol 1998;4:105.

79. Wu JS, Gorbachova T, Morrison WB, Haims AH. Imaging-guided bone biopsy for osteomyelitis: are there factors associated with positive or negative cultures? Am J Roentgenol 2007;188: 1529–34.

80. Zimmerli W. Clinical practice. Vertebral osteomyelitis. N Engl J Med 2010;362:1022–9.

81. Mete B, Kurt C, Yilmaz MH, et al. Vertebral osteomyelitis: eight years' experience of 100 cases. Rheumatol Int 2012;32(11): 3591–7.

82. Colmenero JD, Jiménez-Mejías ME, Sánchez-Lora FJ, et al. Pyogenic, tuberculous, and brucellar vertebral osteomyelitis: a descriptive and comparative study of 219 cases. J Ann Rheum Dis 1997; 56:709–15.

83. Mylona E, Samarkos M, Kakalou E, et al. Pyogenic vertebral osteomyelitis: a systematic review of clinical characteristics. Semin Arthritis Rheum 2009;39:10–17.

84. McHenry MC, Easley KA, Locker GA. Vertebral osteomyelitis: long-term outcome for 253 patients from 7 Cleveland-area hospitals. Clin Infect Dis 2002;34:1342–50.

85. Palestro CJ, Love C, Miller TT. Infections and musculoskeletal conditions: Imaging of musculoskeletal infections. Best Pract Res Clin Rheumatol 2006;20:1197–218.

86. Fitzgerald RH Jr, Kelly PJ. Infections of the skeletal system. In: Howard RJ, Simmons RL, editors. Surgical Infectious Diseases. 3rd ed. London: Appleton & Lange; 1995. pp. 1207–36.

87. Chang MC, Wu HT, Lee CH, et al. Tuberculous spondylitis and pyogenic spondylitis: comparative magnetic resonance imaging features. Spine (Phila Pa 1976) 2006;31:782–8.

88. Pui MH, Mitha A, Rae WI, Corr P. Diffusion-weighted magnetic resonance imaging of spinal infection and malignancy. J Neuroimaging 2005;15:164–70.

89. Chan JH, Peh WC, Tsui EY, et al. Acute vertebral body compression fractures: discrimination between benign and malignant causes using apparent diffusion coefficients. Br J Radiol 2002;75: 207–14.

90. Gemmel F, Rijk PC, Collins JMP, et al. Expanding role of ^{18}F-fluoro-D-deoxyglucose PET and PET/CT in spinal infections. Eur Spine J 2010;19:540–51.

91. Ho EKW, Leong JCY. The pediatric spine: principles and practice. In: Weinstein SL, editor. Tuberculosis of the Spine. 3rd ed. New York: Raven; 1994. pp. 837–49.

92. Moorthy S, Prabhu NK. Spectrum of MR imaging findings in spinal tuberculosis. Am J Roentgenol 2002;179:979–83.

93. Shanley DJ. Tuberculosis of the spine: imaging features. Am J Roentgenol 1995;164:659–64.

94. Jung NY, Jee WH, Ha KY, et al. Discrimination of tuberculous spondylitis from pyogenic spondylitis on MRI. Am J Roentgenol 2004;182:1405–10.

95. al-Mulhim FA, Ibrahim EM, el-Hassan AY, Moharram HM. Magnetic resonance imaging of tuberculous spondylitis. Spine 1995; 20:2287–92.

96. Narlawar RS, Shah JR, Pimple MK, et al. Isolated tuberculosis of posterior elements of spine: magnetic resonance imaging findings in 33 patients. Spine 2002;27:275–81.

97. Khazim RM, Debnath UK, Fares Y. *Candida albicans* osteomyelitis of the spine: progressive clinical and radiological features and surgical management in three cases. Eur Spine J 2006;15:1404–10.

98. Sethi S, Siraj F, Kalra K, Chopra P. *Aspergillus* vertebral osteomyelitis in immunocompetent patients. Indian J Orthop 2012;46: 246–50.

99. Chang HM, Yu HH, Yang YH, et al. Successful treatment of *Aspergillus flavus* spondylodiscitis with epidural abscess in a patient with chronic granulomatous disease. Pediatr Infect Dis J 2012;31:100–1.

Page numbers followed by 'f' indicate figures, 't' indicate tables, and 'b' indicate boxes.

Notes
To simplify the index, the main terms of imaging techniques (e.g. computed tomography, magnetic resonance imaging etc.) are concerned only with the technology and general applications. Users are advised to look for specific anatomical features and diseases/disorders for individual imaging techniques used.
vs. indicates a comparison or differential diagnosis.
To save space in the index, the following abbreviations have been used:
CHD—congenital heart disease
CMR—cardiac magnetic resonance
CT—computed tomography
CXR—chest X-ray
DECT—dual-energy computed tomography
DWI-MRI—diffusion weighted imaging-magnetic resonance imaging
ERCP—endoscopic retrograde cholangiopancreatography
EUS—endoscopic ultrasound
FDG-PET—fluorodeoxyglucose positron emission tomography
HRCT—high-resolution computed tomography
MDCT—multidetector computed tomography
MRA—magnetic resonance angiography
MRCP—magnetic resonance cholangiopancreatography
MRI—magnetic resonance imaging
MRS—magnetic resonance spectroscopy
PET—positron emission tomography
PTC—percutaneous transhepatic cholangiography
SPECT—single photon emission computed tomography
US—ultrasound

A
Abscesses
    para-vertebral abscesses, CT, 220
    subperiosteal, 219
Accessory muscles, tumours, 118, 118f
Acetabulum
    anatomy, 196, 197f
    fractures, 194–200
        anterior column fractures, 192f, 198
        anterior wall fractures, 197
        classification, 194, 196–197, 198f
        complex fractures, 199
        CT, 194

posterior column fractures, 198
        posterior wall fractures, 197–198, 199f
        transverse fractures, 198, 199f
Achilles tendon, 49
    tears, 50, 50f
    tendinopathy, 50
ACL *see* Anterior cruciate ligament (ACL)
ACR *see* American College of Radiology (ACR)
Acromegaly, 152–153
Acrometastases, lung cancer, 82
Acromioclavicular joint (ACJ), 29–30, 31f
    ligaments, 29–30
    trauma, 186
Acute bone infarction, acute osteomyelitis *vs.*, 222
Acute haematogenous osteomyelitis (AHO), 214
Acute intermittent gout, 170
Acute osteomyelitis
    acute bone infarction *vs.*, 222
    children, 214
    paediatric patients, 214
Adamantinoma, 96–97, 97f
Adipose tissue
    MRI, 11, 11f
AHO (acute haematogenous osteomyelitis), 214
Albers–Schönberg disease, 151
ALT (atypical lipomatous tumours), 104, 104f
Amyloidosis, 178
Aneurysmal bone cysts, 55f–56f, 71, 72f
Ankle, 48–52
    anatomy, 48–49
    bones, 50–51
    inversion injury, 209, 209f
    ligaments, 49, 49f
    talar dome, 48–49
    tendons, 49–50
Ankle fractures, 205–209
    bimalleolar, 206, 206f
    trimalleolar, 206, 206f
    unimalleolar, 206
    see also specific bones
Ankylosing spondylitis (AS), 165–167
    peripheral joints, 166–167
        hands and feet, 167
        hip, 166–167, 167f
        shoulder, 167, 167f
    sacriliitis, 165, 165f
    spinal disease, 165–166, 166f
        bone marrow oedema, 165
        fractures, 166, 167f
        MRI, 165
        radiography, 165–166, 166f
Ankylosis
    bony, 168
    rheumatoid arthritis, 163

Anterior column fractures, acetabulum, 192f, 198
Anterior compression injuries, pelvic ring fractures, 195, 195f–196f
Anterior cruciate ligament (ACL), 44–46, 46f
    trauma, 203, 204f
Anterior lesions, tuberculous vertebral osteomyelitis, 243
Anterior talofibular ligament, 49f
    ankle, 49
Anterior tibiotalar ligament, 49
Anterior wall fractures, acetabulum, 197
Antibiotics
    musculoskeletal infection management, 240
Arterial vascular calcification, 12, 12f
Arthritis, 156–181
    asymmetrical distal interphalangeal, 167
    connective tissue diseases, 172–173
        see also specific diseases/disorders
    degenerative, 240
    enteropathy-associated, 169
    HLA-B27, 165
    inflammatory types *see* Inflammatory arthritis
    non-aggressive periosteal reaction, 19
    oligo-arthritis, 167
    psoriatic *see* Psoriatic arthritis
    reactive, 12, 169, 169f
    rheumatoid *see* Rheumatoid arthritis (RA)
    septic *see* Septic arthritis
    sero-negative, 165–169
    see also specific types
Arthritis mutilans, 167
Arthrography, 2–3, 3f
Arthropathy, 177f
    haemophilic *see* Haemophilic arthropathy
    Jaccoud's, 173
    neuropathic, 176, 176t
    pyrophosphate, 171, 171f
Articular cartilage, 122f
AS *see* Ankylosing spondylitis (AS)
Aspergillus fumigatus infection
    musculoskeletal infections, 238
    spinal infections, 245–247
Asymmetrical distal interphalangeal arthritis, 167
Atypical lipomatous tumours (ALT), 104, 104f
Atypical *Mycobacterium* infections *see* Non-tuberculous mycobacteria (NTMB)
Autoimmune diseases/disorders
    soft musculoskeletal tissue calcification, 14–16
    see also specific diseases/disorders
Avascular necrosis (AVN)
    hip, 42, 42t, 43f
    wrist, 35, 35f–36f

AVN *see* Avascular necrosis (AVN)
Avulsion fractures, 183
Avulsion injuries
    pelvis trauma, 199–200, 200*f*
Axotemic osteodystrophy, 143*f*, 148–150
    renal tubular defects, 148–150

B

Bacterial infections
    soft musculoskeletal tissue calcification,
        14, 14*f*
Baker's cyst, 48, 119
Bankart lesion, 184, 184*f*
    bony, 28, 29*f*
    glenohumeral joint instability, 28, 28*f*
Basal multicellular unit (BMU), bone,
        121–122, 122*f*
Bayley triangle, 28
Benign bone tumours *see* Bone tumours,
        benign
Benign fibrous histiocytoma (BFH), 67
Benign osteoid osteoma, 20–21, 21*f*
Bennett's fracture, 192, 194*f*
BFH (benign fibrous histiocytoma), 67
Biceps brachii muscle, 30–31
Bimalleolar ankle fractures, 206, 206*f*
Biopsies
    bone metastases, 83
    musculoskeletal infection management,
        221*f*, 240, 240*f*
    percutaneous *see* Percutaneous biopsy
Bipartite patella, 205, 205*f*
Bizarre parosteal osteochondromatous
        proliferation (BPOP), 111
Blastomycosis
    musculoskeletal infections, 238
BMD *see* Bone mineral density (BMD)
BMU (basal multicellular unit), bone,
        121–122, 122*f*
Bohler's angle, calcaneal fractures, 208
Bone(s)
    ageing, 123
    alignment, joint radiography, 157–158,
        159*f*
    basal multicellular unit, 121–122, 122*f*
    cells, 121
        see also specific types
    CT, 9
    formation, 121–122, 122*f*
    growth and development, 122–124, 122*f*
        age, 123, 123*f*
        length, 123, 123*f*
    MRI, 9–11, 10*f*
    pathophysiology, 121–124
    physiology, 121–124
    radiography, 8
    resorption, 122
    structure, 122*f*, 123
    turnover, 121–122, 122*f*–123*f*
    US, 8
    see also specific bones
Bone disease
    aneurysmal cysts *see* Aneurysmal bone
        cysts
    infarction
        acute osteomyelitis *vs.*, 222
        musculoskeletal infections vs,
            240
    joint disease, 156–157, 158*f*
    joint radiography, 156–157
    metastases *see* Bone metastases
    tumours *see* Bone tumours
Bone marrow disorders
    diabetic foot, 232
    oedemas *see* Bone marrow oedema

Bone marrow oedema
    diabetic foot, 229–230
    knee, 48
    MRI, 221
    spinal ankylosing spondylitis, 165
Bone marrow tumours, 92–95
    malignant, 92–95
    MRI, 10, 10*f*
    see also specific diseases/disorders
Bone metastases, 79–84
    biopsies, 83
    causes, 79
    children, 83–84
    CT, 83
    definition, 79
    diagnosis, 80–83
        MRI, 81
        PET/CT, 81
        radiology, 80–83, 80*f*–81*f*
        ^{99m}Tc-MDP, 81
    distribution, 79–80, 80*f*
    FDG-PET, 83
    Mirels' scoring system, 83, 83*t*
    pathological fractures, 83
    primary malignancies, 79
        breast cancer, 80–82, 80*f*
        kidney cancer, 82, 83*f*
        lung cancer, 81*f*–82*f*, 82
        malignant melanoma, 82–83
        prostate cancer, 80–82, 82*f*
        thyroid cancer, 82
    radiology, 83
    scintigraphy, 83
    SPECT, 83
    see also specific diseases/disorders
Bone mineral density (BMD), 121–122
    osteoporosis, 124
Bone tumours, 54–58, 55*t*
    age at presentation, 54
    assessment, 54–58
        location, 54
        matrix mineralisation, 57, 57*f*
        periosteal reaction, 55, 56*f*
        rate of growth, 54–55, 55*f*–56*f*
    bone scintigraphy, 57–58
    CT, 57–58
    CT-PET, 58
    malignant *see* Bone tumours, malignant
    metastases *see* Bone metastases
    MRI, 57–58
    MRS, 58
    PET, 58
Bone tumours, benign, 58–76
    cartilage tumours, 58–62
    classification, 55*t*, 58
    fibrogenic tumours, 65
    fibrohistiocytic tumours, 65–67
    lipogenic tumours, 70
    neural tumours, 70–71
    osteogenic tumours, 62–65
    rate of growth, 54–55
    vascular tumours, 68–69
    see also specific diseases/disorders
Bone tumours, malignant, 79–98
    adamantinoma, 96–97, 97*f*
    chondroid origin, 84–87
        see also Chondrosarcoma
    classification, 84
    fibrous malignant, 91–92
    fibrous origin, 91–92
    incidence, 84
    metastases *see* Bone metastases
    notochordal origin, 95–96
        chordoma, 95–96
    osteoid origin, 87–91
        see also Osteosarcoma

radiographs, 84
    vascular tumours, 96, 96*f*
    see also specific diseases/disorders
Bony ankylosis, 168
Bony Bankart lesion, 28, 29*f*
Boutonniere deformity, 164, 164*f*
Bowing fractures, 183*f*
BPOP (bizarre parosteal
        osteochondromatous proliferation),
        111
Brachialis muscle, 30–31
Brachioradialis muscle, 30–31
Breast cancer
    bone metastases, 80–82, 80*f*
Brodie's abscess, 213
    MRI, 222, 224*f*
Brown tumours (osteitis fibrous cystica),
        142, 142*f*
Bursitis
    hip, 43
    infective, 219
    trochanteric, 43, 44*f*

C

Caffrey's disease (infantile cortical
        hyperostosis), 19
Calcaneal fractures, 207–208
    tongue type, 207–208, 208*f*
    vertical fracture, 207–208, 208*f*
Calcaneofibular ligament, 49
Calcaneonavicular coalition, 51, 51*f*
Calcification
    malignant, 16, 17*f*
    soft musculoskeletal tissues *see* Soft
        musculoskeletal tissues
Calcific tendinopathy, rotator cuff disease,
        25–26, 28*f*
Calcified cartilage, 122*f*
Calcium hydroxyapatite deposition disease
        (HADD), 13, 171–172
    intra-articular, 172
    periarticular, 171–172, 172*f*
Calcium pyrophosphate deposition disease
        (CPPD), 171
    soft musculoskeletal tissue calcification,
        16
Cam-type femoroacetabular impingement,
        40, 40*f*–41*f*
Cancers/tumours
    musculoskeletal infections *vs.*, 240
    soft musculoskeletal tissues *see* Soft
        musculoskeletal tissues
Candidiasis
    musculoskeletal infections, 238
        in HIV infection, 239–240
    spinal infections, 245–247
Carpal bones, 33–34
    trauma, 189–192
        AP radiograph, 188, 188*f*
        causes, 191–192
        PA radiograph, 191–192,
            192*f*–193*f*
Carpal tunnel syndrome, 39
Carpometacarpal joint, 34
Cartilage
    benign tumours, 58–62
    calcified, 122*f*
    MRI, 6–7
Central osteosarcoma *see* Osteosarcoma
Chauffeur's fracture, 189
Cholecalciferol *see* Vitamin D
        (cholecalciferol)
Chondroblastoma, 61–62
    MRI, 61–62, 62*f*
    radiograph, 61–62, 62*f*

Chondrocalcinosis, 171, 171f, 180, 180f
  hyperparathyroidism, 141, 142f
Chondroma, 60–61
  para-articular (intracapsular), 111
  soft tissue, 111
  see also Enchondroma
Chondromatosis, synovial, 176–177, 177f
Chondromyxoid fibroma, 62
  radiograph, 62, 62f
Chondro-osseous tumours, 111
Chondrosarcoma, 84–86, 84f
  classification, 84
  clear-cell, 87
  clinical presentation, 84–85
  differential diagnosis, 85–86
  enchondroma vs., 60
  hereditary multiple exostoses, 84, 85f
  imaging features, 84f–86f, 85–86
    CT, 85–86
    MRI, 85–86
  Maffucci's syndrome, 84
  mesenchymal, 86–87
  needle biopsy, 84–85
  Ollier's disease, 84
  periosteal, 86
Chordoma, 95–96
Chronic osteomyelitis, paediatric, 214–216,
    217f
Chronic recurrent multifocal osteomyelitis
    (CRMO), 216–217
Chronic renal failure
  soft musculoskeletal tissue calcification,
    12f, 15–16
Chronic tophaceous gout, 170–171, 170f
Clavicle
  fractures, 186
Clear cell chondrosarcoma, 87
Clostridium infections
  musculoskeletal infections in HIV
    infection, 239–240
  paediatric necrotizing fasciitis, 218
Codman's angle
  central osteosarcoma, 87
  Ewing's sarcoma, 94–95
Codman triangle, 22, 22f
COL1A1 gene, 132
COL1A2 gene, 132
Collagen type I, 121
Collateral ligaments, knee, 43–44
Colles' fracture, 189, 190f
Comminuted fractures, 182
Compact bone, 122f
Complex fractures, acetabulum, 199
Compound fractures, 182
Computed tomography (CT)
  high-resolution multi-detector, 139–140
  high resolution peripheral, 139–140
  principles
    'slice wars', 81–82
Condylar fractures
  femur, 203
  phalanges, 193
Coraco–clavicular (C–C) ligaments, 29–30
Coxa profunda, 40–41
CPPD see Calcium pyrophosphate
    deposition disease (CPPD)
CRMO see Chronic recurrent multifocal
    osteomyelitis (CRMO)
Cryptococcus infections
  musculoskeletal infections, 238
Crystal arthritides, 169–172
CT see Computed tomography (CT)
Cushing's disease, 152
Cyst(s)
  aneurysmal bone see Aneurysmal bone
    cysts

kidneys see Renal masses
  popliteal (Baker's) cyst, 119
Cysticercosis
  soft musculoskeletal tissue calcification,
    14, 14f

D

Dedifferentiated liposarcoma, 105, 105f
Dedifferentiated pleomorphic tumours, 104
Degenerative arthritis, musculoskeletal
    infections vs., 240
Delayed gadolinium-enhanced MRI cartilage
    (dGEMRIC), 7
De Quervain's tenosynovitis, 38–39,
    39f
Dermatomyositis (DM), 172, 173f
  soft musculoskeletal tissue calcification,
    14–15
Dermoplastic fibroma, 65
  radiograph, 65, 66f
Desmoid-type fibromatosis, 107–108,
    107f
DEXA see Dual energy X-ray
    absorptiometry (DEXA)
dGEMRIC (delayed gadolinium-enhanced
    MRI cartilage), 7
Diabetes mellitus, foot complications see
    Diabetic foot
Diabetic foot, 227–232
  bone marrow abnormalities, 232
  causes, 228
  clinical presentation, 228
  intra-articular bodies, 232
  intra-osseous fluid collection, 230
  joint effusions, 232
  microangiography, 227
  MRI, 231f
  neuropathic changes, 232
  radiography, 228–229, 230f–231f
  single bone involvement, 232
  skin ulcers, 230
Diaphyseal aclasis, osteochondroma, 58,
    58f
Diaphysis, bones, 122f
Diffuse idiopathic skeletal hyperostosis
    (DISH), 173–175, 174f
  differential diagnosis, 173–174
Diffuse idiopathic skeletal hypoplasia
    (DISH), 137
Diffuse neurofibroma, 114–115
Diffuse-type giant cell tumour (diffuse-type
    pigmented villonodular synovitis),
    108
Diffuse-type pigmented villonodular
    synovitis (diffuse-type giant cell
    tumour), 108
DIP (distal interphalangeal) joints, 163
DISH see Diffuse idiopathic skeletal
    hyperostosis (DISH)
DISI (dorsal intercalated segment
    instability), 35, 37f
Dislocation
  definition, 183
Disseminated staphylococcal disease, 214
Distal biceps tendon, 31, 32f–33f
Distal interphalangeal (DIP) joints, 163
DM see Dermatomyositis (DM)
Dorsal intercalated segment instability
    (DISI), 35, 37f
Dracunculiasis, 14, 15f
Dual energy X-ray absorptiometry (DEXA),
    124, 135–137, 137f
  limitations, 136–137
Dupuytren's disease (palmar fibromatosis),
    107

E

ECU see Extensor carpi ulnaris (ECU)
EF (elastofibroma), 106, 106f
EFOV (extended field-of-view), 4, 5f
Elastofibroma (EF), 106, 106f
Elastography
  musculoskeletal system MRI, 7
  musculoskeletal system US, 4–5, 5f
Elbow, 30–33
  adult trauma, 186–188, 186f
  anatomy, 30
  bones, 31–32, 33f–34f
  cartilage, 31–32, 33f–34f
  flexor muscles, 30–31
  ligaments, 31–33, 34f
  paediatric trauma
    lateral condylar fractures, 187, 187f
    radial head dislocation, 187–188, 187f
    supracondylar fractures, 186–187, 187f
  tendinopathy, 31, 32f
  tendons, 31
Enchondroma, 59–61
  chondrosarcoma vs., 60
  MRI, 60f
  radiograph, 61f
  radiographs, 59, 60f
  see also Ollier's disease
Enchondroma protuberans, 60
Enchondromatosis with haemangiomas
    see Maffucci's syndrome
    (enchondromatosis with
    haemangiomas)
Enteropathy-associated arthritis, 169
Enthesial disease, 157, 158f
Eosinophilic granuloma
  bone, 74
Epiphysis
  bones, 122f
Erosive (inflammatory) osteoarthritis,
    162–163
  seagull wing pattern, 162–163, 163f
Escherichia coli infection
  paediatric necrotizing fasciitis, 218
Ewing's sarcoma, 21f–22f, 22, 93–94, 94f
  Codman angle, 94–95
  FDG-PET, 94–95
  imaging features, 94–95
  MRI, 94–95
  STIR, 94–95, 95f
Extended field-of-view (EFOV), 4, 5f
Extensor carpi ulnaris (ECU)
  tendinopathy, 38–39
  tendon sheath, 34

F

Fasciitis
  necrotizing, 218
  nodular, 105–106
FCD (fibrous cortical defect), 65, 66f
FD see Fibrous dysplasia (FD)
FDL (flexor digitorum longus) tendon, 49
Feet, ankylosing spondylitis, 167
Femoroacetabular impingement, 40
Femur
  dual energy X-ray absorptiometry,
    135
  fractures
    proximal fractures, 201f–202f
    intertrochanteric fractures, 201, 201f–202f
    shaft osteoporosis fractures, 130, 130f
FFD (fixed film focus distance), 139
FHL (flexor hallucis longus) tendon, 49
Fibrodysplasia ossificans progressiva (FOP),
    13–14
Fibrogenic benign bone tumours, 65

Fibrohistiocytic tumours
  benign bone tumours, 65–67
  soft musculoskeletal tissues, 108
Fibroma
  dermoplastic *see* Dermoplastic fibroma
  non-ossifying *see* Non-ossifying fibroma
    (NOF)
Fibroma of the tendon sheath (FTS), 108
Fibromatosis, 106–108
  desmoid-type, 107–108, 107*f*
  superficial, 107
Fibrosarcoma
  bone, 91–92
Fibrous cortical defect (FCD), 65, 66*f*
Fibrous dysplasia (FD), 71–73, 73*f*–74*f*
  CT, 73, 75*f*
  MRI, 73, 75*f*
  scintigraphy, 73, 74*f*
Fibrous histiocytoma, benign, 67
Fibrous malignant bone tumours, 91–92
Fixed film focus distance (FFD), 139
Flexor digitorum longus (FDL) tendon, 49
Flexor hallucis longus (FHL) tendon, 49
Fluorine, periosteal reactions, 19–20
Fluoroscopy
  musculoskeletal system radiography, 2
Fluorosis, 152
Foot, 48–52
  anatomy, 48–49
  diabetes mellitus complications *see*
    Diabetic foot
Foot trauma, 209–210
  Jones' fracture, 209, 210*f*
  Lisfranc injury, 209–210, 210*f*
  paediatric patients, 209, 210*f*
  stress fractures, 210, 211*f*
FOP (fibrodysplasia ossificans progressiva),
  13–14
Forestier's syndrome *see* Diffuse idiopathic
  skeletal hyperostosis (DISH)
Fracture(s)
  acetabulum *see* Acetabulum
  avulsion *see* Avulsion fractures
  butterfly fragments, 182
  calcaneal *see* Calcaneal fractures
  comminuted, 182
  complete, 182
  complex, 199
  compound, 182
  greenstick, 182, 183*f*
  hip *see* Hip
  incomplete *see* Incomplete fractures
  Maisoneuve fracture, 206–207, 207*f*
  Malgane fracture, 195
  malleolar fractures, 206, 206*f*
    Weber classification, 207*f*
  osteoporosis *see* Osteoporosis
  pathological *see* Pathological fractures
  pelvic ring *see* Pelvic ring fractures
  pelvis *see* Pelvic fractures
  segmental, 182
  Segond fracture, 203–204, 204*f*
  shoulder *see* Shoulder
  spinal ankylosing spondylitis, 166, 167*f*
  spine osteoporosis, 125–127, 126*f*
  stress *see* Stress fractures
  subtrochanteric *see* Subtrochanteric
    fractures
  tibial plateau, 203, 203*f*–204*f*
  Tillaux *see* Tillaux fractures
  transverse, acetabulum, 198, 199*f*
  types, 182–183
  wrist, 35
  see also specific bones
Fracture risk prediction tool (FRAX), 135
FRAX (fracture risk prediction tool), 135

FTS (fibroma of the tendon sheath), 108
FTT (full thickness tear), rotator cuff
  disease, 25
Full thickness tear (FTT), rotator cuff
  disease, 25
Fungal infections
  musculoskeletal infections, 238–239, 239*f*
  soft musculoskeletal tissue calcification, 14

G

Gamekeeper's thumb, 39
Gas, in soft musculoskeletal tissues *see* Soft
  musculoskeletal tissues
GCTTS (giant cell tumour of the tendon
  sheath), 108, 110*f*
Generalised osteoporosis, 130–132
GH *see* Glenohumeral joint (GH)
Giant cell tumour (GCT), 67–68
  diffuse-type, 108
  MRI, 68, 69*f*
  radiograph, 68, 68*f*
Giant cell tumour of the tendon sheath
  (GCTTS), 108, 110*f*
Gibbus deformities, 243–244
Glenohumeral joint (GH), 24
Glenohumeral joint (GH) instability, 26–29
  anterior dislocation, 28
  Bankart lesion, 28, 28*f*
  Bayley triangle, 28
  bony Bankart lesion, 28, 29*f*
  Hill–Sachs defect, 28, 29*f*–30*f*
  radiography, 28
Gleno-humeral ligaments, 25
Glenoid fossa, scapula, 24
Golfer's elbow, 31
Gout, 169–171
  acute intermittent, 170
  chronic tophaceous, 170–171, 170*f*
  erosions, 156–157, 158*f*
Granuloma
  eosinophilic *see* Eosinophilic granuloma
Granulomatous disease, musculoskeletal
  infections *vs.*, 240
Greater trochanteric bursae, 43
Greenstick fractures, 182, 183*f*
Growth cartilage, bones, 122*f*

H

HADD *see* Calcium hydroxyapatite
  deposition disease (HADD)
Haemangioma, 68–69, 108–111
  children, 109
  CT, 68–69, 69*f*
  MRI, 68–69, 110–111
  radiographs, 68–69, 69*f*, 109–110, 110*f*
  US, 101*f*, 110
Haemochromatosis, 179–180
  primary, 180
Haemophilia
  arthropathy *see* Haemophilic arthropathy
  pseudotumours, 176
Haemophilic arthropathy, 175–176, 175*f*
  MRI, 175, 176*f*
Haemophilus influenzae infection
  paediatric musculoskeletal infections,
    214
Hand, 33–39
  anatomy, 33–34
  ankylosing spondylitis, 167
  bones, 35
  osteoarthritis, 160*f*, 161
  psoriatic arthritis, 168*f*
Hand–Schuller–Christian disease, 74
Harrison's sulcus, 147

Heart
  sarcoma *see* Sarcoma
Heel, plantar fasciitis, 52*f*
Hereditary multiple exostoses,
  chondrosarcoma, 84, 85*f*
Hibernoma, 104
High-grade surface osteosarcoma, 90,
  91*f*
High-resolution multi-detector computed
  tomography (HR MD-CT),
  139–140
High resolution peripheral computed
  tomography (HR-pQCT), 139–140
Hill–Sachs defect, glenohumeral joint
  instability, 28, 29*f*–30*f*
Hill–Sach's lesion, 185, 185*f*
Hip, 39–43
  ankylosing spondylitis, 166–167, 167*f*
  avascular necrosis, 42, 42*t*, 43*f*
  bone, 42–43
  bursae, 43
  cartilage, 39–41
  fractures, 200–201
    classification, 201
    MRI, 201, 202*f*
  labrum *see* Labrum
  muscles, 41–42, 42*f*
  osteoarthritis, 160–161, 160*f*–161*f*
  pigmented villonodular synovitis, 177–178
  tendon, 41–42
Histiocytoma, benign fibrous, 67
Histology
  musculoskeletal infection management,
    240
HIV infection
  musculoskeletal infections, 239–240
  tuberculous vertebral osteomyelitis, 243
HLA-B27, arthritis, 165
HOA *see* Hypertrophic osteoarthropathy
  (HOA)
HPOA (hypertrophic pulmonary
  osteoarthritis), 179, 180*f*
HR MD-CT (high-resolution multi-detector
  computed tomography), 139–140
HR-pQCT (high resolution peripheral
  computed tomography), 139–140
Humerus fractures
  distal fractures, 188
  head fracture, 185–186
  transverse fractures, 186
Hutchinson's fracture, 189
Hydatid disease
  musculoskeletal infections, 237
Hyperparathyroidism, 140–143
  bone effects, 124
  brown tumours, 142, 142*f*
  chondrocalcinosis, 141, 142*f*
  clinical presentation, 140
  intracortical bone resorption, 141, 141*f*
  metastatic calcification, 143, 143*f*
  osteoporosis, 143
  osteosclerosis, 142–143, 143*f*
  primary, 140
  radiology, 140–143
  secondary, 140, 148
  subperiosteal erosions, 141, 141*f*
  treatment, 140
Hyperphosphatasia, 151–152, 152*f*
Hypertrophic osteoarthropathy (HOA), 19
  primary, 19
Hypertrophic pulmonary osteoarthritis
  (HPOA), 179, 180*f*
Hypertrophy
  ligamentum flavum *see* Ligamentum
    flavum
Hyperuricaemia, 169–170

Hypervitaminosis A, 152
  periosteal reactions, 20
Hypervitaminosis D, 16
Hypocalcaemia
  secondary hyperparathyroidism, 148
  vitamin D deficiency, 147
Hypoparathyroidism, 143–144
  aetiology, 143–144
  radiological abnormalities, 144, 144f
  soft musculoskeletal tissue calcification, 16
Hypophosphataemia
  X-linked, 148–150, 149f
Hypophosphatasia, rickets, 150

I

Idiopathic juvenile osteoporosis (IJO), 132
IJO (idiopathic juvenile osteoporosis), 132
Iliopsoas, bursitis, 43
Image acquisition
  CT optimisation *see* Computed
    tomography (CT)
Image quality, CT *see* Computed
    tomography (CT)
Image reconstruction, CT *see* Computed
    tomography (CT)
Incomplete fractures, 182, 183f
  Salter and Harris classification, 182
Infantile cortical hyperostosis (Caffrey's
    disease), 19
Infection(s)
  gas in soft musculoskeletal tissues, 16–18,
    18f
  musculoskeletal *see* Musculoskeletal
    infections
  soft musculoskeletal tissue
    calcification, 14, 14f–15f
  tumours, 119
Infective bursitis, 219
Inflammation
  soft musculoskeletal tissue tumours, 119
Inflammatory arthritis, 163–180
  joint space, 156, 157f
  musculoskeletal infections *vs.*, 240
Inflammatory osteoarthritis *see* Erosive
    (inflammatory) osteoarthritis
Insall–Salvati ratio, 47
Intermittent gout, acute, 170
Intertrochanteric femoral fractures, 201,
    201f–202f
Intra-articular bodies
  diabetic foot, 232
  elbow, 32, 34f
Intra-articular hydroxyapatite deposition
    disease, 172
Intracapsular chondroma, 111
Intracortical bone resorption,
    hyperparathyroidism, 141, 141f
Intraneural ganglion (nerve sheath
    ganglion), 116–117, 117f
Intra-osseous fluid collection, diabetic foot,
    230
Intraosseous lipoma, 70, 70f
Intrasutural (Wormian) bones, 132
Ischiofemoral impingement, 42, 42f

J

Jaccoud's arthropathy, 173
Joint(s)
  deformity, osteoarthritis, 160, 160f
  effusions, diabetic foot, 232
  internal derangements, 24–53
  MRI, 9–11
  radiography, 156–158
    bone alignment, 157–158, 159f

bone changes, 156–157
distribution of involvement, 158
normal imaging, 8
soft-tissue swelling, 156, 157f
space alteration, 156, 157f
space loss, osteoarthritis, 159, 160f
US, 8
see also specific diseases/disorders; specific joints
Jones' fracture, 209, 210f
Juvenile bone cysts *see* Simple bone cysts
    (SBCs)

K

Kidney(s)
  paediatric patients
    duplex kidneys *see* Duplex kidneys,
      paediatric
Kienbock's disease, 35, 36f
Knee, 43–48
  anterior cruciate ligament, 44–46, 46f
  bone, 47–48
  bursae, 48
  cartilage, 47–48
  collateral ligaments, 43–44
  extensor mechanism, 47
  fractures, 202–205
    lateral view, 202–203, 203f
  lateral collateral ligament, 47
  lateral femorotibial compartment, 43–44
  medial collateral ligament, 46
  medial compartment, 43–44
  menisci, 44
    tears, 44, 44f–45f
  osteoarthritis, 157f, 160, 161f
  patellofemoral compartment, 43–44
  patellofemoral joint, 47, 47f
  pigmented villonodular synovitis, 177–178
  posterior cruciate ligaments, 46, 46f
  posterolateral corner, 47
  Segond fracture, 203–204, 204f
Knuckle pads, 107
Kyphoplasty
  osteoporosis, 127–129

L

Labrum, 39–41
  MRI, 39, 40f
  trauma, 39
Langerhans cell histiocytosis (LCH), 74–76,
    76f
  MRI, 75–76
  radiograph, 75
Lateral collateral ligament (LCL)
  ankle, 49
  knee, 47
Lateral compression injury, pelvic ring
    fractures, 195, 197f
Lateral femorotibial compartment, knee,
    43–44
LCH *see* Langerhans cell histiocytosis
    (LCH)
LCL *see* Lateral collateral ligament (LCL)
Ledderhose disease (plantar fibromatosis),
    107, 107f
Leiomyoma, 70
Lesion margin, bone tumour growth rate, 54
Lethal perinatal osteogenesis imperfecta,
    133
Letterer–Siwe disease, 74
LHB *see* Long head of biceps (LHB) tendon
Ligament(s)
  MRI, 11
  US, 8–9
  see also specific ligaments

Ligamentum flavum
  ossification, 148
Lipoblastoma, 103–104
Lipogenic tumour, 70
Lipoma, 102–103
  CT, 103
  intraosseous, 70, 70f
  MRI, 103, 103f
  parosteal, 70, 70f
  radiography, 102, 102f
  US, 102–103, 103f
Lipoma arborescens, 178, 179f
Lipomatosis
  nerve tumours, 117–118, 118f
Liposarcoma
  dedifferentiated, 105, 105f
  myxoid, 105, 106f
  well-differentiated, 104, 104f
Lisfranc injury, 209–210, 210f
Listeria musculoskeletal infections, 213
Localised neurofibroma, 113
Loiasis, 14
Long head of biceps (LHB) tendon, 25
  tears of, 25
Loose bodies, osteoarthritis, 159–160, 160f
Looser's zone, osteomalacia, 147
Low-grade central osteosarcoma, 89
LPIN2 gene, chronic recurrent multifocal
    osteomyelitis, 216–217
Lumbar spine
  dual energy X-ray absorptiometry, 135
Lunate dislocations, 35, 191–192
Lung cancer
  metastases
    bone metastases, 81f–82f, 82
Lung diseases/disorders
  cancer *see* Lung cancer
Luno-triquetral ligament, 35

M

Maffucci's syndrome (enchondromatosis
    with haemangiomas), 12, 13f, 61
  chondrosarcoma, 84
Maisoneuve fracture, 206–207, 207f
Malgane fracture, 195
Malignant calcification, 16, 17f
Malignant melanoma, bone metastases,
    82–83
Malignant neoplasias
  fibrous histiocytoma, 91–92
  kidney *see* Renal masses
Malignant peripheral nerve sheath tumours
    (MPNSTs), 116, 116f
Malleolar fractures, Weber classification,
    206, 206f–207f
MARS (metal artefact reduction sequences),
    musculoskeletal system MRI, 6
Matrix mineralisation, bone tumour
    assessment, 57, 57f
McCune–Albright syndrome, 71
MCL (medial collateral ligament), 46
MCTD (mixed connective tissue disease),
    173
Medial collateral ligament (MCL), 46
Medial compartment, knee, 43–44
Mesenchymal chondrosarcoma, 86–87
Metabolic soft musculoskeletal tissue
    calcification, 15–16
Metacarpal bones, 33–34
  trauma, 192–194, 193f
    spiral fractures, 192
    transverse fractures, 192
Metachronous multicentric osteosarcoma, 88
Metal artefact reduction sequences (MARS),
    musculoskeletal system MRI, 6

Metaphyseal chondrodysplasia, 147
Metaphysis, bones, 122*f*
Metastases
    calcification, hyperparathyroidism, 143, 143*f*
    lung cancer *see* Lung cancer
Mineralisation, soft tissue tumours, 100
Mirels' scoring system, bone metastases, 83, 83*t*
Mixed connective tissue disease (MCTD), 173
Moderately severe osteogenesis imperfecta, 134–135
Morel–Lavelle lesion, 118–119, 119*f*
Morton's neuroma, 52, 117
MPNSTs (malignant peripheral nerve sheath tumours), 116, 116*f*
Multicentric osteosarcoma, primary, 88
Multicentric reticulohistiocytosis, 179
Muscles
    accessory, tumours, 118, 118*f*
    MRI, 11, 11*f*
    US, 5*f*, 8–9
    see also specific muscles
Musculoskeletal infections, 213–249
    atypical mycobacterial infections, 237
    classification, 214
    clinical features, 218
    clinical presentation, 213
    CT, 219–220, 219*t*, 221*f*–222*f*
    diagnosis, 213
    differential diagnosis, 240
    epidemiology, 213–214
    fungal infections, 238–239, 239*f*
    HIV infection, 239–240
    hydatid disease, 237
    investigations, 218–225, 219*t*
    management, 218–225, 240
    MRI, 219*t*, 221–222, 223*f*–224*f*
    NM, 219*t*
    nuclear medicine, 224–225, 226*f*
    pathogenesis, 218
    PET, 224
    radiograph, 218–219, 219*t*
    sickle cell disease, 237–238
    SPECT, 225
    US, 219
    see also Osteomyelitis; *specific anatomical features; specific diseases/disorders*
Musculoskeletal infections, paediatric, 214–218
    clinical features, 214
    CT, 215
    investigations, 215–216
    management, 215–216
    MRI, 215–216, 216*f*–217*f*
    necrotizing fasciitis, 218
    nuclear medicine, 216
    pathophysiology, 214
    radiography, 215
    sclerosing osteomyelitis of Garre, 217–218
    US, 215, 215*f*
    see also specific diseases/disorders
Musculoskeletal system, 1–23
    CT, 6
        normal tissue, 9
    endocrine disease, 121–155
    fractures *see* fractures
    infections *see* Musculoskeletal infections
    joint disorders, 24–53
        see also specific joints
    metabolic disease, 121–155
    MRI, 6
        cartilage imaging, 6–7
        delayed gadolinium-enhanced MR imaging cartilage, 7

diffusion-weighted, 7
        elastography, 7
        metal artefact reduction sequences, 6
        MR arthrography, 6
        normal tissue, 9–11
        3D T1-weighted spoiled gradient-recalled echo, 7
    nuclear medicine, 7–8, 7*f*
        SPECT, 7–8, 8*f*
    paediatric infections *see* Musculoskeletal infections, paediatric
    radiography, 1–3, 2*f*
        arthrography, 2–3, 3*f*
        benefits, 1
        disadvantages, 1–2
        fluoroscopy, 2
        normal imaging, 8
        picture archiving and storage system, 1
        soft tissue information, 1, 2*f*
        stress views, 2, 3*f*
        tomosynthesis, 3, 3*f*
    soft tissues *see* Soft musculoskeletal tissues
    trauma, 182–212
        fractures *see* Fracture(s)
    US, 3–6, 4*f*–5*f*
        benefits, 4
        contrast-enhanced, 4*f*, 5–6
        disadvantages, 4
        Doppler US, 4, 4*f*
        elastography, 4–5, 5*f*
        extended field-of-view, 4, 5*f*
        normal imaging, 8–9
        power Doppler US, 4
        see also Bone(s)
Musculoskeletal tuberculosis, 234–236, 235*f*
    CT, 235–236
    diagnosis, 235*t*
    MRI, 236, 236*f*–238*f*
    pathogenesis, 235
    radiography, 235
Mycetoma, musculoskeletal infections, 238–239, 239*f*
Mycobacterium avium-intercellulaire infections, 237
    HIV infection, 239–240
Mycobacterium fortuitum infections, 237
Mycobacterium kansasii infections, 237
Mycobacterium scrofulaceum infections, 237
Myelofibrosis
    bone metastases, 81–82
Myositis ossificans, 111
Myxoid liposarcoma, 105, 106*f*
Myxoid pleomorphic tumours, 104
Myxoma, 111–112, 112*f*

N

Necrotizing fasciitis, paediatric, 218
Needle biopsy, chondrosarcoma, 84–85
Neoplasms
    soft musculoskeletal tissue calcification, 15
Nerve(s)
    tumours, 113–118
        benign nerve sheath tumours, 113–115
        lipomatosis, 117–118, 118*f*
        malignant tumours, 116
        Morton's neuroma, 117
        pseudotumours, 116–118
        traumatic neuroma, 117, 117*f*
    US, 9, 9*f*
Nerve sheath ganglion (intraneural ganglion), 116–117, 117*f*
Neural tumours, benign bone tumours, 70–71
Neurilemmoma *see* Schwannoma (neurilemmoma)

Neuroectodermal tumours
    primitive *see* Primitive neuroectodermal tumours (PNETs)
Neurofibroma (NF), 113–114, 115*f*–116*f*
    diffuse, 114–115
    localised, 113
    plexiform *see* Plexiform neurofibroma
Neurofibromatosis type 1 (NF-1), 116
Neuroma, traumatic, 117, 117*f*
Neuropathic arthropathy, 176, 176*t*
Neuropathic changes, diabetic foot, 232
NF *see* Neurofibroma (NF)
NF (nodular fasciitis), 105–106
NF-1 (neurofibromatosis type 1), 116
Nodular fasciitis (NF), 105–106
NOF *see* Non-ossifying fibroma (NOF)
Non-aggressive periosteal reaction, soft musculoskeletal tissues *see* Soft musculoskeletal tissues
Non-ossifying fibroma (NOF), 65–67
    MRI, 67, 67*f*
Non-tuberculous mycobacteria (NTMB)
    spinal infections, 245–247
NTMB *see* Non-tuberculous mycobacteria (NTMB)

O

OCL (osteochondral lesions), talar dome, 50
Oedema
    soft tissue, 222
OFD *see* Osteofibrous dysplasia (OFD)
Oligo arthritis, 167
Ollier's disease, 12
    chondrosarcoma, 84
    see also Enchondroma
Oncogenic osteomalacia, 145–146, 146*f*
OO *see* Osteoid osteoma (OO)
Ossification
    ligamentum flavum, 148
    soft musculoskeletal tissues *see* Soft musculoskeletal tissues
Osteitis fibrous cystica (brown tumours), 142, 142*f*
Osteoarthritis, 158–163
    aetiology, 158–159
    erosive *see* Erosive (inflammatory) osteoarthritis
    hypertrophic pulmonary, 179, 180*f*
    inflammatory *see* Erosive (inflammatory) osteoarthritis
    MRI, 162, 162*f*
    primary, 159
    radiography, 159–160
        hands and wrists, 160*f*, 161
        hip, 160–161, 160*f*–161*f*
        joint deformity, 160, 160*f*
        joint space loss, 159, 160*f*
        knee, 157*f*, 160, 161*f*
        loose bodies, 159–160, 160*f*
        osteophytes, 159, 160*f*
        spine, 161–162
        subchondral bone change, 159, 160*f*
    secondary, 159, 159*t*
    US, 162, 162*f*
Osteoarthropathy
    hypertrophic, 19
    primary hypertrophic, 19
Osteoblastoma, 63–65
    radiograph, 65, 66*f*
Osteoblasts, 121
    bone turnover, 122*f*
Osteochondral lesions (OCL), talar dome, 50

Osteochondritis dissecans
elbow, 31–32, 33*f*
knee, 47–48
Osteochondroma, 58–59
clinical presentation, 58
CT, 58–59
diaphyseal aclasis, 58, 58*f*
MRI, 58–59, 59*f*
radiograph, 58–59, 59*f*
Osteochondromatosis, synovial, 176–177, 177*f*
Osteoclasts, 121
bone turnover, 122*f*
Osteocytes, 121
Osteodystrophy
axotemic *see* Axotemic osteodystrophy
Osteofibrous dysplasia (OFD), 73–74, 76*f*
Osteogenesis imperfecta, 132–135, 134*f*
COL1A1, 132
COL1A2, 132
intrasutural (Wormian) bones, 132
severe progressive, 134
type I, 133
type II (lethal perinatal), 133
type III (severe progressive), 134
type IV (moderately severe), 134–135
Osteoid osteoma (OO), 62–63
CT, 63, 64*f*–65*f*
MRI, 63, 64*f*
periosteal reaction, 63, 64*f*
radiograph, 63, 63*f*
Osteolysis, sickle cell disease, 238
Osteomalacia, 124, 145–150
oncogenic, 145–146, 146*f*
radiology, 147–148, 148*f*
Osteomyelitis
acute *see* Acute osteomyelitis
chronic, paediatric, 214–216, 217*f*
chronic recurrent multifocal *see* Chronic recurrent multifocal osteomyelitis (CRMO)
classification, 214
MRI, 222, 224*f*–225*f*
neonatal, 214
prosthetic devices, 225–227
anti-granulocyte scintigraphy, 227
CT, 226–227, 229*f*
diagnosis, 226–227
MRI, 226–227
PET, 227
skeletal scintigraphy, 227
US, 226–227
pyogenic vertebral *see* Pyogenic vertebral osteomyelitis
tuberculous vertebral *see* Tuberculous vertebral osteomyelitis
vertebrae *see* Vertebral osteomyelitis
Osteopenia
joint disease, 156, 157*f*
Osteopetrosis, 150–151, 151*f*
autosomal dominant type, 151
autosomal recessive type, 150–151
pelvic pathological fractures, 200
Osteophytes
osteoarthritis radiography, 160*f*
Osteoporosis, 124–140
aetiology, 130–132
bone mineral density, 124
causes, 124, 125*t*
dual energy X-ray absorptiometry, 124
epidemiology, 124
fractures, 129–130, 129*f*
femoral shaft, 130, 130*f*
hip fractures, 201
spine, 125–127, 126*f*
subtrochanteric fractures, 130

generalised, 130–132
hyperparathyroidism, 143
idiopathic juvenile, 132
kyphoplasty, 127–129
post-menopausal, 132
post menopausal *see* Post-menopausal osteoporosis
radiology, 124–130, 126*f*
radio-density, 124–125, 125*f*
regional, 130, 131*f*
secondary, 132, 133*f*
senile, 132
spine, 125–127, 126*f*–127*f*
transient, 48, 48*f*
transient, hip, 43, 43*f*, 43*t*
vertebroplasty, 127–129, 128*f*
young adults, 132
Osteosarcoma, 87–91
causes, 87
central, 87–91, 88*f*
Codman's angle, 87
FDG-PET, 87–88
MRI, 87–88
varieties, 88–89
see also specific types
high-grade surface, 90, 91*f*
low-grade central, 89
parosteal, 87–91, 89*f*
periosteal, 90, 90*f*
primary multicentric, 88
secondary, 90
small-cell, 89
surface, 89–91
see also specific types
synchronous multicentric, 88
telangiectatic *see* Telangiectatic osteosarcoma
Osteosclerosis, 142–143, 143*f*

P

Pachydermoperiostosis (primary hypertrophic osteoarthropathy), 19
PACS *see* Picture archiving and storage system (PACS)
Paediatric patients
acute osteomyelitis, 214
osteoid osteoma *see* Osteoid osteoma (OO)
osteosarcoma *see* Osteosarcoma
renovascular hypertension *see* Renovascular hypertension, paediatric
rhabdomyosarcoma *see* Rhabdomyosarcoma (RMS)
Paget's disease, 124
bone metastases, 81–82
pelvic pathological fractures, 200, 201*f*
Paget's sarcoma, 90, 92*f*
MRI, 90
Palmar fibromatosis (Dupuytren's disease), 107
Para-articular (intracapsular) chondroma, 111
Parasitic infections
soft musculoskeletal tissue calcification, 14, 14*f*–15*f*
see also specific infections
Parathyroid gland
disorders, 140–145
see also specific diseases/disorders
Para-vertebral abscesses, CT, 220
Parosteal lipoma, 70, 70*f*
Parosteal osteosarcoma, 87–91, 89*f*
Partial thickness tear (PTT), rotator cuff disease, 25

Patella
bipartite, 205, 205*f*
dislocation, 205, 205*f*
fractures, 204–205, 204*f*–205*f*
tendinopathy, 47, 48*f*
Patellofemoral compartment, knee, 43–44
Patellofemoral joint, knee, 47, 47*f*
Pathological fractures, 183
bone metastases, 83
PB (peroneus brevis) tendon, 50
PCL (posterior cruciate ligaments), knee, 46, 46*f*
Pellegrini–Stieda lesion, 46
Pelvic fractures, 194–200
insufficiency fractures, 200
pathological fractures, 200, 201*f*
stress fractures, 200
CT, 200
MRI, 200, 200*f*
Pelvic ring fractures, 194–196
anatomy, 194–195
anterior compression injuries, 195, 195*f*–196*f*
classification, 195–196, 195*f*
complex injuries, 196
lateral compression injury, 195, 197*f*
vertical shear, 195–196, 197*f*
Pelvis
breast metastases, 80*f*
fractures *see* Pelvic fractures; Pelvic ring fractures
radiography, 80*f*
ring fractures *see* Pelvic ring fractures
trauma, avulsion injuries, 199–200, 200*f*
Penicillium infections, 239–240
Percutaneous biopsy
musculoskeletal infection management, 240
Periarticular hydroxyapatite deposition disease, 171–172, 172*f*
Perilunate dislocations, 35, 191–192, 193*f*
Periosteal reaction
bone tumour assessment, 55, 56*f*
gas in soft musculoskeletal tissues, 18–22, 19*t*
osteoid osteoma, 63, 64*f*
sickle cell disease, 238
Periosteum
anatomy, 18
bones, 122*f*
chondroma, 60–61
MRI, 61*f*
radiograph, 61*f*
chondrosarcoma, 86
osteosarcoma, 90, 90*f*
Periprosthetic infections, CT, 220
Peroneal tendons, 50
Peroneus brevis (PB) tendon, 50
Peroneus longus (PL) tendon, 50
Peyronie's fibromatosis, 107
Phalanges
trauma, 192–194
condylar fractures, 193
proximal interphalangeal joints, 194
Phleboliths, 100
Picture archiving and storage system (PACS)
musculoskeletal system, 1
Pigmented villonodular synovitis (PVNS), 177–178
diffuse-type, 108
hip, 177–178
knee, 177–178
MRI, 178, 178*f*
radiography, 178, 178*f*
Pilon fractures, 207, 207*f*

Pincer-type femoroacetabular impingement, 40–41, 41*f*
PIP (proximal interphalangeal) joints, rheumatoid arthritis, 163
Plantar fasciitis, heel, 52*f*
Plantar fibromatosis (Ledderhose disease), 107, 107*f*
Plantar plate rupture, 52
Plastic bowing, incomplete fractures, 182
Pleiomorphic undifferentiated sarcoma, 112–113
Pleomorphic tumours
  dedifferentiated, 104
  soft tissue tumours, 104
Plexiform neurofibroma, 114
PL (peroneus longus) tendon, 50
PM *see* Polymyositis (PM)
PNETs *see* Primitive neuroectodermal tumours (PNETs)
Polymyositis (PM), 172
Polyostotic fibrous dysplasia, bone, 71
Popliteal (Baker's) cyst, 119
Posterior column fractures, acetabulum, 198
Posterior cruciate ligaments (PCL), knee, 46, 46*f*
Posterior talofibular ligament, ankle, 49
Posterior tibiotalar ligament, 49
Posterior wall fractures, acetabulum, 197–198, 199*f*
Posterolateral corner, knee, 47
Posteromedial ankle tendons, 49
Post-menopausal osteoporosis, 132
  dual energy X-ray absorptiometry, 135
Post-radiation sarcoma (PRS), 90–91, 93*f*
PPHP *see* Pseudo-pseudohypoparathyroidism (PPHP)
Primary haemochromatosis, 180
Primary hyperparathyroidism, 140
Primary hypertrophic osteoarthropathy (pachydermoperiostosis), 19
Primary multicentric osteosarcoma, 88
Primary osteoarthritis, 159
Primitive neuroectodermal tumours (PNETs), 93–94
Progressive systemic sclerosis
  soft musculoskeletal tissue calcification, 15, 15*f*
Prostaglandins, periosteal reactions, 20
Prostate gland cancer
  bone metastases, 80–82, 82*f*
Prosthetic devices, osteomyelitis *see* Osteomyelitis
Prosthetic joint infections, nuclear medicine, 224–225, 227*f*
Protrusio acetabuli, 40–41
Proximal interphalangeal (PIP) joints, rheumatoid arthritis, 163
PRS (post-radiation sarcoma), 90–91, 93*f*
Pseudo-gout, 171
Pseudohypoparathyroidism, 144–145, 144*f*
  soft musculoskeletal tissue calcification, 16
Pseudomonas aeruginosa infection
  paediatric necrotizing fasciitis, 218
Pseudo-pseudohypoparathyroidism (PPHP), 145
  soft musculoskeletal tissue calcification, 16
Pseudotumours
  haemophilia, 176
  subperiosteal, 176
Psoriatic arthritis, 12, 167–169
  hands and feet, 168, 168*f*
  psoriatic spondylitis, 168, 169*f*
  spine, 168–169
  types, 167–168
Psoriatic spondylitis, 168, 169*f*

PTT (partial thickness tear), rotator cuff disease, 25
Pulmonary osteoarthritis, hypertrophic, 179, 180*f*
PVNS *see* Pigmented villonodular synovitis (PVNS)
Pyogenic vertebral osteomyelitis, 215, 241–243
  CT, 241, 243*f*
  MRI, 241–242
  nuclear medicine, 242, 244*f*
  radiographs, 241
  symptoms, 241
  treatment, 243
Pyomyositis, 119
  US, 219, 221*f*
Pyrophosphate arthropathy, 171, 171*f*

Q

Quantitative computed tomography (QCT), 137, 138*f*
  advantages, 137
  limitations, 137
Quantitative ultrasound (QUS), 138

R

RA *see* Rheumatoid arthritis (RA)
Rachitic bone, 147
Radial collateral ligament, 31
Radiogrammetry, 138–139
Radio-ulnar joint, 34
Radius
  paediatric head dislocation, 187–188, 188*f*
  trauma, 189, 191*f*
    Barton's fracture, 189
    Colles' fracture, 189, 190*f*
    distal fracture, 189, 190*f*
    paediatric trauma, 189, 189*f*
    styloid process, 189
Rate of growth, bone tumour assessment, 54–55, 55*f*–56*f*
Reactive arthritis, 12, 169, 169*f*
Regional osteoporosis, 130, 131*f*
Renal cancer *see* Renal masses
Renal masses
  bone metastases, 82, 83*f*
Renal tubular defects, axotemic osteodystrophy, 148–150
Reticulohistiocytosis, multicentric, 179
Rhabdomyosarcoma (RMS), 112–113
Rheumatic fever (Jaccoud's arthropathy), 173
Rheumatoid arthritis (RA), 163–164
  ankylosis, 163
  boutonniere deformity, 164, 164*f*
  distal interphalangeal joints, 163
  proximal interphalangeal joints, 163
  radiography, 164, 164*f*
  synovitis, 163
Rickets, 145–150
  hypophosphatasia, 150
  radiology, 146–147, 146*f*–147*f*
  secondary hyperparathyroidism, 148
  Toni–Fanconi syndrome, 148
  vitamin D deficiency *see* Vitamin D (cholecalciferol)
  X-linked hypophosphataemia, 148–150, 149*f*
RMS *see* Rhabdomyosarcoma (RMS)
Rotator cuff, 24–25
Rotator cuff disease, 25–26
  calcific tendinopathy, 26, 28*f*
  MRI, 25–26, 26*f*
  radiography, 25–26, 25*f*–26*f*
  tendinopathy, 25

tendon tears, 25–26, 27*f*
US, 25–26

S

SAB (subacromial bursa), 24
Sacriliitis, ankylosing spondylitis, 165, 165*f*
Sacrum, osteoporetic fractures, 129
Salmonella infections
  musculoskeletal infections in HIV infection, 239–240
Salter–Harris fracture classification, incomplete fractures, 182
SAPHO (synovitis, acne, pustulosis, hyperostosis and osteitis) syndrome, 217
Sarcoidosis, 178–179, 179*f*
Sarcoma
  pleiomorphic undifferentiated, 112–113
  post-radiation, 90–91, 93*f*
Sarcoma of soft tissue (STS), 112–113, 113*f*
SBCs *see* Simple bone cysts (SBCs)
Scaphoid
  blood supply, 190
  fracture, 190, 191*f*
Scapholunate dislocation, 192, 193*f*
Scapholunate ligament, 35
Scapula
  glenoid fossa, 24
Schwannoma (neurilemmoma), 113
  bone, 70–71
SCJ (sternoclavicular joint), 30
Scleroderma, 172, 173*f*
Sclerosing osteomyelitis of Garre, 217–218
Sclerosis, calcaneal fractures, 208
Screening, lung cancer *see* Lung cancer
SDB (subdeltoid bursa), 24
Seagull wing pattern, erosive osteoarthritis, 162–163, 163*f*
Secondary hyperparathyroidism, 140
Secondary osteoarthritis, 159, 159*t*
Secondary osteoporosis, 132, 133*f*
Secondary osteosarcoma, 90
Segmental fractures, 182
Segond fracture, 203–204, 204*f*
Senile osteoporosis, 132
Septic arthritis, 232–234
  children, 214–215, 216*f*
  CT, 232
  diagnosis, 232, 234
  MRI, 232, 234*f*
  presentation, 232
  progression, 234
  radiography, 232
  US, 219
Sero-negative arthritis, 165–169
Severe progressive osteogenesis imperfecta, 134
Shoulder, 24–29
  anatomy, 24
  ankylosing spondylitis, 167, 167*f*
  disorders, 24–29
    superior labral tears, 29
    see also Glenohumeral joint (GH) instability; Rotator cuff disease
  fracture
    Bankart lesion, 184, 184*f*
    differential diagnosis, 183–184, 184*f*
    greater tuberosity, 184, 184*f*
    Hill–Sach's lesion, 185, 185*f*
  trauma, 183–186
    anterior dislocation, 184–185, 184*f*
    AP radiograph, 183
    posterior dislocation, 185, 185*f*

Sickle-cell disease (SCD)
    musculoskeletal infections, 218, 237–238
Simple bone cysts (SBCs), 71, 73f
Sinus tarsi syndrome, 52, 52f
Skeletal trauma, 182–212
    see also Fracture(s); Musculoskeletal
        system; specific bones
Skeleton
    quantitative assessment, 135–140
        dual energy X-ray absorptiometry,
            135–137
        high-resolution multi-detector CT,
            139–140
        high resolution peripheral CT, 139–140
        quantitative US, 138
        radiogrammetry, 138–139
        vertebral morphometry, 139
    size and shape, 123–124
    see also Musculoskeletal system
Skier's thumb, 39, 194
Skin ulcers, diabetic foot, 230
SLE see Systemic lupus erythematosus (SLE)
Small-cell osteosarcoma, 89
Smooth muscle tumours, 70
Snapping hip, 41
Soft musculoskeletal tissues
    aggressive periosteal reaction, 21f–22f, 22
    calcification and ossification, 11–22, 12t
        autoimmune diseases/disorders, 14–16
        calcium hydroxyapatite deposition
            disease, 13
        congenital causes, 13–14
        dystrophic calcification, 12–16
        infections, 14, 14f–15f
        trauma, 4f, 13, 13f
        see also specific diseases/disorders
    CT, 9
    gas in, 16–22, 18f
        infections, 16–18, 18f
        MRI, 16, 17f
        periosteal reaction, 18–22, 19t
        trauma, 18
    MRI, 9
    non-aggressive periosteal reaction, 19–21
        arthritis, 19
        congenital, 19
        drug-induced, 19–20
        genetic, 19
        metabolic reactions, 19
        trauma, 19, 20f
        tumours, 20–21, 21f
        vascular problems, 21
    radiography, normal imaging, 8
    tumours, 99–120
        atypical lipomatous tumours, 104, 104f
        chondro-osseous tumours, 111
        colour Doppler US, 101
        CT, 100, 100f
        fibroblastic/myofibroblastic tumours,
            105–108
        fibrohistiocytic tumours, 108
        infections, 119
        inflammation, 119
        lipomatous tumours, 102–105
        mineralisation, 100
        MRI, 101
        nerves see Nerve(s)
        non-neoplastic tumour mimics,
            118–119
        phleboliths, 100
        pulsed Doppler US, 101
        radiography, 99–100
        synovial disorders, 119
        trauma, 118–119, 119f
        of uncertain differentiation, 111–113
        US, 100–101

    vascular tumours, 108–111
    well-differentiated liposarcoma, 104,
        104f
    WHO classification, 102–119
    see also specific diseases/disorders
    US, normal imaging, 8–9
    see also specific tissues
Soft tissue chondroma, 111
Soft tissue oedema, 222
Soft-tissue swelling
    joint radiography, 156, 157f
Solitary bone cysts see Simple bone cysts
    (SBCs)
SONK (spontaneous osteonecrosis of the
    knee), 129, 129f
Space alteration, joint radiography, 156, 157f
Spine
    ankylosing spondylitis see Ankylosing
        spondylitis (AS)
    infections, 241–247
        Aspergillus fumigatus infection, 245–247
        atypical Mycobacterium infections,
            245–247
        candidiasis, 245–247
        CT, 220
        pyogenic vertebral osteomyelitis see
            Pyogenic vertebral osteomyelitis
        tuberculous vertebral osteomyelitis see
            Tuberculous vertebral osteomyelitis
        vertebral osteomyelitis, 241
    lumbar see Lumbar spine
    osteoarthritis, 161–162
    osteoporosis see Osteoporosis
    tumours
    see also Lumbar spine; under vertebrae
Spondylitis, psoriatic, 168, 169f
Spontaneous osteonecrosis of the knee
    (SONK), 129, 129f
SPRG (3D T1-weighted spoiled gradient-
    recalled echo), musculoskeletal
    system, 7
Spring ligaments, 49
SPR (superior peroneal retinaculum) tendon,
    50
SS (synovial sarcoma), 113
SSB (subscapularis bursa), 24
SST (supraspinatus tendon), 24–25
Staphylococcal disease, disseminated, 214
Staphylococcus aureus infection
    musculoskeletal infections, 213
        HIV infection, 239–240
    paediatric musculoskeletal infections, 214
    paediatric necrotizing fasciitis, 218
Staphylococcus epidermis infection, 213
Sternoclavicular joint (SCJ), 30
Streptococcus pneumoniae infection
    paediatric musculoskeletal infections, 214
Streptococcus pyogenes infection
    paediatric musculoskeletal infections,
        214
Stress fractures, 183
    foot trauma, 210, 211f
Stress views, musculoskeletal system
    radiography, 2, 3f
STS (sarcoma of soft tissue), 112–113, 113f
Subacromial bursa (SAB), 24
Subcapital femoral fractures, 201f
Subchondral bone change, osteoarthritis,
    159, 160f
Subcutaneous fat, US, 8
Subdeltoid bursa (SDB), 24
Subperiosteal abscesses, US, 219
Subperiosteal erosions, hyperparathyroidism,
    141, 141f
Subperiosteal pseudotumours, 176
Subscapularis bursa (SSB), 24

Subtrochanteric fractures, 201f
    osteoporosis, 130
Superficial fibromatosis, 107
Superior labral tears, 29
Superior peroneal retinaculum (SPR)
    tendon, 50
Supracondylar femoral fractures, 203
Supraspinatus tendon (SST), 24–25
Surface osteosarcoma, 89–91
    see also specific types
Surgical debridement, musculoskeletal
    infection management, 240
Synchronous multicentric osteosarcoma, 88
Synovial chondromatosis, 111, 176–177,
    177f
Synovial disorders, soft musculoskeletal
    tissue tumours, 119
Synovial osteochondromatosis, 176–177,
    177f
Synovial sarcoma (SS), 113
Synovitis, acne, pustulosis, hyperostosis and
    osteitis (SAPHO) syndrome, 217
Synovitis, rheumatoid arthritis, 163
Systemic lupus erythematosus (SLE),
    172–173
    non-erosive arthropathy, 159f, 173
    osteonecrosis, 173
Systemic sclerosis, progressive see
    Progressive systemic sclerosis

T
Taenia solium infection see Cysticercosis;
    Neurocysticercosis
Talar dome
    ankle, 48–49
    fractures, 207, 208f
    osteochondral lesions, 50
Talus
    avulsion fractures, 209
    fractures, 208, 209f
Tarsal coalition, 51
Tarsal tunnel syndrome, 52
Telangiectatic osteosarcoma, 88
    MRI, 88, 89f
Tendinopathy
    elbow, 31, 32f
    patella, 47, 48f
Tendons
    MRI, 11
    US, 5f, 8–9, 9f
    see also specific tendons
Tennis elbow, 31
Tenosynovitis
    De Quervain's, 38–39, 39f
    US, 219, 220f
TFC (triangular fibro-cartilage), 34, 37–38,
    38f
Thoracolumbar junction
    tuberculous vertebral osteomyelitis, 243
3D T1-weighted spoiled gradient-recalled
    echo (SPRG), musculoskeletal
    system, 7
Thyroid disease, 152
Thyroid gland
    bone metastases, 82
Tibialis posterior (TP) tendon, 49, 49f
Tibial plateau, fractures, 203, 203f–204f
Tibio-spring ligament, 49
Tillaux fractures, 207, 207f
Tomosynthesis, 3, 3f
Tongue type, calcaneal fractures, 207–208,
    208f
Toni–Fanconi syndrome, 148
Torus injury, incomplete fractures, 182, 183f
TP (tibialis posterior) tendon, 49, 49f

Trabecular bone, 122f, 123
Trans cervical femoral fractures,
    201f
Transient osteoporosis, knee, 48, 48f
Transient osteoporosis of the hip (TOP), 43,
    43f, 43t
Transverse fractures, acetabulum, 198, 199f
Trauma
    gas in soft musculoskeletal tissues, 18
    non-aggressive periosteal reaction, 19,
        20f
    soft musculoskeletal tissue calcification, 4f,
        13, 13f
Traumatic neuroma, 117, 117f
Triangular fibro-cartilage (TFC), 34, 37–38,
    38f
Trimalleolar ankle fractures, 206, 206f
Triquetral, trauma, 191, 191t, 192f
Trochanteric bursitis, 43, 44f
Trochlea groove, 47
TTD (tubercle–trochlea groove distance),
    47
Tubercle–trochlea groove distance (TTD),
    47
Tuberculosis
    musculoskeletal see Musculoskeletal
        tuberculosis
Tuberculous vertebral osteomyelitis,
    243–245, 244t
    anterior lesions, 243
    central lesions, 243
    CT, 244
    Gibbus deformities, 243–244
    HIV infection, 243
    MRI, 244–245, 245f–247f
    radiographs, 244
    STIR, 245
    thoraco-lumbar junction, 243
Tumoural calcinosis, soft musculoskeletal
    tissue calcification, 16
Tumours see Cancers/tumours

U
Ulna
    paediatric trauma, 189, 189f
    trauma, 189
Ulnar collateral ligament, 31, 39,
    40f
    avulsion injuries, 194, 194f
Ulno-carpal joint, 34
Undifferentiated pleomorphic sarcoma
    (UPS), 91–92
Undifferentiated sarcoma, pleiomorphic,
    112–113
Unicameral bone cysts see Simple bone cysts
    (SBCs)
Unimalleolar ankle fractures, 206
UPS (undifferentiated pleomorphic
    sarcoma), 91–92

V
Vascular disease
    HIV infection see HIV infection
Vasculature
    bone tumours, 96, 96f
Venous malformations (VMs), 109
Venous vascular calcification, 12, 12f–13f
Vertebrae
    morphometry, 139
    osteomyelitis see Vertebral osteomyelitis
    tuberculous osteomyelitis see Tuberculous
        vertebral osteomyelitis
Vertebral osteomyelitis, 241
    causes, 213–214
Vertebroplasty
    osteoporosis, 127–129, 128f
Vertical calcaneal fractures, 207–208,
    208f
Vertical shear, pelvic ring fractures, 195–196,
    197f
VISI (volar intercalated segment instability),
    35

Vitamin D (cholecalciferol)
    deficiency
        hypocalcaemia, 147
        rickets, 145–148
        metabolic disorders, 145
Vitamin D intoxication, 152
VMs (venous malformations), 109
Volar intercalated segment instability (VISI),
    35

W
WDL (well-differentiated liposarcoma), 104,
    104f
Weber classification, malleolar fractures,
    206, 206f–207f
Well-differentiated liposarcoma (WDL),
    104, 104f
Wormian (intrasutural) bones, 132
Wrist, 33–39
    anatomy, 33–34
    bones, 35
        see also specific bones
    ligaments, 35, 37f–38f
    median nerve, 39
    osteoarthritis, 160f, 161
    tendons, 38–39
    trauma, 188–194
        AP radiograph, 188, 188f
        lateral radiograph, 188, 188f
        MRI, 190, 191f
        triangular fibro-cartilage, 37–38, 38f

X
X-linked hypophosphataemia, 148–150, 149f

Y
YOP (transient osteoporosis of the hip), 43,
    43f, 43t

Printed in the United States
By Bookmasters